This report contains the collective views of an international group of experts and does not necessarily represent the decisions or the stated policy of the International Commission on Non-Ionizing Radiation Protection, the International Labour Organization, or the World Health Organization.

Environmental Health Criteria 232

STATIC FIELDS

Published under the joint sponsorship of
the International Labour Organization,
the International Commission on
Non-Ionizing Radiation Protection, and
the World Health Organization.

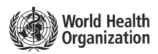
**World Health
Organization**

WHO Library Cataloguing-in-Publication Data

Static fields.

(Environmental health criteria ; 232)

1. Electromagnetic fields - adverse effects   2. Magnetic resonance imaging - adverse effects 3. Radiometry - standards 4. Environ-mental exposure   5. Risk assessment   I. International Programme for Chemical Safety II. Working Group on Static Electric and Magnetic Fields. Meeting (2002 : Vlaardingen, Netherlands) III. Task Group on Static Electric and Magnetic Fields. Meeting (2004 : Geneva, Switzerland) IV. Series

ISBN 92 4 157232 9   (LC/NLM classification: QT 34)
ISSN 0250-863X

© World Health Organization 2006

Printed in China

Environmental Health Criteria
STATIC FIELDS

CONTENTS

NOTE TO READERS OF THE CRITERIA MONOGRAPHS

Every effort has been made to present information in the criteria monographs as accurately as possible without unduly delaying their publication. In the interest of all users of the environmental health criteria monographs, readers are kindly requested to communicate any errors that may have occurred to the Coordinator, Radiation and Environmental Health, World Health Organization, Geneva, Switzerland, in order that they may be included in corrigenda, which will appear in subsequent volumes.

Environmental Health Criteria

PREAMBLE

The WHO Environmental Health Criteria Programme

In 1973 the WHO Environmental Health Criteria Programme was initiated, with the following objectives:

(i)   to assess information on the relationship between exposure to environmental pollutants and human health, and to provide guidelines for setting exposure limits;

(ii)   to identify new or potential pollutants;

(iii)   to identify gaps in knowledge concerning the health effects of pollutants;

(iv)   to promote the harmonization of toxicological and epidemiological methods to have internationally comparable results.

The first Environmental Health Criteria (EHC) monograph, on mercury, was published in 1976. Since that time, an ever-increasing number of assessments of chemical and physical agents have been produced. In addition, many EHC monographs have been devoted to evaluating toxicological methodology, e.g., for genetic, neurotoxic, teratogenic and nephrotoxic agents. Other publications have been concerned with epidemiological guidelines, evaluation of short-term tests for carcinogens, biomarkers, effects on the elderly and so forth.

The original impetus for the Programme came from World Health Assembly resolutions and the recommendations of the 1972 UN Conference on the Human Environment. The work subsequently became an integral part of the International Programme on Chemical Safety (IPCS), a cooperative programme of UNEP, ILO and WHO. With the strong support of the new partners, the importance of occupational health and environmental effects became fully recognized. The EHC monographs have become widely established, used and acknowledged throughout the world.

Electromagnetic Fields

Three monographs on electromagnetic fields (EMF) have addressed possible health effects from exposure to extremely low frequency (ELF) fields, static and ELF magnetic fields, and radiofrequency (RF) fields (WHO, 1984; WHO, 1987; WHO, 1993). They were produced in collaboration with the United Nations Environment Programme (UNEP), the International Labour Office (ILO) and the International Non-Ionizing Radiation Committee (INIRC) of the International Radiation Protection Association (IRPA), and from 1992 the International Commission on Non-Ionizing Radiation Protection (ICNIRP).

EHC monographs are usually revised if new data are available that would substantially change the evaluation, if there is public concern for health or environmental effects of the agent because of greater exposure, or if an appreciable time period has elapsed since the last evaluation. The EHCs on EMF are being revised and will be published as a set of three monographs spanning the relevant EMF frequency range (0 - 300 GHz); static fields (this volume), ELF fields (up to 100 kHz) and RF fields (100 kHz - 300 GHz).

WHO's assessment of any health risks produced by EMF emitting technologies falls within the responsibilities of the International EMF Project. This Project was established by WHO in 1996 in response to public concern over health effects of EMF exposure and is managed by the Radiation and Environmental Health Unit (RAD), which is coordinating the preparation of the EHC Monograph on static fields.

The WHO health risk assessment exercise includes the development of an extensive database comprising relevant scientific publications. Interpretation of these studies can be controversial, as there is a spectrum of opinion within the scientific community and elsewhere. To achieve as wide a degree of consensus as possible, the health risk assessment also draws on reviews already completed by other national and international expert review bodies. With regard to static fields in particular, these reviews include:

-        the IARC Monograph on static and extremely low frequency (ELF) fields (IARC, 2002). In June 2001 IARC formally evaluated the evidence for carcinogenesis from exposure to static and ELF fields. The review concluded that static fields were not classifiable as to their carcinogenicity to humans because there was inadequate evidence in humans and no relevant data available in experimental animals,

-        reviews on physics/engineering, biology and epidemiology commissioned by WHO to the International Commission on Non-Ionizing Radiation Protection (ICNIRP), a non-governmental organization in formal relations with WHO (ICNIRP, 2003), and

-        the WHO workshop on 'Effects of Static Magnetic Fields relevant to Human Health', co-sponsored with ICNIRP and the UK National

Radiological Protection Board (NRPB), and hosted by NRPB on 26-27 April 2004 (Noble et al., 2005).

Scope

The EHC monographs are intended to provide critical reviews on the effect on human health and the environment of physical, chemical and biological agents. As such, they include and review studies that are of direct relevance for the evaluation. However, they do not describe *every* study that has been carried out. Worldwide data are used and are quoted from original studies, not from abstracts or reviews. Both published and unpublished reports are considered, but preference is always given to published data. Unpublished data are only used when relevant published data are absent or when the unpublished data are pivotal to the risk assessment. A detailed policy statement is available that describes the procedures used for unpublished proprietary data so that this information can be used in the evaluation without compromising its confidential nature (WHO, 1990).

In the evaluation of human health risks, sound human data, whenever available, are generally more informative than animal data. Animal and *in vitro* studies provide support and are used mainly to supply evidence that is missing from human studies. It is mandatory that research on human subjects be conducted in full accord with ethical principles, including the provisions of the Helsinki Declaration.

All studies, with either positive or negative effects, need to be evaluated and judged on their own merit, and then collectively evaluated and judged in a weight of evidence approach. It is important to determine how much a set of evidence changes the probability that exposure causes an outcome. Generally, studies must be replicated or be in agreement with similar studies. The evidence for an effect is further strengthened if the results from different types of studies (epidemiology or laboratory) point to the same conclusion.

The EHC monographs are intended to assist national and international authorities in making risk assessments and subsequent risk management decisions. They represent a thorough evaluation of risks and are not, in any sense, recommendations for regulation or standard setting. These latter are the exclusive purview of national and regional governments. However, the EMF EHCs do provide bodies such as ICNIRP with the scientific basis for reviewing their international exposure guidelines.

Procedures

The general procedures that result in the publication of this EHC monograph are discussed below (for more information, see van Deventer et al., 2005).

A first draft, prepared by consultants or staff from a RAD Collaborating Centre, is initially based on data provided from reference databases, such as Medline and PubMed. The draft document, when received by RAD, may require an initial review by a small panel of experts to determine its scientific quality and objectivity. Once the document is acceptable as a first draft, it is distributed, in its unedited form, to well over 150 EHC contact points throughout the world who are asked to comment on its completeness and accuracy and, where necessary, provide additional material. The contact points, usually designated by governments, may be Collaborating Centres, or individual scientists known for their particular expertise. Generally, some months are allowed before the comments are considered by the author(s). A second draft incorporating comments received and approved by the Coordinator (RAD) is then distributed to Task Group members, who carry out the peer review at least six weeks before their meeting.

The Task Group members serve as individual scientists, not as representatives of their organization. Their function is to evaluate the accuracy, significance and relevance of the information in the document and to assess the health and environmental risks from exposure to the part of the electromagnetic spectrum being addressed. A summary and recommendations for further research and improved safety aspects are also required. The composition of the Task Group is dictated by the range of expertise required for the subject of the meeting (epidemiology, biological and physical sciences, medicine and public health) and by the need for a balance in gender, geographical distribution and the range of opinions on the science.

The membership of the WHO Task Groups is approved by the Assistant Director General of the Cluster on Sustainable Development and Healthy Environments. These Task Groups are the highest level committees within WHO for conducting health risk assessments. They are similar to the Working Groups established by the International Agency for Research on Cancer (IARC) that conduct 'carcinogen identification and classification' of various physical, chemical and biological agents.

Task Groups conduct a critical and thorough review of the scientific literature and assess any risks to health from exposure to both static electric and magnetic fields, reach agreements by consensus, and make final conclusions and recommendations that cannot be altered after the Task Group meeting.

The World Health Organization recognizes the important role played by non-governmental organizations (NGOs). Representatives from relevant national and international agencies may be invited to join the Task Group as observers. While observers may provide a valuable contribution to the process, they can only speak at the invitation of the Chairperson. Observers do not participate in the final evaluation, since this is the sole responsibility of the Task Group members. When the Task Group considers it to be appropriate, it may meet *in camera.*

All individuals who participate as authors, consultants or advisers in the preparation of the EHC monograph must, in addition to serving in their personal capacity as scientists, inform WHO if at any time a conflict of interest, whether actual or potential, could be perceived in their work. They are required to sign a conflict of interest statement. Such a procedure ensures the transparency and probity of the process.

When the Task Group has completed its review and the Coordinator (RAD) is satisfied as to the scientific consistency and completeness of the document, it is then subjected to language editing, reference checking, and a camera-ready copy is then prepared. After approval by the Director, the monograph is submitted to the WHO Office of Publications for printing. A copy of the final draft is then sent to the Chairperson and Rapporteur of the Task Group to check the proofs.

Static Fields Environmental Health Criteria

This EHC addresses the possible health effects of exposure to static electric fields and exposure to static magnetic fields. However, only a few animal and human laboratory studies have investigated the effects of exposure to static electric fields. The majority of studies reviewed here concern the effects of exposure to static magnetic fields. For completeness, studies of the effects of exposure to magnetic resonance imaging (MRI) fields have also been reviewed. In this case, however, the effects of static magnetic fields may well be confounded by possible effects of the pulsed gradient and radiofrequency (RF) magnetic fields. Other possible confounding variables, such as noise and vibration, may not have been adequately controlled in many experiments. These studies therefore contribute little to the static magnetic field health risk assessment.

The first draft of the EHC was written by a working group that met in Vlaardingen in the Netherlands (November 18-19, 2002). At this meeting, hosted by the Health Council of the Netherlands, it was decided that papers identified through literature searches performed in PubMed and other databases, including the reference lists and personal databases of working group members, would be reviewed by two reviewers and, on the basis of predefined criteria, considered informative or uninformative in the context of the EHC. These criteria included publication in a peer-reviewed journal, adequate description of the exposure, adequate description of the tests performed and of the biological system and materials used, appropriate statistical analysis of the data, and inclusion of adequate controls. Papers in languages other than English have been included as far as they could be read by at least one reviewer. All reviewed papers have been included in tables. Relevant information and comments from the reviewers are shown in the tables of those papers considered informative for health risk assessment. These have also been described in the text and form the basis of the health risk assessment and the recommendations. Any papers considered inadequate for health risk assessment requirements have been listed at the end of each table.

The final draft EHC was subsequently distributed for external review. The comments received were processed by Dr Colin Roy (ARPANSA, Australia), Dr Rick Saunders (WHO, Switzerland) and Dr Eric van Rongen (Health Council of the Netherlands). The resulting modified draft EHC was then sent to the Task Group members.

The Task Group met from December 6-10, 2004, at WHO headquarters in Geneva, Switzerland. A full review of the draft EHC was made and changes incorporated into the text. The Task Group carried out a static field health risk assessment, summarized the EHC and formulated recommendations for further research.

Participants in the working group and Task Group meetings on static electric and magnetic fields

Members

Dr Igor Y. Belyaev, Department of Genetics Microbiology, and Toxicology, Stockholm University, Stockholm, Sweden [c]

Professor Donald Chakeres, College of Medicine and Public Health, The Ohio State University Medical Center, Columbus, Ohio, USA [c]

Professor Stuart Crozier, The School of Information Technology and Electrical Engineering, The University of Queensland, Brisbane, Australia[c]

Dr Stefan Engstrom, Vanderbilt University Medical Center, Neurology Department, USA [a]

Dr Maria Feychting, Institute of Environmental Medicine, Division of Epidemiology, Karolinska Institute, Stockholm, Sweden [a, c]

Dr Lawrence Goldstein, private consultant, California, USA [a]

Professor Leeka Kheifets, Department of Epidemiology, UCLA School of Public Health, Los Angeles, California, USA [a, c]

Dr Isabelle Lagroye, Laboratoire de Bioélectromagnétisme EPHE, Bordeaux, France [c]

Mr Rüdiger Matthes, Federal Office for Radiation Protection, Bundesamt für Strahlenschutz, Oberschleissheim, Germany [c]

Dr Alastair McKinlay, National Radiological Protection Board, Chilton, Didcot, Oxfordshire, United Kingdom [c]

Dr Chiyoji Ohkubo, National Institute of Public Health, Department of Environmental Health, Tokyo, Japan [a, c]

Dr Eric van Rongen, Health Council of the Netherlands, The Hague, The Netherlands [a, b, c]

Dr Martin Röösli, Department of Social & Preventive Medicine, University of Bern, Switzerland [a, c]

Dr Colin Roy, Australian Radiation Protection and Nuclear Safety Agency, Victoria, Australia [a,b,c]

Dr Paolo Vecchia, Department of Technology and Health, National Institute of Health, Rome, Italy [c]

Professor Barney de Villiers, University of Stellenbosch, Faculty of Health Sciences, Cape Town, South Africa [c]

Dr Jakub Wiskirchen, University Hospital Tübingen, Germany [a]

Professor Zhengping Xu, Zhejiang University School of Medicine, Hangzhou, People's Republic of China [c]

Observers

Dr Hans Engels, Philips Medical Systems, The Netherlands [a]

Dr Daniel J. (Joe) Schaefer, GE Healthcare, Milwaukee, Wisconsin, USA [c]

Secretariat

Dr Michael Repacholi, Radiation & Environmental Health, World Health Organization, Geneva, Switzerland [c]

Dr Rick Saunders, Radiation & Environmental Health, World Health Organization, Geneva, Switzerland [b, c]

Dr Emilie van Deventer, Radiation & Environmental Health, World Health Organization, Geneva, Switzerland [c]

Dr Elisabeth Cardis, International Agency for Research on Cancer (IARC), Lyon, France [c]

[a] Participated in the working group meeting on the initial draft of the Static Fields EHC (Vlaardingen, the Netherlands, November 2002).

[b] Met in Geneva in September 2004 to review the draft monograph in preparation for the WHO Task Group meeting.

[c] Participated in the WHO Task Group meeting on static fields (World Health Organization, Geneva, Switzerland, 6 - 10 December 2004).

Acknowledgements

This monograph represents the most thorough health risk assessment ever undertaken for the static magnetic fields that are being increasingly used in medicine, industry and commerce. WHO acknowledges and thanks all contributors to this important monograph. Particular thanks go to Dr Eric van Rongen, Dr Colin Roy and Dr Richard Saunders for their continuing work throughout the development of this monograph. WHO also acknowledges the generous support from the Health Council of the Netherlands in providing the time of Dr van Rongen, and for providing the scientific and language editing.

Dr Michael Repacholi
Coordinator, Radiation and Environmental Health
World Health Organization
23 August 2005

Abbreviations

AC	Alternating Current
ADPR	ADP Ribosylation
AGNIR	Independent Advisory Group on Non-ionising Radiation (United Kingdom)
AP	Action Potential
ARPANSA	Australian Radiation Protection and Nuclear Safety Agency
ASTM	American Society for Testing and Materials
BMD	Bone Mineral Density
CA	Chromosomal Aberrations
CERN	European Organization for Nuclear Research (Switzerland)
CGS	Centimetre – Gram – Second-based system of units (obsolete)
DC	Direct Current
DNA	Deoxyribonucleic Acid
DSV	Diameter Spherical Volume
EC	European Commission
ECG	Electrocardiogram
HVDC	High Voltage Direct Current
IARC	International Agency for Research on Cancer
ICNIRP	International Commission on Non-Ionizing Radiation Protection

INIRC	International Non-Ionizing Radiation Committee
IRPA	International Radiation Protection Association
ILO	International Labour Office
IPCS	International Programme on Chemical Safety
EHC	Environmental Health Criteria
ELF	Extremely Low Frequency
EMF	Electromagnetic Fields
EPSP	Excitatory Postsynaptic Potentials
GOT	Glutamic Oxalacetic Transaminase
GTP	Glutamic Pyruvic Transaminase
HIAA	Hydroxyindoleacetic Acid
HT	Serotonin
IFN	Interferon
LDH	Lactate Dehydrogenase
LEP	Large Electron Positron Collider
MAG	Metal Active Gas
MagLev	Magnetic Levitation
MEPP	Miniature End-plate Potential
MIG	Metal Inert Gas
MN	Micronuclei
MRI	Magnetic Resonance Imaging
MRS	Magnetic Resonance Spectroscopy
NAT	Serotonin-N-acetyltransferase
NGO	Non-governmental Organization
NIR	Non-ionizing Radiation
NMR	Nuclear Magnetic Resonance
NRPB	National Radiological Protection Board (United Kingdom)
PAF	Platelet Activating Factor
PBMC	Peripheral Blood Mononuclear Cells
PHA	Phytohaemagglutinin
PMNL	Polymorphonuclear Leucocytes
RNA	Ribonucleic Acid
RF	Radiofrequency
SCE	Sister Chromatid Exchange
SI	System International
SMF	Static Magnetic Fields
TNF	Tumour Necrosis Factor
US FDA	US Food and Drug Agency
UN	United Nations
UNEP	United Nations Environmental Program
UV	Ultraviolet
VDU	Visual Display Unit
WHO	World Health Organization

1 SUMMARY AND RECOMMENDATIONS FOR FURTHER STUDIES

1.1 Summary

1.1.1 Natural and Human-made sources

Static electric fields occur naturally in the atmosphere. Values of up to 3 kV m-1 can occur under thunderclouds, but otherwise are of order of 100 V m-1 in fair weather. The next most common cause of human exposure is charge separation as a result of friction. For example, charge potentials of several kilovolts can be accumulated while walking on non-conducting carpets, generating local fields of up to 500 kV m-1. Direct current (DC) power transmission can produce static electric fields of up to 20 kV m-1, rail systems using DC can generate fields of up to 300 V m-1 inside the train, and VDUs create electric fields of around 10 - 20 kV m-1 at a distance of 30 cm.

The geomagnetic field varies over the Earth's surface between about 35 - 70 µT and is implicated in the orientation and migratory behaviour of certain animal species. Man-made static magnetic fields are generated wherever DC currents are used, such as in some transportation systems powered by electricity, industrial processes such as aluminium production and in gas welding. Magnetic flux densities of up to 2 mT have been reported inside electric trains and in developmental magnetic levitation (MagLev) systems. Workers are exposed to larger fields of up to around 60 mT in the electrolytic reduction of alumina, and electric arc welding produces around 5 mT at 1 cm from the welding cables.

The advent of superconductors in the 1970s and 1980s facilitated the use of much larger magnetic fields in medical diagnosis through the development of magnetic resonance imaging (MRI) and spectroscopy (MRS)[1], and nuclear magnetic resonance (NMR), for research. It is estimated that some 200 million MRI scans have been performed worldwide. The static magnetic field of MRI scanners in routine clinical systems is generated by permanent magnets, superconducting magnets and combinations thereof in the range of 0.2 - 3 T. In research applications, higher magnetic fields up to 9.4 T are used for whole body patient scanning. The stray magnetic fields around the magnets for MRI studies are well defined and can be minimized in the shielded magnet versions. In terms of exposure, at the operator's console the magnetic flux density is typically about 0.5 mT, but may be higher. However,

---

[1] This document refers throughout to MRI; exposures experienced during MRS are essentially similar.

occupational exposure up to and exceeding 1 T can occur during the construction and testing of these devices, and during medical procedures carried out in interventional MRI. Various physics research and high-energy technologies also employ superconductors where workers can be exposed regularly and for long periods to fields as high as 1.5 T.

1.1.2 Interaction Mechanisms

The following three classes of physical interactions of static magnetic fields with biological systems are well established on the basis of experimental data:

(1)   Electrodynamic interactions with ionic conduction currents. Ionic currents interact with static magnetic fields as a result of Lorentz forces exerted on moving charge carriers. These effects lead to the induction of electrical (flow) potentials and currents. Flow potentials are generally associated with ventricular contraction and the ejection of blood into the aorta in animals and humans. The Lorentz interaction also results in a magnetohydrodynamic force opposing the flow of blood. The reduction of aortic blood flow has been estimated to reach about 10% at 15 T.

(2)   Magnetomechanical effects, including the orientation of magnetically anisotropic structures in uniform fields and the translation of paramagnetic and ferromagnetic materials in magnetic field gradients. Forces and torques on both endogenous and exogenous metallic objects are the interaction mechanism of most concern.

(3)   Effects on electronic spin states of reaction intermediates. Spin-correlated radical pair chemistry has long been a consideration for magnetic field effects in chemistry and biology. Several classes of organic chemical reactions can be influenced by static magnetic fields in the range of 10 to 100 mT as a result of effects on the electronic spin states of the reaction intermediates. A spin-correlated radical pair may recombine and prevent the formation of a reaction product if two conditions are met: (a) the pair, formed in a triplet state, must be converted into a singlet state by some mechanism and (b) the radicals must physically meet again in order to recombine. Step (a) can be sensitive to magnetic fields. Most research has been on the use of radical pair magnetic field effects as a tool to study enzyme reactions. However, neither physiological effects on cellular functions, nor long-term mutagenic effects from magnetic-field induced changes in free radical concentrations or fluxes appear possible.

Dosimetry

To understand the biological effects of electric and magnetic fields, it is important to consider the fields directly influencing cells in different parts of the body and tissues. A dose can then be defined as an

2

appropriate function of the electric and magnetic fields at the point of interaction. The establishment of a relationship between the external non-perturbed fields and internal fields is the main objective of dosimetry. Computational studies using voxel-based models of humans and animals, and experimental studies of exposure are important aspects of dosimetry.

The interactions of tissue with static magnetic fields are likely to be parametric of physical properties of the field including the magnetic field vector, the gradient of the magnetic field, and/or the product of those quantities, often termed the 'force product'. Some of the larger interactions are characterized by motion through these field quantities, such as body motion or blood flow.

Appropriate dosimetric parameters depend on the physical mechanism for the safety concern. Clearly, ferromagnetic objects must be restricted from the vicinity of the magnet. Screening for such objects and for implants that may move either due to forces or torques is imperative. Measures of peak magnetic induction vector and peak magnetic force product are appropriate. Field maps may be used to estimate these at various locations near the magnets where workers may be exposed, but personal dosimetry may be more useful.

Movement of the whole or part of the body, e.g. eyes and head, in a static magnetic field gradient will also induce an electric field and current during the period of movement. Dosimetric calculation suggests that such induced electric fields will be substantial during normal movement around or within fields > 2 - 3 T, and may account for the numerous anecdotal reports of vertigo and occasionally magnetic phosphenes experienced by patients, volunteers and workers during movement in the field.

There are many sources of exposure and one of the most prolific is that of magnetic resonance imaging (MRI) equipment. In the past decade, there has been a concerted effort to enable MRI to operate at very high field strengths. The most common system in current clinical use has a 1.5 T central field. However, 3.0 T systems are now accepted for routine clinical work and more than 100 systems were operational worldwide by 2004. Research systems from 4 - 9.4 T are now being developed for clinical imaging. As the field strength of the MRI system increases, so does the potential for a variety of types of tissue/field interactions. Understanding the interactions between the electromagnetic fields generated by MRI systems and the human body has become more significant with this push to high field strengths.

1.1.3 *In vitro studies*

The results of *in vitro* studies are useful for elucidating interaction mechanisms, and for indicating the sorts of effects that might be investigated *in vivo*. However, they are not sufficient to identify health effects without corroborating evidence from *in vivo* studies.

A number of different biological effects of static magnetic fields have been explored *in vitro*. Different levels of organization have been investigated, including cell free systems (employing isolated membranes, enzymes or biochemical reactions) and various cell models (using both bacteria and mammalian cells). Endpoints studied included cell orientation, cell metabolic activity, cell membrane physiology, gene expression, cell growth and genotoxicity.

Positive and negative findings have been reported for all these endpoints. However, most data were not replicated. The observed effects are rather diverse and were found after exposure to a wide range of magnetic flux densities. There is evidence that static magnetic fields can affect several endpoints at intensities lower than 1 T, in the mT range. Thresholds for some of the effects were reported, but other studies indicated non-linear responses without clear threshold values.

Effects of static magnetic fields on cell orientation have been consistently found above 1 T, but their *in vivo* relevance is questionable. A few studies suggested that combined effects of static magnetic field with other agents such as genotoxic chemicals seem to produce synergistic, both protective and stimulating, effects. The current information is inadequate and needs to be confirmed before any firm conclusions on human health can be drawn.

Besides possible complicated dependence on physical parameters such as intensity, duration, recurrence and gradients of exposure, biological variables appear to be important for the effects of static magnetic fields. Variables such as cell type, cell activation, and other physiological conditions during exposure have been shown to affect the outcome of the experiments. The mechanisms for these effects are not known, but effects on radicals and ions may be involved. *In vitro* studies provide some evidence for this.

If the very few studies employing MRI signals or other combined fields show any biological effects, they do not show any that are different from those of static magnetic fields alone.

Taken together, the *in vitro* experiments do not present a clear picture of specific effects of static magnetic fields, and they consequently also do not indicate possible adverse health effects.

1.1.4 Animal studies

Few animal studies on the effects of static electric fields have been carried out. No evidence of adverse health effects have been noted, other than those associated with the perception of the surface electric charge.

A large number of animal studies on the effects of static magnetic fields have been carried out. Most of those considered relevant to human health have examined the effects of fields considerably larger than the natural geomagnetic field. A number of studies have been carried out of fields in the millitesla region, comparable to relatively high industrial exposures. More recently, with the advent of superconducting magnet technology and MRI, studies of behavioural, physiological and reproductive effects have been carried out at flux densities around, or exceeding, 1 T. Few studies, however, have examined possible chronic effects of exposure, particularly in relation to carcinogenesis.

The most consistent responses seen in neurobehavioural studies suggest that the movement of laboratory rodents in static magnetic fields equal to or greater than 4 T may be unpleasant, inducing aversive responses and conditioned avoidance. Such effects are thought to be consistent with magnetohydrodynamic effects on the endolymph of the vestibular apparatus. The data are otherwise variable.

There is some evidence that several vertebrate and invertebrate species are able to use static magnetic fields, at levels as low as geomagnetic field strengths, for orientation. However, these responses are not thought to have any significance for health.

There is good evidence that exposure to fields greater than about 1 T (0.1 T in larger animals) will induce flow potentials around the heart and major blood vessels, but the physiological consequences of this remain unclear. Several hours of exposure to very high flux densities of up to 8 T in the heart region did not result in any cardiovascular effects in pigs. In rabbits, short and long exposures to fields ranging from geomagnetic levels to the millitesla range have been reported to affect the cardiovascular system, although the evidence is not strong.

The results from one group suggest that the static magnetic fields of mT intensities may suppress early blood pressure elevation via hormonal regulatory system. The same group has reported that low-intensity static magnetic fields of up to 0.2 T may induce local effects on blood flow that may lead to improvement of microcirculation. In addition, another group reported that high static magnetic field flux densities of up to 10 T may lead to reduced skin blood flow and temperature. In all these cases, however, the endpoints are rather labile, a situation that may have been complicated by pharmacological manipulation, including anaesthesia in some cases, and immobilisation. In general, it is difficult to reach any firm conclusion without some independent replication.

Several studies described possible effects of magnetic field exposure on blood cells and the haemopoietic system. However, the results are equivocal, limiting the conclusions that can be drawn. The available evidence regarding effects of static magnetic field exposure on enzymatic and ionic constituents in serum comes primarily from one laboratory. These findings need to be confirmed by independent laboratories before conclusions can be drawn.

In terms of effects on the endocrine system, several studies from one laboratory suggest that static magnetic field exposure can affect pineal synthesis and melatonin content. However, some studies performed at other laboratories have been unable to demonstrate an effect. The finding of a suppressive effect of static magnetic field exposure on melatonin production needs to be confirmed in further research before firm conclusions can be drawn. On the whole, few studies have investigated static magnetic field effects on endocrine systems other than the pineal. No consistent effects have emerged.

Reproduction and development are very important issues in MRI exposure of both patients and clinical staff. In this respect, only a few good studies of static magnetic fields are available at field values above 1 T. MRI studies *per se* are uninformative because the effect of the static field cannot be distinguished from the possible general effects of the radiofrequency and pulsed gradient fields. Further examination is urgently needed to assess the health risk.

In general, so few animal studies have been carried out with regard to genotoxicity and cancer that it is not possible to draw any firm conclusions.

1.1.5 Laboratory studies on humans

Static electric fields do not penetrate electrically conductive objects such as the human body; the field induces a surface electric charge and is always perpendicular to the body surface. A sufficiently large surface charge density may be perceived through its interaction with body hair and by other effects such as spark discharges (microshocks). The perception threshold in people depends on various factors and can range between 10 - 45 kV m^{-1}. Annoying sensation thresholds are probably equally variable, but have not been systematically studied. Painful microshocks can be expected when a person who is well insulated from the ground touches a grounded object, or when a grounded person touches a conductive object that is well insulated from ground. However, the threshold static electric field values will vary depending on the degree of insulation and other factors.

Endpoints investigated in human experimental studies have included peripheral nerve function, brain activity, neurobehavioural and cognitive function, sensory perception, cardiac function, blood pressure, heart rate, serum proteins and hormone levels, body and skin temperature, and therapeutic effects. Exposure levels up to 8 T have been investigated, and both pure static fields and MRI imaging have been studied. The exposure duration ranged from a few seconds up to nine hours, but was usually less than one hour. The data available are limited for several reasons, including the facts that generally convenience samples of patients or healthy volunteers have been studied and the numbers of subjects have usually been small.

The results do not indicate that there are effects of static magnetic field exposure on neurophysiological responses and cognitive functions in stationary volunteers, nor can they rule out such effects. A dose-dependent induction of vertigo and nausea was found in workers, patients and volunteers during movement in static fields greater than about 2 T. One study suggested that eye-hand coordination and near visual contrast sensitivity are reduced in fields adjacent to a 1.5 T MRI unit. Occurrence of these effects is likely to be dependent on the gradient of the field and the movement of the subject. A small change in blood pressure and heart rate was observed in some studies, but were in the range of normal physiological variability. There is no evidence of effects of static magnetic fields on other aspects of cardiovascular physiology, or on serum proteins and hormones. Exposure to static magnetic fields of up to 8 T does not appear to induce temperature changes in humans.

Note, however, that most of the studies were very small, were based on convenience samples, and often included non-comparable groups. Thus, it is not possible to draw any conclusions regarding the wide variety of end-points examined in this report.

1.1.6 Epidemiological studies

Epidemiological studies have been carried out almost exclusively on workers exposed to static magnetic fields generated by equipment using large DC currents. Most workers were exposed to moderate static magnetic fields of up to several 10's mT either as welders, aluminium smelters, or workers in various industrial plants using large electrolytic cells in chemical separation processes. However, such work is also likely to have involved exposure to a variety of potentially hazardous fumes and aerosols, thus confounding interpretation. Health endpoints studied in these workers include cancer, haematological changes and related outcomes, chromosome aberration frequency, reproductive outcomes, and musculoskeletal disorders. In addition, a few studies examined fertility and pregnancy outcome in female MRI operators, where the potential to have been exposed to relatively large static fields of up to ~ 1 T may have existed. Two studies examined pregnancy outcome in healthy volunteers exposed to MRI examinations during pregnancy.

Increased risks of various cancers, e.g. lung cancer, pancreatic cancer, and haematological malignancies, were reported, but results were not consistent across studies. The few epidemiological studies published to date leave a number of unresolved issues concerning the possibility of increased cancer risk from exposure to static magnetic fields. Assessment of exposure has been poor, the number of participants in some of the studies has been very small, and these studies are thus able to detect only very large risks for such rare diseases. The inability of these studies to provide useful information is confirmed by the lack of clear evidence for other, more established carcinogenic factors present in some of the work environments. Other non-cancerous health effects have been considered even more sporadically. Most of these studies are based on very small numbers and have numerous methodological limitations. Other environments with a potential for high fields have not been adequately evaluated, e.g. those for MRI operators. At present, there is inadequate data for a health evaluation.

1.1.7 Health risk assessment

Static electric fields

There are no studies on exposure to static electric fields from which any conclusions on chronic or delayed effects can be made. IARC (IARC, 2002) noted there was insufficient evidence to determine the carcinogenicity of static electric fields.

Few studies of the acute effects of static electric field effects have been carried out. On the whole, the results suggest that the only adverse acute health effects are associated with direct perception of fields and discomfort from microshocks.

Static magnetic fields

The available evidence from epidemiological and laboratory studies is not sufficient to draw any conclusions with regard to chronic and delayed effects. IARC (IARC, 2002) concluded that there was inadequate evidence in humans for the carcinogenicity of static magnetic fields, and no relevant data available from experimental animals. Their carcinogenicity to humans is therefore not at present classifiable.

Short-term exposure to static magnetic fields in the tesla range and associated field gradients induce a number of acute effects. Cardiovascular responses, such as changes in blood pressure and heart rate, have been occasionally observed in human volunteer and animal studies. However, these were within the range of normal physiology for exposure to static magnetic fields up to 8 T.

Although not experimentally verified, it is important to note that calculations suggest three possible effects of induced flow potentials. These include minor changes in heartbeat (which may be considered to have no health consequences), the induction of ectopic heartbeats (which may be more physiologically significant), and an increase in the likelihood of re-entrant arrhythmia (possibly leading to ventricular fibrillation). The first two effects are thought to have thresholds in excess of 8 T, and threshold values for the third are difficult to assess at present because of modelling complexity. Some 5 - 10 per 10,000 people are particularly susceptible to re-entrant arrhythmia, and the risk to such people may be increased by exposure to static magnetic fields and gradient fields.

The limitations of the available data are such, however, that it is not possible to put them all together to draw firm conclusions about the effects of static magnetic fields on the endpoints considered above.

Physical movement within a static field gradient induced sensations of vertigo and nausea, and sometimes phosphenes and a metallic taste in the mouth, for static fields in excess of about 2 - 4 T. Although only transient, such effects may adversely affect people. Together with possible effects on eye-hand coordination, the optimal performance of workers executing delicate procedures (e.g. surgeons) could be reduced, with a concomitant impact on safety.

Effects on other physiological responses have been reported, but it is difficult to reach any firm conclusion without independent replication.

1.1.8 Recommendations for national authorities

National authorities are recommended to implement programs that protect both the public and workers from any untoward effects of static fields. However, given that the main effect of static electric fields is discomfort from electric discharge to tissues of the body, the protective program could merely be to provide information on situations that could lead to exposure to large electric fields and how to avoid them. A program is needed to protect against established acute effects of static magnetic fields. Because sufficient information on possible long-term or delayed effects of exposure is currently unavailable, cost-effective precautionary measures such as those being developed by WHO (www.who.int/emf) may be needed to limit the exposures of workers and the public.

National authorities should adopt standards based on sound science that limit the exposure of people to static magnetic fields. Implementation of health-based standards provides the primary protective measure for workers and the public. International standards exist for static magnetic fields (ICNIRP, 1994) and are described in Appendix 1. However, WHO recommends that these be reviewed in light of more recent evidence from the scientific literature.

National authorities should establish or complement existing programs that protect against possible effects of exposure to static magnetic fields. Protective measures for the industrial and scientific use of magnetic fields can be categorized as engineering design controls, the use of separation distance, and administrative controls. Protective measures against ancillary hazards from magnetic interference with emergency or medical electronic equipment, and for surgical and dental implants, are a special area of concern regarding possible adverse health effects of static magnetic fields. Precautions must be taken because of the mechanical forces imparted to ferromagnetic implants and loose objects in high-field facilities.

National authorities should consider licensing MRI units in order to ensure that protective measures are implemented. This would also allow additional requirements for MRI units with strengths in excess of local national standards or 2 T to be complied with. Such requirements relate to provision of information on patients, workers and any incidents or injuries resulting from the strong magnetic fields.

National authorities should fund research to fill the large gaps in knowledge that pertain to the safety of people exposed to static magnetic fields. Recommendations for further research form part of this document (see below) and are posted on the WHO web site: www.who.int/emf. Researchers should be funded to conduct studies recommended in this WHO research agenda.

National authorities should fund MRI units to collect information on worker exposure to static magnetic fields and patient exposure to MRI. These should be available for future epidemiological studies. They should also fund databases collecting information on exposures to workers where high long-term exposures occur, such as those involved in the manufacture of MRI or similarly high strength magnets and new technologies such as MagLev trains.

1.2 Recommendations for further study

Identifying gaps in our knowledge of the possible health effects of static field exposure is an essential part of this health risk assessment. The following recommendations for further research have been made.

1.2.1 Static electric fields

There appears to be little benefit in continuing research into the effects that static electric fields have on health. None of the studies conducted to date suggest any untoward health effects, except for possible stress resulting from prolonged exposure to microshocks. Thus, there are no recommendations for further research concerning biological effects from exposure to static electric fields. In addition, there is only limited opportunity for significant exposure to these fields in the workplace or living environment and this therefore does not warrant any epidemiological studies.

1.2.2 Static magnetic fields

In general terms, research carried out to date has not been systematic and has often been performed without appropriate methodology and exposure information. Coordinated research programs are recommended as an aid to a more systematic approach. There is also a need to investigate the importance of physical parameters such as intensity, duration and gradient on biological outcome.

Following a discussion of the limitations of existing studies, further research is recommended covering epidemiology, volunteer studies, animal and *in vitro* biology, studies into mechanisms of interaction, and theoretical and computational investigations. These recommendations are summarized in Table 1.

1.2.2.1 Theoretical and computational studies

Computational dosimetry provides the link between an external static magnetic field and the internal electric fields and induced currents caused by movement of living tissues in the field. Such theoretical techniques allow the fields to be characterised in specific tissues and organs. There are 4 fine resolution, anatomically realistic, voxel phantoms of adult men available, and these have been widely used in studies with time-varying electromagnetic fields. However, very little work has been done with static fields, and further work is considered necessary using these models. In particular, the use of different sized phantoms, and the use of female phantoms, is considered important, as is the use of pregnant phantoms with fetuses of differing ages. Similar studies could be performed with phantoms of pregnant animals to aid interpretation of the results of developmental studies with these models. (**Medium priority**)

A very fine resolution head-and-shoulder phantom should be developed and used to investigate the electric fields and currents associated with visual phosphenes and vertigo. This model could also be used to investigate the fields and currents generated by head and eye movements in a static magnetic field. The latter is considered of particular relevance to interventional MRI procedures where reduced head movements of surgeons and other clinical staff may necessitate increased movement of the eyes. Gross body movement by staff around the interventional system should also be simulated. (**High priority**)

Computations using a detailed model of the heart and modelling of common cardiac pathologies are considered important. This model should include the micro-architecture of the heart as well as the smaller blood vessels within the heart that might produce fields and currents that could have some influence on pacemaker rhythm generation and the propagation of depolarisation. In addition, calculations are necessary to estimate the magnitude and spatial distribution of currents that are induced in the heart as a consequence of field and field gradient exposure. Multiple orientations to the field should be studied. These would allow comparison with the currents that have been calculated to induce cardiac effects. Supportive experimental and laboratory studies are recommended. (**High priority**)

Although there is a reluctance to use high field MRI on pregnant women at the moment, it is acknowledged that this situation may change. It would therefore be advisable to carry out modelling studies investigating the currents induced in a fetus by maternal or intrinsic fetal movement in a high field. These calculations (and similar studies with gradient and radiofrequency fields) would allow an estimate to be made of the likelihood of possible effects on the fetus. (**High priority**)

1.2.2.2 In vitro studies

Static magnetic fields may interact with biological systems in a number of ways, although the most likely means of causing health effects are via field-induced effects on charged molecules and alterations in the rate of biochemical reactions.

Further studies are needed on possible mechanisms and targets for biological effects of static magnetic fields. It is recommended to investigate the effects of static magnetic fields of 0.01 - 10 T on interaction of ions (e.g. Ca^{2+} or Mg^{2+}) with enzymes and radical pair formation. Although it is considered difficult to do, there is merit in searching for more enzymatic reactions that proceed through radical pair mechanisms in model systems that are relevant for human health. Another suggestion is to concentrate on toxic radical species, such as the superoxide, which are known to be damaging and are produced by free radical mechanisms. (**Medium priority**)

Reports of a co-mutagenic effect in various cells are of particular interest concerning the carcinogenic potential of static magnetic fields. This type of study should be performed using human primary cells and extended to include transformation and genetically-modified systems. (**High priority**)

Static magnetic fields might affect gene expression and relevant functions in human and mammalian cells under specific conditions of exposure, but there is only little information available on this. Studies with techniques such as proteomics and genomics should be performed with primary human cells to search for possible molecular markers for effects of static magnetic fields relevant to human health issues. (**Low priority**)

1.2.2.3 Animal experimental studies

The effects of long-term exposure to static magnetic fields can be addressed using animal models. In the absence of specific information regarding the carcinogenic potential of static magnetic fields, long-term (including life-time) studies are recommended. Both normal and genetically-modified animals could be used. For example, if an amplification of free radicals was considered a possible route whereby cancer risk may be increased, a mouse model with deletion of the superoxide dismutase gene could be used. The susceptibility to tumours and other free radical related diseases is greatly enhanced in this model. The use of microarray techniques allows the effects of many different exposure parameters to be readily assessed and quantified on the genome and proteome. (**High priority**)

The possibility of increased risk of developmental abnormalities and teratological effects needs to be addressed in a systematic fashion. The developing brain may be particularly susceptible to the effects of movement-induced currents since orientation effects are very important for guiding the normal growth of neuronal dendrites. It is also possible that long-lasting changes could be induced by relatively short exposures. The study of neurobehavioural parameters can provide a rapid and sensitive assay to explore the effects of exposure on developing brain function, and such studies are recommended. Studies to chart the subtle morphological changes that occur during development of specific regions of the brain, such as the cortex or hippocampus, are also of value. The use of appropriate transgenic models should be considered. (**High priority**)

Although there are data indicating that exposure of animals (and human) to fields of around 2 T does not cause electrophysiological effects, it would be useful to know the effects of higher fields. Thus the effects of exposure up to and above 10 T could usefully be explored in animals. (**Medium priority**)

A variety of other endpoints have been investigated in animals that have so far provided only limited information. While a series of single studies for each of those endpoints might not be cost-effective, a broad animal study to cover different endpoints might be worthwhile. (**Low priority**)

1.2.2.4 Human experimental studies

The cognitive and behavioural effects of static magnetic fields should be investigated further. However, the available data do not suggest particular risks to specific aspects of cognition nor do they suggest which parameters should be tested in the laboratory. In the absence of a clear direction, a possible approach would be to investigate the effects of exposure on the performance of a battery of cognitive tasks that encompass standard tests of attention, reaction time and memory, if only to act as an initial screen pending more focused work. The initial work could be done with volunteers as part of experimental studies. (**Medium priority**)

With a wider utilization of MRI studies where support staff are in close proximity to patients within a magnet, such as in MRI interventional procedures, additional studies are needed of head and eye coordination, cognitive performance and behaviour in a gradient field. Further investigation of mechanisms and intensity of field-induced vestibular dysfunction including vertigo is considered of special interest because of the increasing likelihood that medical staff will be performing complicated tasks for extended periods of time within a magnetic field. (**High priority**)

Similarly, additional studies on cardiac function would be useful and could investigate effects on the cardiovascular system. These studies may also need to be performed at higher than 3 T to evaluate potential risks beyond those in the routine clinical environment. (**Low priority**)

1.2.2.5 Epidemiological studies

There are a number of categories of workers with elevated exposures to static magnetic fields, including MRI technicians, workers at aluminium smelting plants, and certain transportation workers (those on subways, MagLev trains, commuter trains, and light rail). For rare chronic diseases such as cancer, feasibility studies are needed to identify the highly exposed occupational groups that could be assessed for participation in epidemiological studies. Feasibility studies also need to determine which other exposures are present in these occupations. If sufficient numbers of workers can be identified, then a nested case-control approach is probably the most appropriate, since detailed information about the exposure and important confounding variables, such as ionizing radiation, needs to be obtained. International collaborative studies will probably be necessary to obtain sufficient numbers of exposed subjects. (**High priority**)

For other more common health outcomes with short latency periods, specific highly exposed occupational groups (for example, workers in industries where MRI systems are manufactured) can be identified and followed over time. Information about different health outcomes may already be available from routinely performed health examinations of these workers, but this can only be used if similar information is also available for a comparable unexposed group. A health survey of surgeons, nurses and other workers using interventional MRI would provide useful information as to levels, durations and frequency of exposures of workers to static fields in these systems. Similarly, patient records may exist in some hospitals from which it might be possible to obtain data on people who were exposed, but whose condition was subsequently found to be benign. (**High priority**)

There is also merit in performing a prospective study of pregnancy risks associated with occupational static magnetic field exposure, as well as follow-up studies of pregnancy outcomes of pregnant women who had to undergo MRI examinations. (**High priority**)

Experience with other frequencies has shown that obtaining reliable estimates of exposure to electromagnetic fields for use in epidemiological studies can be very difficult, and surrogate measures of exposure, such as job title or distance from a particular source, may not always provide sufficiently accurate assessments. The use of specific instruments is thus required to measure exposure. Relatively small personal dosimeters have proved very useful in research on ELF fields. Personal dosimeters would therefore greatly improve exposure assessment in epidemiological studies. Numerical and experimental validation of the dosimeters should be performed. Magnetic field strength, magnetic field gradients, exposure durations and, ideally, the rate of change of the magnetic due to motion should be recorded. (**High priority**)

Table 1. Recommendations for research

Interaction mechanisms

    Chemistry of radical pair reactions (0.1 - 10 T)

    Co-mutagenic effects using human cells

Theoretical and computational studies

    Dosimetric studies with male/female/pregnant voxel phantoms

    Induced currents in the eye

    Flow potentials in the heart

***In vitro* studies**

    Interaction mechanisms: radical pair reactions and enzymatic activity

    Influence of physical parameters (intensity, duration, recurrence, SMF gradients)

    Mutagenicity and transformation in primary human cells

    Gene expression in primary human cells

Experimental studies with animals

    Cancer

    Developmental/neurobehavioural effects

    Cardiac function (~20 T)

Experimental studies with volunteers

    Vestibular function, head and eye coordination

    Cognitive performance and behaviour

    Cardiovascular effects

Epidemiological studies

    Feasibility study of exposure sources, confounding factors, no. exposed

    Nested case-control study of chronic disease, e.g. cancer (if feasible)

    Pregnancy outcomes in relation to occupational exposure and MRI examinations

    Cohort study of short-term effects in highly exposed occupations

---

2   PHYSICAL CHARACTERISTICS

When a voltage is applied to an object such as an electrical conductor, the conductor becomes charged and forces start to act on other charges in the vicinity. Two types of forces may be distinguished: that which arises from stationary electric charges, known as the electrostatic force, and that which appears only when charges are moving (as in an electric current in a conductor), known as the magnetic force. The concept of field has been created to describe the existence and spatial distribution of these forces. Reference is then made to field of force, or simply electric and magnetic fields.

The term static refers to a situation where all charges are fixed in space, or move as a steady flow, so that both charges and current densities are constant in time. For fixed charges there is an electric field whose strength at any point in space depends on the value and geometry of all the charges. For a steady current in a circuit, both the electric and magnetic field are constant in time (static fields), since the charge density at any point of the circuit is constant.

Static electric and magnetic fields are characterized by steady, time independent strengths and correspond to the zero-frequency limit of the extremely low frequency (ELF) band. Electricity and magnetism are distinct phenomena as long as charges and current are static (ICNIRP, 1996).

2.1   Quantities and Units

A magnetic field refers to the fields of force, produced by moving electric charges (electric currents), that act on other moving charges. The field from a 'permanent' magnet results from the subatomic spin of electrons. A magnetic field is a vector field, and the fundamental vector quantities describing the magnetic field are the field strength (H) and the magnetic flux density (B) (or equivalently, the magnetic induction). The magnetic flux density is related to the magnetic field strength by the formula $H=B/\mu$. The value of μ (the magnetic permeability) is determined by the properties of the medium. In biological material, the magnetic permeability is equal to μ_0, the value of the permeability of free space (air). Thus, the values of B and H for biological materials are related by this constant.

An electric field refers to a region near an electric charge in which a force is exerted on a charged particle. The force between two point charges is described by Coulomb's law. The electric field is denoted by E and is a vector quantity. The SI unit for E is newton per coulomb (N C^{-1}).

However it is easier to measure the electric potential, V, rather than the force and charge, and the unit of volt per metre $(V\ m^{-1})$ is used in practice. As electric fields exert forces on charged particles, this will cause an electric current to flow in an electrically conductive material. This current is specified by the current density, J, with a unit of ampere per square metre $(A\ m^{-2})$.

The quantities, units, and symbols used in describing electric and magnetic fields are provided in Table 2.

Table 2. Electric and magnetic field quantities and units in the SI system

Quantity	Symbol	Unit
Electric field strength	E	volt per metre $(V\ m^{-1})$
Electric flux density	D	Coulomb per square metre $(C\ m^{-2})$
Current	I	ampere (A)
Current density	J	ampere per square metre $(A\ m^{-2})$
Magnetic field strength	H	ampere per metre $(A\ m^{-1})$
Magnetic flux	φ	weber (Wb) = V s
Magnetic flux density	B	tesla[a] (T) = $Wb\ m^{-2}$
Permeability	μ	henry per metre $(H\ m^{-1})$
Permeability of vacuum	μ_0	$\mu_0 = 1.257 \times 10^{-6}\ H\ m^{-1}$

[a] 1 T = 10^4 gauss (G), a unit in the CGS unit system

3   NATURAL BACKGROUND AND HUMAN-MADE SOURCES AND EXPOSURE

3.1   Natural Electric and Magnetic Fields

3.1.1   Natural electric fields

The natural electric field encountered above the surface of the Earth varies greatly with time and location. The primary cause of the field is the charge separation that occurs between the Earth and the ionosphere, which acts as a perfect conductor separated by air of negligible conductivity (König et al., 1981). The field near the surface typically has a fair weather strength of about 130 V m^{-1} (Dolezalek, 1979). The field strength decreases with height, with values of about 100 V m^{-1} at 100 m elevation, 45 V m^{-1} at 1 km, and less than 1 V m^{-1} at 20 km. Actual values vary widely, depending upon the local temperature, the humidity profile and the presence of ionized contaminants. Large field variations occur at ground level beneath thunderclouds, and even as thunderclouds are approaching, because the lower part of a cloud is normally negatively charged while the upper part contains a positive charge. In addition, space charge is present between the cloud and ground. As the cloud approaches, the field at ground level may first increase and then reverse, with the ground becoming positively charged. Fields of 100 V m^{-1} to 3 kV m^{-1} may be observed during this process, even in the absence of local lightning. Field reversals may take place very rapidly, within 1 min, and high field strengths may persist for the duration of the storm. Ordinary clouds, as well as thunderclouds, contain electric charge and therefore have a strong effect on the electric field at ground level. Large deviations from the fair-weather field of up to 200% are also to be expected in the presence of fog, rain, and naturally occurring small and large ions. Electric field diurnal changes can even be expected in completely fair weather. Fairly regular changes in local ionization, temperature or humidity and the resulting changes in the atmospheric electrical conductivity near the ground, as well as mechanical charge transfer by local air movements, are probably responsible for these diurnal variations.

3.1.2   Natural magnetic fields

The natural magnetic field is the sum of an internal field due to the Earth acting as a permanent magnet and an external field generated in the environment from such factors as solar activity and atmospheric processes.

The Earth's magnetic field changes continually at periods ranging from a few milliseconds to up to several million years for a field reversal.

The main feature of the geomagnetic field is its close resemblance to a dipole field aligned approximately with the spin axis of the earth (Gauss, 1839). The dipole field is explained by electrical currents flowing in the core. There are significant local differences in the strength of this field, whose average magnitude varies from about 28 A m^{-1} at the equator (corresponding to a magnetic flux density of about 35 µT in a non-magnetic material such as air) to about 56 A m^{-1} over the geomagnetic poles (corresponding to about 70 µT in air). Changes of the dipole field with periods of approximately 100 years constitute the secular variation, and are explained by eddy currents located near the core boundary (Bullard, 1948). Most other changes are due to processes occurring in the ionosphere and magnetosphere, where typical magnetic field amplitudes are very small and are generally only a fraction of 1 µT.

See Table 3 for a summary of natural electric and magnetic fields.

Table 3. Natural static electric and magnetic fields

Description/activity	Field average value
Static electric field (kV/m)	
Surface (fair weather)	0.13
Altitude of 1,000 m	0.045
Approaching storm	0.1 - 3
Static magnetic field (µT)	
Magnetic equator	35
Magnetic poles	70
Atmospheric processes	< 1

3.2   Human-made fields

3.2.1 Electric fields

3.2.1.1 Power transmission

Since the late 1950's direct current has been used in several countries to efficiently transmit electricity over long distances. Voltages of up to 800 kV have been used in commercial systems. In Europe, maximum static electric field strengths of up to 20 kV m^{-1} have been recorded directly beneath a 500 kV DC transmission line, and field levels decayed only slowly with distance, to about 2 kV m^{-1} at 400 m and 1 kV m^{-1} at 800 m from the line (EC, 1996). Blondin et al. (Blondin et al., 1996) quoted average values of 13.7 kV m^{-1} and a maximum value of 23.3 kV m^{-1} beneath a Canadian ± 450 kV high voltage direct current (HVDC) line.

3.2.1.2 Transportation

Static electric fields are also produced by the many conventional electrical rail systems, including rapid transit and light rail systems that use DC electricity. Static field strengths of around 30 V m^{-1} have been reported at 5 m from the lines on 600 V DC underground systems or tramways. Static fields of up to 300 V m^{-1} can occur inside trains that operate at 1.5, 3 and 6 kV DC. In general, regardless of category, electric fields associated with transportation systems have not been reported in any great detail, nor have concerns about them been consistently expressed. Voltages are low to moderate (generally less than a few kV), energized conductors are sufficiently well separated from passengers or workers and located overhead or as a third rail and, most importantly, shielding is provided by the intervening metallic structures of the passenger and operator compartments. Excluding sources that might be carried in by occupants, electric fields within vehicles are typically highest near windows and do not exceed a few tens of V m^{-1}.

3.2.1.3 Other

The main cause of man-made static electric fields in the environment is charge separation as a result of friction. Charge potentials of several kilovolts can be accumulated by walking on non-conductive carpets, producing field strengths near the body in the range 10 - 500 kV m^{-1} (EC, 1996). Visual display units (VDUs) produce static electric fields, the strength depending on humidity, the grounding conditions of the screen, and the electric potential between the VDU and the operator. Electric field strengths in the range 100 - 300 kV m^{-1} have been measured at 5 cm from screens, typically falling to 10 - 20 kV m^{-1} at 30 cm. A grounded electrically conductive surface on the outside of a VDU screen can significantly reduce the field strength to levels of a few hundred volts per metre at a distance of a few centimetres (AGNIR, 1994). The handling and treating of plastics can produce static field strengths near the body of up to several hundred kilovolts per metre (EC, 1996).

See Table 4 for a summary of human-made electric fields.

Table 4. Human-made static electric field in a variety of situations

Description/activity	Static electric field Average value (kV m^{-1})	Static electric field Maximum value (kV m^{-1})
Walking on non-conductive carpets[a]	10 - 500	
Video display terminals[b]		
5 cm from screen	100 - 300	
30 cm	10 - 20	
Plastic welding and moulding	100 - 300	
DC electric transmission lines[a]		176.3
500 kV (directly below)	20	
at 400 m	2	
at 800 m	1	
Electrical railway system[c]		
600 V (at 5m)	0.03	
15 - 6 kV (inside)	0.3	

[a] (EC, 1996); [b] (AGNIR, 1994); [c] (ICNIRP, 2003)

3.2.2 Magnetic fields

There may be man-made magnetic fields of significantly higher strength that are superimposed on the Earth's magnetic field.

3.2.2.1 Transportation

Dietrich and Jacobs (Dietrich & Jacobs, 1999) in the USA have reported static magnetic field levels in a range of transport environments. In general, electrified railway systems produce some of the largest static field levels encountered by the general public. Magnetic flux densities of up to 1 mT have been reported inside Italian high-speed trains operating at 30 kV DC at a maximum speed of 250 km/h (Grandolfo, 1989). Modern magnetic levitation (MagLev) systems use very high fields (around 1 T) directly on the rails. However fields inside the trains vary between 50 μT and 1 - 2 mT, depending on the design. Static fields up to several tens of microtesla have been reported inside trams operating at 500 A DC (EC, 1996).

See Table 5 or a summary of magnetic fields in transportation systems.

Table 5. Static field magnetic flux densities (µT) measured in US and European transportation systems.

Mode of transport	Static magnetic field Average value (µT)	Static magnetic field Range of values (µT)
Ferry boat (diesel powered)[b]	55.9	47.6 - 67.9
Escalator[b]	57.6	30.9 - 84.9
Moving walkway[b]	61.7	23.6 - 121.8
Conventional cars, light trucks and buses[c]	33.9	2.7 - 87.5
Electric cars & light trucks[c]		
Test facility	40.8	10.6 - 104.4
Test track	38.8	12.5 - 104.1
Electric shuttle bus	37.4	15.1 - 61.0
Shuttle Tram (AC)[b]	48.6	24.3 - 73.4
Commuter Train (AC)[d]	53.8	19.4 - 196.9
US railway system		
25 Hz version	60.6	176.3
60 Hz version	63.0	103.9
Non-Electrified	56.9	103.3
New Jersey Long Branch	73.4	101.6
TGV-A	54.5	96.2
UK railway system[e]		
London underground		
Driver's cabin		200
Passenger car – floor level		100 - 2,000
Suburban & mainline railways		
Passengers		25
Equipment car		2,000

23

German Transrapid MagLev System[f]

TR07	61.1	111.0
TR08 – passenger location	46.2	108.4
TR08 – platform (1 m from car)	52.9	71.8

Japan Railways developmental MagLev system[g]

4 m outside guideway	190	
8 m under bridge section	20	
Inside passenger cabin		80 - 1060
Between passenger cars		60 - 1330

[a] Dietrich and Jacobs (Dietrich & Jacobs, 1999) on behalf of US Department of Transportation, Federal Railroad Administration DOT-VNTSC-FRA-02-11
[b] Measured at a height of 3 feet (0.9m)
[c] Average of all sensor positions (i.e. driver and passenger head, waist and ankle)
[d] Includes all locations and sensor positions (head, waist & ankle)
[e] Chadwick and Lowes (Chadwick & Lowes, 1998)
[f] Experimental vehicles
[g] (IEEJ - Institute of Electrical Engineers of Japan, 1998)

3.2.2.2 Industry

Static fields formed by rectifying an intense alternating current are used in several industrial processes, including gas welding and the production of aluminium and chlorine.

Aluminium is produced by the electrolytic reduction of alumina in Soderberg reduction cells or 'pots'. The workers involved in this operation are called 'potroom' or 'potline' workers and are exposed to static magnetic fields. Measurements at eleven factories in France (Mur et al., 1998) found that the fields near the pots were ~ 4 - 30 mT, but the workers were generally exposed to < 20 mT. Measurements at a Norwegian plant (Moen et al., 1996) showed a maximum level of 63 mT, but results were otherwise similar to Mur et al. (1998). This corresponds to measurements made in a Californian aluminium production test facility, where magnetic fields up to 57 mT were determined by Tenforde (1986a).

There are many different electric arc welding processes involving direct alternating or pulsed current that produce magnetic fields. Metal inert gas (MIG) or metal active gas (MAG) welding produce static magnetic field strengths up to 5 mT at the distance of 1 cm from the welding cables (Skotte & Hjollund, 1997). Static magnetic field strength in MIG/MAG welding is roughly one order of magnitude higher than the ELF magnetic field.

3.2.2.3 Magnetic resonance imaging (MRI)

MRI systems have proliferated in recent years and there are currently many thousands worldwide. The technique utilizes a strong homogeneous static magnetic field, much smaller time-varying gradient magnetic fields, and radiofrequency radiation. The static magnetic field is generated by permanent magnets, superconducting magnets and combinations thereof in the range of 0.2 - 3 T for systems for routine clinical use. In research applications, higher magnetic fields of up to 9.4 T are used for whole body patient scanning. The stray magnetic fields around the magnets for MRI studies are well defined and can be minimized in the shielded magnet versions – unfortunately very few surveys have been published. Stuchly and Lecuyer (1987) mapped the static fields around four MRI machines (the units ranged from 0.15 - 1.9 T). Magnetic flux densities of up to about 1 T were measured close to the magnet, but these had dropped to less than 30 mT at 2 m. Measurements at the operator console position were less than 5 mT. Nevertheless, the operator will be exposed to magnetic flux density up to the maximum field strength of the magnet, which still exists just outside the bore of the magnets. Apart from the static magnetic field, the other parameters likely to be important for static magnetic field effects are the gradient field, $\partial B/\partial z$, and the 'force product' given by $B(\partial B/\partial z)$. Typical values of the gradient field and force product for a 4 T system are 2.8 T m^{-1} and 8.8 T^2 m^{-1} (Schenck et al., 1992) and 7.9 T m^{-1} and 42.9 T^2 m^{-1} for a 8 T system (Kangarlu & Robitaille, 2000).

Modern applications for the MRI systems include the use of the system in the operating theatre for interventional applications. The magnetic field strength of these systems varies from low field open (vertical field) systems, 0.2 - 0.6 T, up to medium or high field cylindrical (horizontal field) systems, 0.5 - 1.5 T. These systems have openings between the poles so theatre staff can access patients. Peak static field exposures may approach or even exceed the static field for the scanner. Force products (see section 6.1) for such designs may be higher than for solenoidal designs at the same field strength. Systems are also being introduced whereby the patient can be transported from the MRI system into an X-ray system and vice versa, using one patient table positioning device. In this way, both imaging modalities can be used for optimal diagnosis and treatment of the patient. Such systems typically operate at 1.5 T and above. However, workers will generally not be closer than the magnet opening and magnetic field exposures are not likely to exceed the rated field strength. For actively shielded magnets, the peak force product may occur close to the magnet opening. Appropriate controls to limit exposure of theatre staff are still being developed. Medical applications with the potential of using fields up to 10 T and higher are also being developed (Simon & Szumowski, 1992; Polk et al., 1996; Gowland, 2005).

A new medical system that applies strong static (inhomogeneous) magnetic fields has been recently introduced. The system, referred to as the 'magnetic navigator system' applies an inhomogeneous 0.5 T static magnetic field to navigate the ferromagnetic tip of a catheter under X-ray control to the correct anatomical position in a patient's body.

3.2.2.4 Research and energy technologies

Large superconducting magnets are used in a variety of research applications including:

- Particle accelerators like the LEP (Large Electron Positron Collider) at CERN in Geneva that can consist of thousands of magnets, including large superconducting magnets.
- Thermonuclear fusion research requires large magnets (~ 4 T) for plasma containment. Worldwide efforts in fusion research are now being combined in an international project currently under design, but which will include the largest tokamak (chamber in which a plasma is heated and confined by magnetic fields) ever constructed.
- Magnetohydrodynamic research involving superconducting magnets of up to 5 T.
- Bubble chambers for subatomic particle detection, which have largely been replaced by different detectors, such as the multiwire chamber.
- Nuclear magnetic resonance (NMR) spectroscopy, used to obtain physical and chemical properties of molecules, can involve the use of large superconducting magnets (12 - 22 T).

See Table 6 for typical static magnetic fields in industrial, research and medical environments.

Table 6.   Major technologies involving the use of large static magnetic fields, and corresponding exposure levels

Procedures	Static magnetic field Typical value (mT)
Energy technologies[g]	
Thermonuclear fusion reactors	
Hot cell areas	45
Accessible areas	5
Outside reactor site	0.1
Magnetohydrodynamic systems	10 (at about 50 m)
	0.1 (at distances greater than 250 m)
Superconducting magnet energy storage systems	50 (max) at accessible locations
Superconducting generators and transmission lines	< 0.1 (projected)
Research facilities	
Bubble chambers[g, h]	600 - 1,500 (for several minutes during changes of film cassettes)
Superconducting spectrometers[a, h]	1,000 at operator-accessible locations
Particle accelerators[a]	Exposure only during maintenance
Isotope separation units[a]	1 (typical) and 50 (occasionally)
Nuclear Magnetic Resonance	2,000 (24 cm radially from 18.8 T magnet)
	600 (52 cm radially from 18.8 T magnet)
Industry	
Aluminium production[e,f,h]	up to 100 in accessible locations < 20 (generally)
Electrolytic processes[a]	10 (average) and 50 (maximum)
Magnet production[a]	0.3 - 0.5 (chest and head) & 2 - 5 (hands)
Welding[b]	5 (submerged arc)
	0.9 - 1.9 (MIG/MAG)

	5 (1 cm from cables – MIG/MAG)
Heavy manufacturing industries[c]	< 0.13 (maximum value)
Medicine[a]	
Magnetic resonance imaging and spectroscopy	0.5 (unshielded I T magnet at 10 m)
	0.5 (unshielded 2 T magnet at 13 m)
MRI[d]	850 (next to 1.9 T unit)
	< 30 at 2 m
	0.5-< 5 at operator console
	~ 1,000 next to a shielded 4 T system

[a] (ICNIRP, 1996)
[b] (Skotte & Hjollund, 1997)
[c] (Bowman & Methner, 2000)
[d] (Stuchly & Lecuyer, 1987)
[e] (Moen et al., 1996)
[f] (Mur et al., 1998)
[g] (Stuchly, 1986)
[h] (Tenforde, 1986a)

3.2.2.5 Other

Variations of up to 20% in the Earth's static magnetic field have been observed both within and between homes (Swanson, 1994). These observations point to steel construction materials as important contributors to local field variation in homes. Static magnetic field sources within homes otherwise tend to be small and only generate high levels very locally.

Steel-belted radial tyres are magnetic and produce static and low-frequency alternating magnetic fields in the passenger compartments of cars. Milham et al. (1999) measured static fields of about 150 μT 10 mm from a tyre. At 50 km/h, the static magnetic field measured within the car did not exceed about 0.01 μT.

Headphones and telephone speakers produce magnetic flux densities of 0.3 - 1.0 mT at their surfaces (EC, 1996). The static magnetic fields from battery-powered devices are very small compared with the natural background. Magnetic plasters, blankets and mattresses for alleged therapeutic properties have surface magnetic flux densities of about 50 mT, but these decay quickly within a few millimetres or so (EC,

1996). Small bar magnets can produce 1 - 10 mT magnetic flux densities within a centimetre of the magnet.

High voltage DC transmission lines produce magnetic fields of up to a few tens of microtesla. Bracken (1979) reported 22 µT under a 500 kV line. For an underground transmission line buried at 1.4 m and carrying a maximum current of about 1 kA, the maximum field was less than 10 µT at ground level (Hassenzahl et al., 1978). These are still relatively uncommon sources of exposure.

4   MEASUREMENT OF STATIC ELECTRIC AND MAGNETIC FIELDS

Measurements of static electric and magnetic fields are used to characterize emissions from sources and exposure of persons or experimental subjects. Early epidemiological and laboratory studies used simple survey instruments that displayed the maximum static electric or magnetic field measured along a single axis. Most fields that are encountered will have a linear polarization vector whose direction is unknown. This requires the measurement of three orthogonal components of the electric or magnetic field, at each location of interest. This can be done with either a single sensor or with a multiple sensor instrument. If a single sensor is used, then each of the three orthogonal components must be measured sequentially. The preferred method is the use of an instrument with three mutually orthogonal sensors housed in a common, small volume. This allows the simultaneous measurement of each component of a field. Irrespective of whether a single or three sensor instrument is used, the total field vector must be obtained by squaring the magnitude of each field component, summing the three squared values, and then taking the square root of the sum as indicated in Eq. 4.1 for magnetic flux density.

$$B_{total} = \sqrt{B_x^2 + B_y^2 + B_z^2} \tag{4.1}$$

where:

B_{total} is the magnitude of the magnetic flux density
B_x, B_y, B_z are the magnitudes of the components of the magnetic flux density along the axes in a rectangular coordinate system.

It is not necessary to measure each of the components of the field if its polarization is linear and the orientation of the field vector is known. For example, the electric field orientation is known near the boundary of a conducting object, such as the ground (if it is highly conductive). The electric field vector here must be perpendicular to the conducting object. Therefore, only a vertical component of the electric field need be measured near a highly conducting surface (ICNIRP, 2003).

4.1   Electric fields

Static electric-field-strength sensors that are commercially available include the electric field mill, the vibrating plate, and the vibrating probe sensors. All are used to measure static fields with respect to a reference object (usually electrical ground). All of these instruments interrupt or 'chop' the static voltage detected by the sensor. This provides a time-varying (AC) voltage that is easier to process and calibrate than a static (DC) voltage. The field strengths that are measured by field mill, vibrating plate, and vibrating probe sensors involve the quantification of the AC current across known, high impedance between the sensing electrode and the ground (ICNIRP, 2003).

The electric field mill can determine the static electric field strength by measuring modulated, capacitively induced charges sensed by metal electrodes. The time-varying charge and the current are proportional to the electric field strength (E). Sensitivity of the electric field mill is on the order of a few hundred V m^{-1}, with a maximum measurement capability of up to 100 kV m^{-1} or more.

The vibrating plate sensor consists of a faceplate with an aperture and a central vibrating plate or probe. The faceplate is placed parallel to, and in contact with, the ground plane. A mechanical driver moves the vibrating plate or probe up and down in the direction normal to the faceplate. The position of the vibrating electrode oscillates from one extreme position that is flush with the faceplate aperture to the other extreme position where it is separated a fixed distance below the ground plane (usually, the ground plane is the earth beneath a HVDC power line). Sensitivity of the vibrating plate sensor is on the order of a few hundred V m^{-1}.

During the measurement procedure, other objects and persons operating the equipment must be removed from any area that will perturb the field at the location of the measurement instrument. E-field meters that operate in contact with the ground plane need only measure the vector component that exists close to ground (the component that is perpendicular to the ground plane). Fields mills and vibrating plate/probe sensors are intended to be placed on a 'ground plane', but can be elevated above the physical source of the earth if electrical connection to the earth is provided by a grounding wire (ICNIRP, 2003).

4.2   Magnetic fields

Magnetic flux densities that are of interest range from approximately 20 µT (the Earth's magnetic flux) to more than 20 T (high field NMR and MRI devices). The instrument for measuring the magnitude and direction of a magnetic field is called a magnetometer. Two types of magnetometers (Fluxgate and Hall effect) are practical for the measurement of static magnetic fields. Both are capable of determining a single vector component of the magnetic field. The Fluxgate magnetometer is a sensitive device based on the magnetic saturation effect in ferromagnetic materials. It is constructed of two parallel cores of a ferromagnetic material placed closely together. It measures an alternating current that is induced in a secondary coil wrapped around the cores. The secondary coil signal is proportional to the strength of any external magnetic field that is aligned in the proper orientation with respect to the cores. Current (AC) is passed through coils that are wrapped separately around each core. AC voltage Fluxgate magnetometers are capable of measuring the strength of the magnetic field from 1.0 nT to 0.01 T. They can be used in a mode that subtracts the constant value of the Earth's static field so that other static fields weaker that this field can be measured.

Hall effect devices consist of a thin square or rectangular plate or film of gallium arsenide and indium arsenide to which four electrical contacts are made. An electrical current is passed through the length of the semiconductor and the voltage across the width of the semiconductor is measured. The Hall voltage, V_h, is directly proportional to the number of flux lines passing through the foil, the cosine of the angle at which they pass through it (i.e. they are polarization dependent), and the amount of current passing through the device. Hall effect instruments can measure flux density from 100 µT to up to 100 T.

5   INTERACTION MECHANISMS

Many biological processes are affected by electromagnetic fields. Even small changes in internal fields caused by external magnetic fields can affect that biology. Human tissues respond in radically different ways to applied electric and magnetic fields. Electric fields are experienced as a force by electrically charged objects. The electric field at the surface of an object, particularly where the radius is small (for example, at the limit, a point), can be larger than the unperturbed electric field. However, because of the high conductivity of body tissues relative to air, exposure to a static electric field does not produce a significant internal field, but leads to the build up of surface charge on the body. The induced surface charge may be perceived if discharged to a grounded object. In contrast, the magnetic field strength is virtually the same inside the body as outside. Such fields will interact directly with magnetically anisotropic materials and moving charges. These interactions are subtle and difficult to observe in living tissues. Several excellent reviews of the possible physical interactions of static magnetic fields have been published, including Azanza and del Moral (1994); Goodman et al. (1995); Grissom (1995); Frankel and Liburdy (1996); Valberg et al. (1997); Beers et al. (1998); Adair (2000); Zhadin (2001); Binhi (2002); and Binhi and Savin (2003).

Biological effects of static magnetic fields are studied in several specialized fields of research, each with specific objectives and applications. These studies cover a wide range of static field strengths and it is possible that different physical mechanisms are relevant in the different areas, which include:

- animal navigation and the general study of animal behaviour influenced by magnetic fields;
- static magnetic fields as an alleged therapeutic modality, either alone or in conjunction with pharmacological agents;
- static magnetic fields as a component in biological detection of relatively weak environmental and occupational magnetic fields resulting from the distribution and use of direct current electric power; and
- the use of strong magnetic fields for magnetic resonance clinical diagnostic procedures, such as magnetic resonance imaging (MRI), and in chemical analysis and spectroscopy (NMR).

Outline

A number of physical and chemical effects can occur as a result of exposure of living tissues to static magnetic fields. At the level of macromolecules and larger structures, interactions of stationary magnetic

33

fields with biological systems can be characterised as electrodynamic or magnetomechanical in nature. Electrodynamic effects originate through the interaction of magnetic fields with electrolyte flows, leading to the induction of electrical potentials and currents. Magnetomechanical phenomena include orientation effects on macromolecular assemblies in fields, and the movement of paramagnetic and ferromagnetic molecular species in strong field gradients. Several types of magnetic field interactions have been shown to occur at the atomic and subatomic levels in biological systems. Two such interactions are the nuclear magnetic resonance and the effects on electronic spin states, and their relevance to certain classes of electron transfer reactions in living tissues. These interaction mechanisms will be considered in some detail in this section. Because static electric fields barely penetrate human bodies, they will not be considered further in this chapter.

5.1   Electrodynamic interactions

With some minor exceptions, all chemistry and biology acts exclusively through forces produced by electromagnetic fields acting on electric charges. The science of electromagnetism has had many famous contributors, but it was James Maxwell (1831 - 1879) who placed the laws of electromagnetism into the form in which they are now known. Maxwell's equations are a set of four equations that describe the behaviour of both electric and magnetic fields as well as their interaction with matter. The equations express:

• how electric charges produce electric fields (Gauss' law);
• the absence of magnetic charges (i.e. the impossibility of creating an isolated magnetic pole);
• how currents produce magnetic fields (Ampère's law); and
• how changing magnetic fields produce electric fields (Faraday's law of induction).

The first physical interaction mechanism follows directly from Maxwell's equations (Jackson, 1999).

5.1.1   Magnetic induction of electric fields and currents

The Lorentz force, F, exerted on a charged particle in an electromagnetic field is given by the Lorentz force equation (5.1).

$$F = q(E + v \times B) \qquad (5.1)$$

where:
E is the electric field (vector)
B is the magnetic field (vector)
q is the charge of the particle
v is the particle velocity (expressed as a vector).

34

The electric field is proportional to that part of the force that is independent of its motion. The magnetic field is proportional to the velocity of the charge.

Just as static magnetic fields exert forces on moving electric charges, due to Galilean relativity, changing magnetic fields produce forces on stationary electric charges. The forces on stationary charges are a measure of the electric field. The induced electric field generated by a changing magnetic field can be calculated using the integral form of Faraday's law:

$$\oint_C \bar{E} \cdot d\bar{l} = -\frac{d}{dt} \int_S \bar{B} \cdot d\bar{A} \tag{5.2}$$

where the left-hand side is a line integral over a closed loop C, and the right hand side is the time derivative of a surface integral of the normal component of the magnetic flux through the area S enclosed by C. Equation (5.2) only calculates the average electric field over the loop C, but it is often the only measure available when the actual local field in a complex system can only be estimated with numerical methods that require very detailed knowledge about the fields on the system boundary and its material properties. If we assume that the bulk conductivity of the material is relatively homogeneous, then we can also infer the average induced current by Ohm's law.

Equation (5.2) will register an average electric field when the integral changes with time. If we consider the loop to be of fixed dimensions, this can happen in several different ways:

- the magnetic field itself varies with time. This is the typical situation for many field studies in which a spatially homogenous field modulated, e.g. with a sine wave;
- by motion in a field that has spatial variation. This is, for instance, relevant when transporting a person into or out of a MRI machine that has very strong gradients at the coil entrance; and
- the relative orientation between the loop and the field vector is changed. This is what happens if we rotate the loop in a static field.

A very detailed analysis of these possibilities is available in Ptisyna et al. (1998). The rate of change directly determines the induced field, so that the frequency of the field application, the speed of the motion in a gradient, and the rotation frequency enter directly into the value of the induced fields.

5.1.2 Lorentz force

Ionic currents interact with static magnetic fields as a result of the Lorentz forces exerted on moving charge carriers (equation 5.1). This phenomenon is the physical basis of the Hall effect (see below) in solid-state materials, and it also occurs in several biological processes that involve the flow of electrolytes in an aqueous medium. Examples of such processes are the ionic currents associated with the flow of blood in the circulatory system, nerve impulse propagation, and visual photo-transduction processes.

5.1.2.1 Flow potentials

A well-studied example of electrodynamic interactions that leads to measurable biological effects is the induction of electrical potentials as a result of blood flow in the presence of a static magnetic field (Tenforde, 2005). These are a direct consequence of the Lorentz force exerted on moving ionic currents, so that blood flowing through a cylindrical vessel of diameter, d, will develop an electrical potential, ψ given by the equation:

$$\psi = |E_i|\, d = |v|\, |B|\, d \sin \theta \tag{5.3}$$

where θ is the angle between B and the velocity vector. That is, the induced electrical potential is proportional to the velocity of the blood flow and to the magnetic field strength. This equation was originally shown by Kolin (1945) to describe the interaction of blood flow with an applied magnetic field, and it forms the theoretical basis for analysing the rate of blood flow using an electromagnetic flow meter (Kolin, 1952).

There have been numerous accounts of flow potentials being recorded in the ECGs of animals and volunteers placed in strong static magnetic fields (see chapters 7.2 and 8.1). These effects are largest in the blood vessels around the heart and in the heart itself (see Tenforde, 2005). It has been suggested that this effect may place a limit on the magnetic field strength that can be safely tolerated by human beings (Schenck, 1992). The possible consequences for human health have been reviewed by Holden (2005).

Several early models of aortic blood flow in magnetic fields relied on an approximate solution of the Navier-Stokes equation describing the dynamic properties of an electrically conductive fluid flowing in the presence of a strong magnetic field (Hartmann, 1937; Hartmann & Lazarus, 1937). The results of these theoretical calculations indicated that static magnetic fields should produce only small magnetohydrodynamic effects on blood flow in the aorta at field levels up to 2 T (Belousova, 1965; Vardanyan, 1973; Abashin & Yevtushenko, 1974; Sud et al., 1978;

Kumar, 1978; Tenforde et al., 1983; Chen & Saha, 1985; Sud & Sekhon, 1989). An exact solution of the Navier-Stokes equation was later obtained by Keltner et al. (1990), and led to a similar conclusion. All of these models made the simplifying assumption that the wall of the aorta is not electrically conductive.

Kinouchi et al. (1996) developed a theoretical model assuming finite conductivity of the arterial wall. In this model, a complete solution of the Navier-Stokes equation for aortic blood flow was obtained by a finite element analysis method for static magnetic fields of arbitrarily high intensity under the condition that the wall of the aortic vessel is electrically conductive. This model was used to obtain quantitative estimates as a function of the applied magnetic field of the magnetically-induced fields and currents in the aorta, magnetohydrodynamic slowing of the aortic blood flow rate and the leakage currents passing from the aorta into the thoracic region, including those present at the sino-atrial pacemaker node of the heart. In a 5 T field, the predicted current density at the sino-atrial node was about 110 - 120 mA m^{-2}, rising to about 220 mA m^{-2} at 10 T and 300 mA m^{-2} at 15 T. Theoretically, the greatest effects should occur for flow in long blood vessels orthogonal to the static magnetic field, while no effect should be seen for flow aligned with the field. Orientation of the patient with respect to the magnetic field may be a consideration for any bio-effects, but this has not been considered in detail.

5.1.2.2 A theoretical study of the possible effects of flow potentials on the heart

Holden (2005) assessed the effects of the electric fields and currents induced by the flow potentials on cardiac function using virtual cardiac tissues – computational models of cardiac electrophysiology. These models are used to understand the normal and pathological electrophysiology of the heart and how this can be modified by pharmacological intervention. The author noted that, although the flow potential generated by blood flow in the aorta will be the largest, a greater fraction of the smaller potentials generated in blood vessels on or in the myocardium of the heart have less distance over which to decay, and so may have the largest effect. Three possibilities were considered, including changing the rate of excitation of the heart by acting on the sino-atrial pacemaker tissues, inducing the ectopic initiation of activity at sites that are not normally endogenously active, and triggering arrhythmias by altering the pattern of action potential propagation through the ventricular myocardium.

Electrical currents generated by flow potentials will have either a depolarising or hyperpolarising effect on myocardial tissue, depending on the orientation of the induced current relative to the myocardial tissue. Holden (2005) noted that, in the sinoatrial node, a greater fraction of external current would flow into the peripheral cells, whereas the pacemaker function resides primarily in cells located at the centre. This possibly may contribute to the lack of any effect of 8 T static fields on heart rate {Chakeres, 2003 736 /id /ft "; see below"}, although a change in rate would, however, be considered benign. Such current flow may also initiate ectopic activity, if action potentials are excited in a sufficiently large volume of myocardial cells. This could be induced by relatively small changes in membrane potential, if the cell parameters are very close to a critical value (one that produces an early after-depolarisation during an action potential). However, the initiation of activity at an ectopic focus would be suppressed by a higher rate of activity driven by the sinoatrial node. In addition, ectopic beats are also considered relatively benign. These two effects are thought to have thresholds in excess of 8 T.

The situation is more complex with regard to ventricular fibrillation. The flow potentials induced in coronary arteries and branches (but not those induced by the aorta) will have opposite polarities on opposite sides of the left ventricle. This would increase the electrical heterogeneity of the ventricle and so may enhance or establish spatial gradients in action potential duration between different parts of the ventricle. This is likely to increase the probability of the initiation of re-entrant arrhythmias, which can be lethal. However, the author noted that such re-entrant arrhythmias are very rare events, so that even a large increase in their probability leaves them remaining very unlikely in an individual during an exposure period of up to a few hours. Nevertheless, a more precise indication of the risk, and threshold, which Holden (2005) notes is lower than that for pacemaker modulation and ectopic beat induction, would be of value. This is especially the case in people that are more susceptible to re-entrant arrhythmias, such as people with enlarged (hypertrophic cardiomyopathy) or damaged (postinfarct) hearts, and carriers of some rare inherited disorders in repolarisation, including the long QT syndrome. Similar simulations in non–homogeneous magnetic fields are yet to be completed.

5.1.3 Magnetohydrodynamic model

Flow-induced electric currents also act through magnetohydrodynamic (MHD) forces to produce a retarding force on blood flow. It has been estimated that there is a 5% reduction in humans in the flow rate at 10 T, rising to 10% at 15 T (Kinouchi et al., 1996), compared to Keltner's estimate (Keltner et al., 1990) of 0.2% pressure change at 10 T for worst-case conditions (magnetic field orthogonal to flow in long blood vessels). Kangarlu et al. (1999) observed no blood pressure changes in dogs exposed to 8 T fields for 3 hours. In contrast, studies of blood pressure changes in volunteers indicated that systolic pressure rose by about 4 mm Hg in an 8 T static field, which is consistent with a haemodynamic compensation for a magnetohydrodynamic reduction in blood flow (Chakeres & de Vocht, 2005), see section 8.1.2.2.1.

Schenck (2005) has suggested that the mild sensations of vertigo and nausea often experienced by MRI patients might be related to a magnetic interaction with the vestibular apparatus of the inner ear. There are three semicircular canals in this structure that are roughly orthogonal to one another. Each is sensitive to a different component of the angular acceleration of the head. Each of these canals is filled with a conducting fluid called the endolymph and contains structures at one end referred to as neuromast organs. These consist of sensory (hair) cells and supporting cells covered by a gelatinous cupula. When the head undergoes angular acceleration, the inertia of the endolymph produces a force on the cupulas, which are slightly deflected by it. This transfers to the hair cells in the neuromast organs and initiates a signal that is eventually interpreted within the central nervous system as a head motion. Any excitation of hair cells by the magnetic field would be perceived as an extraneous head rotation that would not correspond to other sensory inputs. A field-induced excitation could result from direct depolarization of sensory cells or from diamagnetic anisotropy in the cupula, which would produce torque and deflection of this structure when the head was turned. Another possibility (Schenck, 1992) is that the changing magnetic flux through the semicircular canals when the head is turned leads to an additional force, of magnetohydrodynamic origin, on the endolymphatic fluid.

The mild vertigo and nausea is analogous to similar symptoms associated with motion sickness. According to the conflict hypothesis (Brandt, 2003) motion sickness is the consequence of discordant inputs to the brain information about the position and motion of the body from the vestibular and the visual systems, and from other sensory sources. Further work is necessary to determine if these field-related sensory effects can be explained by magnetohydrodynamic forces acting on the semicircular canals or by other induced current effects.

5.2   Magnetomechanical interactions

There are two basic mechanisms through which static magnetic fields exert mechanical forces and torques on objects. In the first type of magnetomechanical interaction, rotational motion of a substance occurs in a uniform field until it achieves a minimum energy state. The second mechanism involves the translational force exerted on a paramagnetic or ferromagnetic substance placed in a magnetic field gradient, although in theory the only requirement is that the object has a different magnetic susceptibility to its surroundings.

Other less understood mechanisms are related to rotations and vibrations of ions and charged molecules in static magnetic fields. These mechanisms have not been established.

Another important aspect of magnetomechanical interactions with biological systems are the forces exerted by the geomagnetic field on magnetotactic bacteria and in the tissue structures in various organisms that contain deposits of biogenic magnetite (see section 5.4).

5.2.1 Magnetomechanics (torque on magnetic dipole moment)

Macromolecules and structurally ordered molecular assemblies with a high degree of magnetic anisotropy will experience a torque in a uniform magnetic field and rotate until they reach an equilibrium orientation that represents a minimum energy state.

A magnetic dipole with moment $\vec{m}$ in an external magnetic field $\vec{B}$ experiences a torque

$$\vec{N} = \vec{m} \times \vec{B} \tag{5.4}$$

and the potential energy associated with the system is:

$$U = -\vec{m} \cdot \vec{B} \tag{5.5}$$

Hence, the effect of the field is a tendency to rotate the dipole towards alignment with the field. This is the basis for various interaction mechanisms. Note that this does not occur for magnetic dipoles that are formed in isotropic diamagnetic or paramagnetic materials in response to an applied magnetic field, since their magnetic moments would be aligned parallel (or anti-parallel) with the local field. If we have a material with intrinsic magnetization or with anisotropic susceptibility, then there is a possibility for a physical mechanism (see section 5.2.3 on anisotropic diamagnetism).

In living systems, the effect of thermal noise will tend to randomize the dipole's orientation. The energy U has to be compared to $k_B T$ (where k_B is Boltzmann's constant) for typical temperatures of living systems ($T \sim 310$ K). For protons with a nuclear magneton of magnetic moment ($\mu_B = e\hbar / 2m_e$), the comparison leaves a very slight alignment even at high (> 1 T) fields, although it is large enough to be technologically useful for MRI.

An example of an intact cell that can be oriented magnetically is the deoxygenated sickle erythrocyte. It has been shown that these cells, in which the deoxygenated haemoglobin is paramagnetic, will align in a 0.35 T static field with the long axis of the sickle cell oriented perpendicular to the magnetic flux lines (Murayama, 1965). Another example of systems that overcome the thermal drive to isotropy is that of magnetic moments created by diamagnetic anisotropy in relatively large structures (see section 5.2.3).

5.2.2 Magnetophoresis (force on magnetic dipole moment)

The second mechanism through which static magnetic fields exert mechanical forces and torques on objects involves a translational force. A magnetic dipole ($\bar{m}$) in a static gradient magnetic field experiences a (lowest order) force of:

$$F = (m \cdot \nabla)B \qquad\qquad (5.6)$$

The magnetic dipole can be a permanent dipole or its magnetization can be induced by the field itself. An example of the latter is diamagnetic levitation in which the force is sufficiently large to oppose the gravitational pull (Beaugnon & Tournier, 1991; Valles, Jr. et al., 1997). The magnetic moment of an object of volume V and magnetic susceptibility χ in a field B is:

$$m = \chi V B / \mu_0 ,$$

where μ_0 is the permeability of vacuum. To balance the force of gravity, $(g\rho V)$ we need $B \nabla B > 1000$ T^2 m^{-1} for typical tissue parameters.

This effect is possible for ferromagnetic materials in high gradients, such as those encountered in magnetic resonance imaging. A realistic example (Kangarlu & Robitaille, 2000) shows how typical MRI conditions can accelerate a steel wrench to over 40 m/s^2. In addition, significant magnetic forces are exerted on many types of implanted medical devices, including aneurysm clips, dental amalgam, prostheses, and pacemaker cases (Tenforde & Budinger, 1986; ASTM, 2003a; ASTM, 2003b).

Some alleged therapeutic applications of magnets claim that strong gradients are required for efficacy (McLean et al., 1995), with a threshold gradient observed somewhere in the region of 1 T m^{-1} (Cavopol et al., 1995). The corresponding threshold force on a Bohr magneton is approximately 10^{-23} N. As a comparison, the electric field required to apply this force on a unit charge is $E = 1.7$ x 10^{-4} V m^{-1}. This is a very small field, but it is in within range of another threshold $E = 4 \times 10^{-4}$ V m^{-1} suggested by other experimental studies (Blank & Soo, 1992; Blank & Soo, 1996). The mechanism of magnetophoresis of diamagnetic materials is the only proposed mechanism for gradient specific effects, but it probably does not provide an explanation of the experimental evidence at this relatively weak end of exposures.

Experiments on the rate of myosin phosphorylation in a gradient magnetic field (Engström et al., 2002) suggest that a combination of field and gradient are required to explain the mechanism producing the effect on this biochemical enzyme system.

The forces exerted on paramagnetic and ferromagnetic substances by strong static magnetic field gradients provide the physical basis for a number of useful biological and biochemical processes (ICNIRP, 2003). Examples of the application of magnetic forces include the targeting of drugs encapsulated in magnetic microcarriers (Widder et al., 1982), the separation of deoxygenated erythrocytes from whole blood (Melville, 1975; Paul et al., 1978), the separation of antibody-secreting cells from a suspension of bone marrow cells (Poynton et al., 1983), and the removal of micro-organisms from water (De Latour, 1973; Kurinobu & Uchiyama, 1982). It has also been observed that strong magnetic field gradients can influence the distribution of deoxygenated, paramagnetic erythrocytes in a flowing suspension of blood cells (Shiga et al., 1993). It has been suggested (Ichioka et al., 2000) that this effect could retard the rate of blood flow when the product of the flux density and the field gradient exceeds 100 T^2 m^{-1}.

5.2.3 Anisotropic diamagnetism

If a material has anisotropic diamagnetic susceptibility, then a static magnetic field will apply a torque on the system, since the orientations parallel and perpendicular become differentially magnetized. Orientation with respect to the field becomes energetically differentiated and we have the basis for a physical transduction mechanism (Maret & Dransfeld, 1977). The energy of a cylindrical molecule with magnetic susceptibility χ_p and parallel and perpendicular to the cylinder axis, respectively, is:

$$E = -VB^2 (\chi_p - \chi_q) / 2\mu_0 \qquad (5.7)$$

where V is the molecular volume.

Substantial fields are typically needed to take advantage of this mechanism, and large, elongated, structured molecules do better in the competition with thermal noise. For example, a 5 μm long microtubule is estimated to be completely aligned by a magnetic field in the 10 T range (Bras et al., 1998). When material is organized so that the diamagnetic anisotropies align over some volume, larger induced magnetic moments can be achieved. This effect is sometimes called superdiamagnetism (Braganza et al., 1984).

This mechanism is the basis for some detailed models of effects in lipid bilayers (Helfrich, 1973; Gaffney & McConnel, 1974; Tenforde & Liburdy, 1988), subsequent effects on calcium liberation (del Moral & Azanza, 1992; Azanza & del Moral, 1994), and an explanation of how mitotic structures may be affected by large fields (Denegre et al., 1998; Valles, Jr. et al., 2002), resulting in abnormal embryonic development.

5.3   Radical recombination rates

Spin-correlated radical pair chemistry has long been a consideration for magnetic field effects in chemistry and biology. Several classes of organic chemical reactions can be influenced by static magnetic fields in the range of 10 - 100 mT as a result of effects on the electronic spin states of the reaction intermediates (Schulten, 1982; McLauchlan, 1989; Cozens & Scaiano, 1993; Grissom, 1995; Hore, 2005). A spin-correlated radical pair may recombine and prevent the formation of reaction product if two conditions are met: 1) the pair, formed in a triplet state, must be converted into a singlet state by some mechanism and 2) the radicals must physically meet again in order to recombine. Step 1, the singlet-triplet interconversion, is the step that can be magnetic field sensitive. The probability of having a re-encounter is dependent on how constrained the diffusive motion of the two radicals is. There are several mechanisms outlined within this framework, for example, by McLauchlan and Steiner (1991).

If the two radicals have different g-factors, they will differentially precess and oscillate in and out of triplet and singlet states, allowing for a high rate of re-conversion in the short interval after the pair generation when the re-encounter probability is high. This process becomes dominant at high fields (> 1 T) and is generally referred to as the Δg - mechanism.

At intermediate field strengths (down to the mT range), spin mixing due to hyperfine interactions dominates the singlet-triplet interconversion. The rate of this type of spin conversion is higher when the involved nuclear states are significantly different. The magnetic field has an effect in this regime because it separates the degenerate energy levels of the triplet state, leading to enhanced spin conversion as the T_{-1} state experiences an enhanced ability to mix into the singlet state. At higher field strengths the T_{+1} states become decoupled from any interaction with the singlet state and a reduction in the interconversion rate occurs. This mechanism is fairly well understood and is experimentally supported by detailed experiments (Harkins & Grissom, 1995).

There is also a low field effect based on the fact that the selection rules of hyperfine-induced mixing are more restrictive in zero fields and that one might see a reduction in spin conversion rates for low fields (McLauchlan & Steiner, 1991). Given a reaction environment that imposes spatial constraints on the radical pair diffusion so that long recombination times can be possible, this free radical low field effect is predicted to achieve significant responses to magnetic fields in the μT region (Timmel et al., 1998; Till et al., 1998). Further structure in the response to varying magnetic field amplitude has been predicted if anisotropic hyperfine structures are considered (Timmel et al., 2001).

It should be noted that the radical pair mechanism requires the two radicals to be spin-correlated or geminate (twins). If they are not statistically correlated with each other, then a magnetic field will still rotate the spin angular momentum, but no coherent change in recombination rates will occur. This applies to freely diffusing radicals, and it is important to exclude these chemical species from consideration as a magnetic field target (Brocklehurst & McLauchlan, 1996).

Since the radicals stay spin-correlated for a relatively short time, it has been argued that an effect of low frequency magnetic fields should be equivalent to a static field with appropriate amplitude. However, this may not be true if the dynamics of the biological system responding to the time-varying field has any frequency specificity in the appropriate range (Walleczek, 1995; Eichwald & Walleczek, 1998). The property of timescale of the transductive mechanism can be investigated with appropriate experiments (Engström, 1997; Engström & Fitzsimmons, 1999).

Radical pair magnetic field effects have been used as a tool to study enzyme reactions, in part because more than 60 enzymes use radicals or other paramagnetic molecules as reaction intermediates. It has been established (Hore, 2005) that two (non-mammalian) enzyme reactions are magnetic-field sensitive under appropriate, non-physiological, conditions: 1) the conversion of ethanolamine to acetaldehyde by the bacterial enzyme ethanolamine ammonia lyase (Harkins & Grissom, 1994) and 2) the reduction of hydrogen peroxide by horseradish peroxidase (Taraban & Leshina, 1997). Changes in catalytic rates of up to 30% were found for fields of up to 0.3 T. Although there remain biological systems worthy of further investigation, there is, based on the evidence at present, no strong likelihood of major effects of physiological consequence on cellular functions or of long-term mutagenic effects arising from magnetic-field induced changes in free radical concentrations or fluxes (Hore, 2005).

5.4   Biogenic magnetite

Biogenic magnetite is the basis of a well-documented mechanism explaining how some bacteria can use the magnetic field to an evolutionary advantage (Blakemore, 1975). A chain of magnetosomes provides a large enough magnetic moment that the whole organism orients and swims along geomagnetic flux lines (magnetotaxis), providing a reliable source of direction for swimming up or down as this bacterium's circumstances require.

The large magnetic moment associated with a magnetite grain results in the potential energy for rotation in a magnetic field having a magnitude comparable to kT at biological temperatures.

Kirschvink et al. (2001) reviewed the development of magnetite-based magnetoreception and argued that a highly evolved sensory system capable of explaining the observed sensitivities to very small variations in the geomagnetic field should be expected (Fischer et al., 2001; Phillips et al., 2002). An interesting requirement for high-resolution observation of the magnetic vector orientation is an equally sensitive measurement of the gravitational vector, as well as integration/comparison of these two senses.

Magnetite-based mechanisms are modelled in bio-electromagnetic research (Phillips, 1996; Deutschlander et al., 1999b; Ritz et al., 2000) and there are data in various forms for several different animal models (Beason & Semm, 1996; Brassart et al., 1999; Deutschlander et al., 1999a; Lohmann & Johnsen, 2000; Hanzlik et al., 2000; Phillips et al., 2001; Wiltschko & Wiltschko, 2002).

5.4.1 Single-domain crystals

Single domain magnetite crystals can only be magnetized along one axis (with positive or negative polarity), and the crystal maintains the magnetization, unlike superparamagnetic magnetite (see below). Single domain magnetite or greigite are the elements of magnetotactic bacteria. It has been suggested that these are functional components of higher magnetosensitive animals. Remagnetization experiments provide good reasons to believe that permanent ferromagnets are involved in the physical transduction (Beason et al., 1997; Munro et al., 1997). Physical models utilizing single domain crystals have been discussed in the literature (Kirschvink et al., 1992).

45

Edmonds (1996) proposed a sensitive biological magnetic compass by examining the behaviour of a cluster of needle-shaped magnetite crystals in a nematic fluid. The argument is that this system would be able, given enough crystals in the cluster, to respond to the orientation of the magnetic field with relatively high resolution and that useful detection could be achieved optically.

5.4.2 Superparamagnetic magnetite

Superparamagnetism is a phenomenon by which magnetic materials may exhibit behaviour similar to paramagnetism at temperatures below the Curie or the Neel temperature. Superparamagnetic magnetite grains are too small to have a stable magnetic moment impressed, but they do respond to an externally applied field. Clusters (1 - 3 μm in diameter) of superparamagnetic nanocrystals (2 - 5 nm in diameter) have been reported in the upper beak of homing pigeons (Hanzlik et al., 2000; Winklhofer et al., 2001). Single domain features were ruled out in these studies.

5.4.3 Other ferromagnetic inclusions

There are suggestions of possibilities other than magnetite for ferromagnetic inclusions in bacterial and archaeal cells (Vainshtein et al., 2002). These reported structures were detected by magnetophoresis in a tesla-level field. The structures did not show the crystalline signatures of magnetite.

5.4.4 Local amplification due to ferromagnetic material

It is conceivable that magnetotransduction could occur in the immediate vicinity of a magnetite grain, if this would provide a local amplification of the applied field. If a particle has magnetic permeability larger than one, it will produce a locally enhanced field and this secondary field could be detected. Another possibility is that a permanently magnetized single domain grain could be rotated by the magnetic field and 'shine' its own relatively large local field onto a nearby magnetic field sensitive structure.

5.5 Mechanistic co-factors and other mechanisms

There are co-factors in some experimental work of static and low frequency magnetic field studies that might provide clues about low level mechanisms. These are discussed below.

5.5.1 *Light as a co-factor*

One recurring theme is light sensitive magnetic field detection (Ritz et al., 2002). It has been shown that wavelength specific effects occur in avian and reptile magnetic navigation (Deutschlander et al., 1999b) and in magnetic field detection (Deutschlander et al., 1999a). A model is proposed in salamanders in which two separate and antagonistic magnetic field sensitive systems are activated by short and long-wavelength light (Phillips et al., 2001).

Animal models are used to investigate the relation between magnetic field detection and light by forming hypotheses that can be tested by training, and later testing, behavioural responses in various light conditions varying with respect to wavelength (Deutschlander et al., 1999a) and polarization (Able & Able, 1993). The presence of light is also required in a snail behavioural model in which nociceptive responses are modulated only by magnetic fields (Prato et al., 1997).

It is not known whether the light dependent part of the biological mechanism at work is integrated with the magnetic field transduction. It is uncommon in sensory physiology for two independent detectors to become tightly integrated, but one model for the avian magnetic field detection embeds the detection organ in the bird's eye (Ritz et al., 2000). It could also be that light is enabling a physical detection mechanism, either on a behavioural level, or directly, as suggested by Leask (1977).

5.5.2 *State dependence*

State/activation dependent factors have been theoretically examined in a model of free radical responses in enzyme systems (Eichwald & Walleczek, 1996). It has been experimentally observed that the sign of the response of Na-K-ATPase depends upon its activation state (Blank & Soo, 1996).

5.6 Constraints on physical detection

For either the direct magnetic fields or the magnetically induced electric fields to affect the biology of systems, the interactions with such systems must generally be larger than the interactions with endogenous physiological and thermal noise. The disruptive effects of thermal noise puts limits on what signals can be detected in simple biological systems (Adair, 1991; Adair, 2000). Much work on the possible lower limits of detection has focused on energetic comparisons to the average thermal energy of the environment encountered by any detection mechanism operating in a living biological setting. It should however be noted that the magnetic interactions involved in the radical pair mechanism are weak compared to thermal energy (Hore, 2005).

5.7 Conclusions

It has been shown in this chapter that the following three classes of physical interactions of static magnetic fields with biological systems are well established on the basis of experimental data:

(1)   electrodynamic interactions with ionic conduction currents;

(2)   magnetomechanical effects, including the orientation of magnetically anisotropic structures in   uniform fields and the translation of paramagnetic and ferromagnetic materials in magnetic   field gradients; and

(3)   effects on electronic spin states of reaction intermediates.

Forces and torques on both endogenous and exogenous metallic objects are the interaction mechanism of most concern. The induction of electric fields and currents in tissue is also of concern. Other interaction mechanisms do not appear to be of concern at this stage. None of the mechanisms discussed to date would seem to indicate differences in effects from acute or chronic exposures, although no suitable epidemiological studies are available in this regard.

6   DOSIMETRY

To understand the biological effects of electric and magnetic fields, it is important to consider the fields directly influencing cells in different parts of body and tissues. A dose can then be defined as an appropriate function of the electric and magnetic fields at the point of interaction. The establishment of a relationship between the external non-perturbed fields and internal fields is the main objective of dosimetry. Microscopic dosimetry is the quantitative study of the induced electric environment on size scales comparable to, or smaller than, the living cell. Macroscopic dosimetry deals with dosimetric quantities averaged over volumes or areas where the dimensions are greater than the dimensions of most individual cells (ICNIRP, 2003).

6.1   Static electric fields

The distortion of fields due to bodily presence is characteristic of exposure to static electric fields. External perturbed electric field strength near the skin is the most relevant dosimetric quantity when studying skin surface effects, such as hair vibrations and static discharges, caused by extremely intense electric fields.

Relatively few experimental studies of static electric fields effects have been undertaken. A discussion of dosimetric aspects of static fields can be found in ICNIRP (2003) and in section 9.1 of this monograph.

6.2   Static magnetic fields

Chapter 3 discussed the sources of static fields while the focus in this section is mostly on static magnetic fields relevant to the health risk assessment provided in section 9.1. A main concern with respect to exposure of static magnetic fields is the proliferation of magnetic resonance systems, but the following discussion applies equally to any static magnetic source.

In the case of exposure to static magnetic fields, the human body has very little influence on the magnetic field. External magnetic field strength or magnetic flux density can be used for both dosimetry and exposure assessments.

In terms of MRI or NMR systems, the magnetic sources mostly used are superconductor solenoids. Typically, the magnetic field vector inside solenoidal magnets is aligned with the patient's long axis. Many lower field magnets have the static magnetic field vectors aligned with the anterior/posterior patient axis, though some magnets place the field along the left/right axis. In general, magnets (not just MRI magnets) may be actively shielded to limit the spatial extent of the fringe field, but many are not. In MRI applications, magnets up to about 4 T can be actively shielded, but current technology prohibits active shielding above this level. Therefore, significant fields are present around 7 T magnets, for example, but actively shielded magnets may in fact have large gradients near the ends of magnets due to the effect of active shielding. In NMR, which is used for chemical analysis and spectroscopy, small bore magnets are used to house test tube sized samples. These magnets are routinely 12 to 21 T and workers are exposed to stray fields and field gradients when changing samples or the probes within the magnet.

Static magnetic field effects are likely to be caused by the magnetic field vector, B, the gradient of the magnetic field, $\partial B/\partial z$, the 'force product', or by motion or flow induced magnetic fields. The force product, P_F, may be expressed as:

$$P_F = B . \frac{\partial B}{\partial z} \tag{6.1}$$

where z is taken as the direction of B. Note, however, that B is a vector and that all components should be considered. Flow induced electric fields, E_f, depend on the product of flow velocity, v, the magnetic field vector, B, and the angle, θ, between them:

$$E_f = v B \sin(\theta) \tag{6.2}$$

The motion-induced electric field, E_m, depends on the geometry and on the time rate of change of the magnetic field:

$$\oint \overline{E}_m \bullet d\overline{l} = - \int \frac{d\overline{B}}{dt} \bullet d\overline{s} \tag{6.3}$$

where $d\overline{l}$ is the incremental length vector of the body part enclosing the changing magnetic field and $d\overline{s}$ is the normal vector to the incremental area. It is clear from equation 6.3 that electric fields may be induced when the dot product of B and s changes with time. For static magnetic fields, this happens because the area vector changes with time or because the magnetic field vector changes with location due to motion in a static field gradient or both.

Forces, and even torques, on ferromagnetic, paramagnetic, or diamagnetic objects are proportional to the force product (see section 5.2.2). This effect is a primary concern with static magnetic fields. Affected objects (e.g., tools and implants) may move with sufficient force to be hazardous. Force products depend on the field gradient and the field. Thus, even low field magnets could have high force products.

Flow and motion-induced electric fields may result in vertigo or, potentially, nerve or muscle stimulation. Flow-induced cardiac

50

stimulation has not been reported in the literature. However, it is a potential concern for sufficiently high static magnetic fields. It is not clear whether the orientation of the body with respect to B will affect flow potentials.

Past exposure standards and guidelines have included time-weighted magnetic field exposure limits. It is, however, currently unclear which form of dose is the most appropriate to monitor. Dosimetry for future exposure limits must depend on a realistic effects mechanism. Limiting forces and torques requires restricting ferromagnetic objects from the vicinity of magnets and limiting the peak force product that an object may experience. Protection from nerve and muscle stimulation during patient exposure requires limiting peak dB/dt, either by limiting motion or by limiting peak B. Flow potential concerns require limiting peak B or at least peak v B $\sin(\theta)$ - see equation (6.2). Some mechanism may require limiting the root mean square of the static field vector, though this is not clear.

6.3 Motion induced effects in MRI

The example presented in the following section details theoretical investigations into the spatial distribution of induced currents and electric fields in a tissue equivalent human model when moving at various positions around a magnet. The numerical calculations are based on a quasistatic, finite difference scheme (Liu et al., 2003b; Liu & Crozier, 2004).

Three dimensional field profiles from an actively shielded 4 T magnet system are used as an example and the body model is projected through the field profile with normalised velocity. Most clinical MRI systems are actively shielded in that the stray field emanating from the MRI system is restricted by the use of a counterwound coil exterior to the main or primary magnet windings. The methodology presented herein is not restricted to MRI, but can be used to calculate induced fields due to patient or occupationally exposed worker movement around a magnetic field source.

There has been a concerted effort in the past decade to enable MRI to operate at very high field strengths. The most common system in current clinical use has a 1.5 T central field. However, 3 T systems are now accepted for routine clinical work and more than 100 systems were operational worldwide by 2004. Research systems from 4 - 9.4 T are now being developed for clinical imaging. As the field strength of the MRI system increases, so does the potential for tissue/field interactions of a variety of types. Understanding the interactions between the electromagnetic fields generated by MRI systems and the human body has

51

become more significant with this push to high field strengths (Schmitt et al., 1998; Schenck, 2000; Kangarlu & Robitaille, 2000; Liu et al., 2003b).

The static magnetic fields used in MRI may be associated, in varying degrees, with biological influences such as diamagnetic and paramagnetic effects (Kangarlu & Robitaille, 2000). Another concern in high-field MRI is related not to the strength of the static field, but to electromagnetic induction. The 3D pattern of the static magnetic field can induce current in moving conductive objects, such as the body. Systematic study using volunteers (Schenck et al., 1992) and anecdotal evidence that some patients experience uncomfortable sensations when moved into MRI or when moving their head during entry to the scanner or once in the system, has motivated the study of the induced fields inside a patient model (Liu et al., 2003a). Reported sensations included phosphenes (light flashes), vertigo, and a metallic taste in the mouth. The motion-induced effects in patients, and the eddy currents induced in an occupationally exposed worker (radiographer or MRI technician) moving around the magnet, are discussed below. These calculations provide assistance in the evaluation of the risks involved for health workers and patients when moving through intense, static magnetic fields.

6.3.1 Numerical calculations of the induced fields

The human model used for the calculations represents a large male and was obtained from the United States Air Force Research Laboratory (http://www.brooks.af.mil/AFRL/HED/hedr/). The original spatial resolution of the model was 1 mm, but the model was mapped onto a 4-mm grid with volume-averaged conductive properties.

The simulations presented here are based on the fields generated by a 4 T, actively-shielded MRI magnet (Crozier & Doddrell, 1997). This magnet has a length of 1.5 m with a homogeneous imaging region (or Diameter Spherical Volume [DSV]) of 50 cm. The shielding area (to 0.5 mT) is 4.5 m in the z direction and 4.0 m in the radial direction from the magnet iso-centre. The numerical method for the calculation of the static magnetic field was based on Forbes et al. (1997). The vector magnetic potential components are used to calculate the induced fields inside the body.

The calculation of the E-fields induced by the relative movement of the body inside the static magnetic field is based on a finite difference scheme (Liu et al., 2003b). The time-varying magnetic flux is expressed by the difference of vector potentials of two neighbouring cells divided by the time difference. The formulation supports multi-direction translation using vector analyses of velocity. To simulate a realistic human movement, the velocity of different parts of the body can be set to different values.

During the period when the body is moving around the magnet, the transient induced fields at each position in the body relative to the magnet centre are registered. The peak values and their positions in the human body are obtained for further evaluation. A variety of movement directions and velocities were modelled.

Figure 6.1 provides curves describing the peak E-fields and current densities induced in the human model for all the positions near the magnet. In Fig. 6.1(a,c), the E-field and current density curves are both shown. These curves depict the obviously stronger electromagnetic induction when the body moves near a magnet end, where the magnetic field gradient is large. Fig. 6.1(b,d) shows the amplitudes of the E-fields for maximum induction at various layers within the body.

An example of histogram distributions for the front-back movement along the end of the magnet is shown in Fig 6.2(a,b). For the skin/subcutaneous fat regions of the body (*i.e.* those parts expected to be most sensitive to peripheral nerve stimulation (Dawson & Stuchly, 1998; Stuchly & Dawson, 2000)) the largest induced E-field (1% threshold) was 2.0 V m^{-1}. For deeper structures in the chest, however, the value was 3.1 V m^{-1}.

Detailed calculations have been made of induced field during patient movement and head-shake while in the magnet. Fig 6.3a shows typical induced field results for movement at 0.5 m s^{-1} in the 4 T magnet, which indicates E-fields around the 2.0 V m^{-1} range at maximum, and Fig 6.3b shows extrapolated results to higher fields and velocities. Note that at higher fields, magnets are unshielded and significantly longer, and that the curves in Fig 6.3b do not account for that because they only provide indicative values. Importantly, the threshold induced current density for peripheral nerve stimulation is estimated to be about 0.48 A m^{-2}, (Kangarlu & Robitaille, 2000) but this is frequency dependent, and so Fig 6.3b gives a rough indication of the field strengths and patient velocities capable of such induction. At 7 T, for example, it is estimated that a body velocity of about 0.8 m s^{-1} would result in induced current density at the peripheral nerve stimulation level. No reports of peripheral nerve stimulation due to table motion have appeared in the literature. Note, however, that recommended restrictions on occupational exposure to low frequency EMFs where weak electric fields and currents are also induced in the body are based on effects on neural tissue in the central nervous system where thresholds are considerably lower than those for peripheral nerve stimulation (e.g. (ICNIRP, 1998); see (ICNIRP, 2003) for a full discussion).

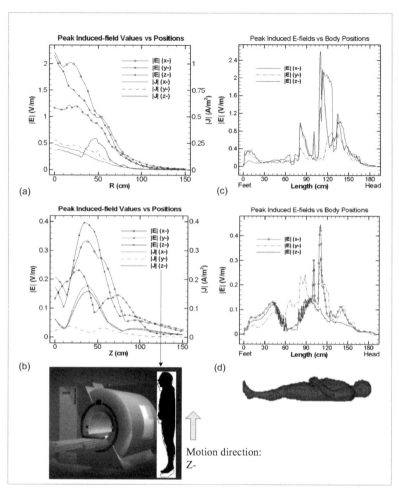

Figure 6.1.   Curves of the induced fields for the body moving around
the magnet. (a,b): peak E-fields and current densities in the
human model for all the positions (0 ~ 1.5 m) when the
body is moving around the 4 T magnet (a: near the magnet
end; b: along the cylinder); (c,d): the amplitudes of the E-
fields for various layers of the human body model. These
induced values are calculated when peak E-fields occur in
(a,b). In all the figures, 'x-, y-, z-' denotes the body motion
direction: 'x-': left-right direction, 'y-': front-back direction
and 'z-': up-down direction. (Crozier & Liu, 2005)

54

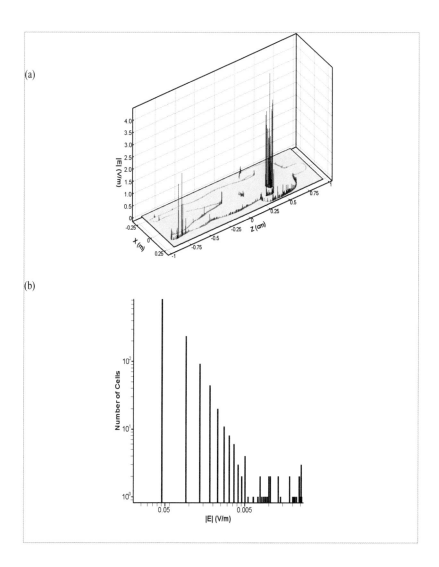

Figure 6.2.   Histogram distribution of induced electric field in different voxels (cells) of the phantom for front-back movement at 1.0 m s^{-1} along the end of the 4 T magnet. For the skin/subcutaneous fat regions of the body, the largest induced E-field was 2.0 V m^{-1}. For deeper structures in the chest, however, the value was 3.1 V m^{-1}. (Crozier & Liu, 2005)

55

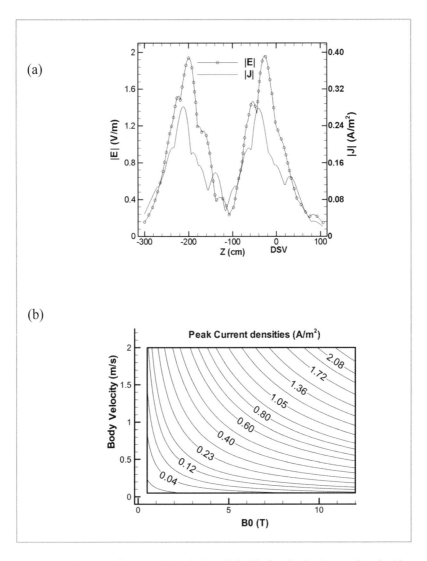

Figure 6.3.   Curves of the induced fields for the body moving inside the magnet. (a) shows typical induced field results for movement at 0.5 m s-1 in the 4 T magnet, which indicates E-fields around the 2.0 V m-1 range at maximum, and (b) gives peak induced current densities in the skin as a function of body velocity and field strength. (Crozier & Liu, 2005)

6.4   Personal dosimetry

To assess health risks in relation to static fields, measurements of exposure are useful. Occupationally exposed workers and patients alike may be monitored for exposure using personal dosimeters (Fujita & Tenforde, 1982) or estimates from field plots. In the case of occupationally exposed workers, exposure to either instantaneous or cumulative fields may be monitored, as appropriate. Although the quantities to be measured are not exactly clear, at least the instantaneous B field vector and the B field time derivative should be considered in the static magnetic field case. While a number of commercial products exist for personal dosimetry in ELF electromagnetic regime, this is not the case for personal static magnetic field dosimetry, where there is currently only one instrument available (Wave Instruments, see http://www.waveinstruments.com.au/). It is also noted that the measurement devices themselves must be able to withstand strong magnetic fields and must not alter the local field in any significant manner.

6.5   Conclusions

Appropriate dosimetric parameters depend on the physical mechanism for the safety concern. Clearly, ferromagnetic objects must be restricted from the vicinity of the magnet. Screening is imperative for such objects and for implants that may move either due to forces or torques. Measures of peak magnetic induction vector, B, and peak magnetic force product are appropriate. Field maps may be used to estimate these at various locations near the magnets where workers may be exposed, but personal dosimetry may be useful.

Movement of the whole or part of the body, e.g. eyes and head, in a static magnetic field gradient will also induce an electric field and current during the period of movement. Dosimetric calculation suggests that such induced electric fields will be substantial during normal movement around or within fields > 2 - 3 T, and may account for the numerous anecdotal reports of vertigo and occasionally magnetic phosphenes experienced by patients, volunteers and workers during movement in the field.

7 CELLULAR AND ANIMAL STUDIES

7.1 *In vitro* studies

Studies carried out at the cellular level are often used to investigate mechanisms of interaction with EMFs, but these are not generally taken alone as evidence of *in vivo* effects. There are a number of reasons for this. Cells in culture are removed from the normal constraints of *in vivo* growth, and quite often the cell lines used are derived from various types of cancer because of their ability to grow for long periods in culture. AGNIR (2001) noted that cellular studies are often used as a pre-screen to identify agents that are relatively inexpensive and rapid and are thus suitable for entry into long-term testing on animals or in human studies.

The studies reviewed in this section concern static magnetic field effects, including, for completeness, studies carried out in combination with time varying magnetic fields. Static electric fields generate a surface electric charge (see chapter 5, introduction) and are not appropriately studied *in vitro*.

7.1.1 Cell free systems

The number of options available for biological systems to detect magnetic fields increases with larger, more complex structures and the consequent greater possible specialization of putative transduction processes. As sub-systems of cells are addressed, or even cell-free biochemical reactions, it is necessary to consider strictly molecular-based interaction mechanisms, particularly in experiments conducted in suspension or in solution.

7.1.1.1 Membrane structure

Liburdy et al. (1986) studied lipid membrane breakdown as a function of temperature and magnetic field exposure. They found that a threshold field of 15 mT was able to shift the phase transition point to slightly lower temperatures, but the study is weakened by the lack of sham exposure. A direct application of a model based on diamagnetic anisotropy suggests that this threshold is about two magnitudes too low for overcoming the thermal noise. A theoretical paper (Tenforde & Liburdy, 1988) suggested a catastrophic model of membrane breakdown at close to the lipid phase transition temperature that accounts for this sensitivity to the magnetic field.

7.1.1.2 Enzyme activity

The possibility that magnetic field exposure might directly affect enzyme kinetics has long been of interest, but such studies are fraught with difficulty. The dependence of Ca^{2+}-calmodulin-dependent myosin phosphorylation on calcium concentration and various magnetic field characteristics was extensively studied by Markov and co-workers (1992; 1993) in a model originally developed by Shuvalova et al. (1991). The study by Bull et al. supported the observation that static magnetic fields affect Ca^{2+}-calmodulin-dependent reactions (Bull et al., 1993). A replication of some of these results was attempted (Coulton et al., 2000), but was not successful. The causes of the failure to reproduce the magnetic field effect are not known. It is possible that the calcium concentration in the reaction is a confounding variable between experiments, but other explanations are also possible. Engström et al. (2002) used this assay and found that a combination of static magnetic field intensity and gradient was able to influence the rate of phosphorylation.

A related experiment investigating cyclic nucleotide phosphodiesterase (Liboff et al., 2003) also appeared to be sensitive to very low magnetic fields, although this report may have used inappropriate statistical methods for evaluating exposure/control measurements.

Nossol et al. (1993) studied effects of static magnetic fields in the range of 50 μT - 100 mT on the redox activity of cytochrome-C oxidase. Static magnetic fields resulted in significant changes of up to 90% of overall activity only at 300 μT and 10 mT. No effects were observed at other flux densities. The observed effects were reversible. These data suggested that effects of static magnetic fields might be observed only at specific 'flux density windows'.

Taraban and Leshina (1997) investigated the reduction of hydrogen peroxide by horseradish peroxidase. Changes in catalytic rates of up to 30% were found for fields up to 0.3 T.

Small changes were also observed in plasmin activity at fields of 8 T, with a threshold of around 4 T for the magnetic field effects (Iwasaka et al., 1994).

7.1.1.3 Radical pair chemistry

Some clear demonstrations are available of how enzyme-catalysed metabolic reactions that involve a short-lived radical pair as an intermediate can be modulated with magnetic fields (Harkins & Grissom, 1994; Mohtat et al., 1998). (See section 5.3.) Demonstrations of the field effect of free radical recombination rates have also been reported by Eveson et al. (2000). Two of these studies used laser flash photolysis to show consistency with free radical theory for the field effect at approximately 2 mT (Eveson et al., 2000) and for hyperfine interactions in the 100 mT range (Mohtat et al., 1998).

Radical chemistry also offers clear mechanistic options as demonstrated in B12 ethanolamine ammonia lyase by Harkins and Grissom (1994). The basic result was replicated, but two other coenzyme B_{12}-dependent enzymes (human and bacterial-derived, respectively) were found not to be magnetic field sensitive (Taoka et al., 1997) despite broad similarities between the chemical structures.

7.1.1.4 Crystallization of biologically relevant molecules

Some clear demonstrations are available that static magnetic fields, in the range of 0.1 - 10 T, affect crystallization of proteins and cholesterol (Sato et al., 2000; Sundaram et al., 2002). It is important to note that the crystallisation may be relevant to biology because some cellular structures such as complexes of DNA-protein–RNA in nuclei may possess the properties of liquid crystals.

Table 7. Cell free systems

Authors	System	Endpoint	Exposure	Results	Comments
Static magnetic field effects					
(Liburdy et al., 1986)	Liposome vesicles	Permeability	0.01 - 7.5 T 15 min	Increased permeability ED_{50} = 15 mT. Threshold two orders of magnitude too low for a mechanism based on diamagnetism.	
(Markov et al., 1993) (Markov et al., 1992)	Myosin light chain kinase and calmodulin isolated from turkey gizzard	Myosin phosphorylation	0 - 200 µT 2 - 15 min	Differential response for controls, AC, DC, and AC+DC exposure. Dose response to fine scan of vertical DC field.	Assay of interest, because Ca^{2+}-calmodulin binding is a probable field target.

(Coulton et al., 2000)	Myosin	Radiolabeled ATP into 20 kDa light chain myosin. Myosin phosphorylation	0 - 400 µT 5 or 10 min	No effect of magnetic fields on rate of phosphorylation	Not clear what calcium concentration was required to observe the phos-phorylation effect.
(Engström et al., 2002)	Myosin light chain (and kinase) from turkey gizzard	Myosin phosphorylation	0.7 - 86 mT 5 min	Increased phosphorylation, but not fully explained by SMF.	Magnetic field gradients played a specific role in the outcome of this experiment.
(Liboff et al., 2003)	Chemicals from commercial providers	Calmodulin-dependent cyclic nucleotide phosphodiesterase activity	17 - 24 µT 30 min	Calmodulin-dependent cyclic nucleotide phosphodi-esterase activity is activated by 19.8 µT SMF. Field and Ca2+ concentration consistent with previous experiments.	Data are very noisy. Incorrect statistical analysis used to test data.
(Nossol et al., 1993)	Cytochrome-C oxidase isolated from beef heart	Cytochrome-C oxidase activity	50 µT - 100 mT up to 100 sec	Significant changes up to 90% of overall activity only at 300 µT or 10 mT.	Effects observed in specific 'windows' of magnetic intensity around 0.3 and 10 mT.
(Taraban & Leshina, 1997)	Horseradish peroxidase	H_2O_2 reduction	up to 0.3 T	Changes in catalytic rates of up to 30%.	
(Iwasaka et al., 1994)	Plasmin	Enzymatic activity	0 - 8 T 5 - 80 min	Slight changes (5 -10%) in plasmin activity. Threshold of observed effects at 4 T.	Neither statistical analysis, nor amount of independent experiments provided.

(Harkins & Grissom, 1994)	B_{12} ethanol-amine ammonia lyase	Free radical recombination rates, enzyme kinetics	0.1 - 0.15 T	~25% decrease of V_{max}/K_m for B_{12} ethanol-amine ammonia lyase around 0.1 T with unlabelled ethanol-amine; decrease ~60% around 0.15 T with perdeuterated ethanolamine.	Neither statistical analysis, nor amount of independent experiments provided.
(Mohtat et al., 1998)	Human and bovine serum albumin, calf thymus DNA	Benzophenone recombination, ketyl radicals	up to 150 mT up to 10 μs	Change in lifetime of radicals. Consistent with theory of free radical recombination in containment.	
(Eveson et al., 2000)	Purely chemical experiment	Benzophenone ketyl radical concentration after flash stimulation	0 - 11 mT 9 μsec	Observation of predicted low field effect in free radical recombination rates. Maximum response at 2 mT.	A pulsed magnetic field was applied.
(Taoka et al., 1997)	Coenzyme B_{12} – dependent enzymes	Coenzyme B_{12}-dependent rearrangement reactions catalysed by bacterial enzyme, ethanolamine ammonia lyase and human enzyme, methylmalonyl-CoA mutase	0 - 250 mT up to 5 h	No effect on enzyme kinetics greater than about 15%. B_{12}-dependent methyl-malonyl-CoA mutase not a likely transduction target for SMF in the studied field range.	Small differences between controls and SMF at some flux densities. However, no statistical analysis described and number of experiments not reported.
(Sato et al., 2000)	Chicken egg-white lysozyme	Crystallization	10 T 11 d	Enhancement in the perfection of lysozyme crystals.	No statistical analysis.

(Sundaram et al., 2002)	Anhydrous cholesterol	Cholesterol solubility and supersaturation in various solvents	100 mT up to 8 h	Induction time of cholesterol crystallization decreases in a magnetic field for all examined solvents. No changes in morphology due to field exposure.	Counter changes in induction period times did not result in change in the interfacial energy. Neither statistical analysis nor sham-exposure performed.
(Bull et al., 1993)	Calmodulin-dependent cyclic nucleotide phospho-diester-ase (PDE)	Activity of PDE	16.9 - 23.7 µT 30 min	13% stimulation of PDE activity in samples exposed to SMF in the range from 19.2 to 20.4 µT.	No statistical analysis described.

Studies considered to be uninformative

(Chiles et al., 1989)

(Bras et al., 1998)

(Liu et al., 2005)

7.1.2 Magneto-mechanical effects on macromolecules and cells

Macromolecules and structurally ordered molecular assemblies with a high degree of magnetic anisotropy will experience a torque in a uniform magnetic field and they will rotate until they reach an equilibrium orientation that represents a minimum energy state (ICNIRP, 2003). Macromolecules that exhibit this property, such as DNA, generally have a cylindrical symmetry. Magneto-orientation occurs as a result of the anisotropy of the diamagnetic susceptibility tensor along the axial and radial coordinates. The extent to which these molecules orient is a function of their magnetic interaction energy relative to the Boltzmann thermal energy.

The extent of orientation of individual molecules in strong magnetic fields is very small for individual macromolecules. For example, optical birefringence measurements on calf thymus DNA in solution have demonstrated that a field of 13 T is required to produce orientation of 1% of the molecules (Maret et al., 1975). In contrast, there are several examples of molecular assemblies that can be completely oriented by fields on the order of 1 T (Tenforde, 1985). These assemblies behave as structurally coupled units in which the summed magnetic anisotropy is large, thus giving rise to a large magnetic interaction energy.

An example of an intact cell that can be oriented magnetically is the deoxygenated sickle erythrocyte. It has been shown that these cells, in which the deoxygenated haemoglobin is paramagnetic, will align in a 0.35 T static field with the long axis of the sickle cell oriented perpendicular to the magnetic flux lines (Murayama, 1965). In a follow-up to this experiment, Brody et al. (1985) investigated the magnetic resonance imaging of patients with sickle-cell disease. They studied flowing sickle erythrocytes in the presence and absence of a magnetic field of 0.38 T and found that sickle erythrocytes that were maintained under full deoxygenation exhibited a marked alignment, perpendicular to the magnetic field, even while flowing. It was suggested that orientated sickle erythrocytes could have difficulty negotiating capillary branch points.

In a series of experiments, Higashi and co-workers (1993; 1995; 1996) also studied the orientation of erythrocytes in the presence of a magnetic field of up to 8 T. They found that the erythrocytes were oriented with their disk plane parallel to the magnetic field direction. These erythrocytes were even influenced by 1 T and almost 100% of them were oriented when exposed to 4 T. The degree of orientation was not influenced by the state of haemoglobin (oxygenated haemoglobin is diamagnetic; deoxygenated haemoglobin and methaemoglobin are paramagnetic). The data concurred with the theoretical equation for the magnetic orientation of diamagnetic substances. In contrast, glutaraldehyde-fixed erythrocytes were oriented perpendicular to the magnetic field. This was attributed to the paramagnetism of the membrane-bound methaemoglobin.

Emura et al. (2001) studied fixed bull sperm in a magnetic field of up to 1.7 T. The sperm became increasingly oriented perpendicular to the field, reaching 100% at about 1 T. Diamagnetic cell components (cell membrane, DNA in the head, microtubule in the tail) were thought to contribute to the orientation.

Hirose et al. (2003a) exposed human glioblastoma cells to a 10 T magnet in the presence and absence of collagen. Only cells embedded within the collagen gel and the collagen fibres were affected, and these were oriented perpendicular to the magnetic field. The effect was attributed to the arrangement of microtubules under the influence of magnetically oriented collagen fibres. The orientation of both rat Schwann cells and mouse osteoblasts was influenced by 8 T, in the presence as well as in the absence of collagen fibres (Eguchi et al., 2003). Without collagen fibres, it took 60 h to orient the cells parallel to the magnetic flux lines. Exposure in the presence of fibres resulted in perpendicular alignment after only 2 h. This resulted from perpendicular orientation of the collagen fibres, followed by growth of the cells along the fibres. This mechanism is thought to be potentially helpful in tissue regeneration.

Iwasaka et al. (2003) investigated the orientation of rat smooth muscle cells after exposure to 8 - 14 T for 60 h. Effects were seen for fields > 8 T, where circular spots of proliferating cells became elliptical. The same researchers (Iwasaka & Ueno, 2003) studied the effect on intracellular components in another study. A 2 - 3 h exposure to 14 T induced a change in transmission of polarized light, indicating an orientational effect on macromolecules in the cells. This agrees with the above-described observed effects on collagen molecules.

Okazaki and co-workers (1988; 1991) studied the flow and sedimentation rate of erythrocytes in the presence of a magnetic field. The presence of the magnetic field (up to 0.3 T) redistributed the flow of erythrocytes (depending on the magnetic properties of the solution) and caused an increase in the sedimentation rate of erythrocytes in a vertical cylinder.

Iino (1997; 2001) found an increased erythrocyte sedimentation rate specifically for anisotropic erythrocytes in the presence of a 6.3 T field. This was attributed to an increased cell aggregation and was said to result from an increase in intermembrane adhesive area due to the magnetic orientation of the anisotropic erythrocytes.

Pacini et al. (1999b) investigated the effect of a 0.2 T static field on human neurons (FNC-B4), using human breast carcinoma cells (MCF-7) and murine leukaemia cells (WEHI-3) as non-neuron controls. Following a short exposure (0.25 h), the neuron cells became elongated and formed vortexes of cells. Exposed cells showed branched neurites and an increase of synaptic connections. Controls did not show any changes.

Exposure of human malignant melanoma cells (Short et al., 1992) to a 4.7 T superconducting magnet resulted in a decrease in adhesion of the cells. Normal human fibroblasts showed no effects. The magnetic field had no effect on cell numbers or viability of either the melanoma cells or the non-tumour controls. Danielyan et al. (1999) also investigated the effect of a magnetic field (0.2 T) on cancer tissue (breast cancer) and found that the magnetic field had a dehydrating effect on the cancer cells.

No changes in orientation, distribution or activity (alkaline phosphatase production) were observed by Papadopulos et al. (1992) in osteoblast cell cultures exposed to a static field of 178 mT.

Testorf et al. (2002) studied exposure of melanophores to both 8 and 14 T fields for times of up to 5 h. They found no statistically significant changes in aggregation.

Yano et al. (2001) exposed roots of radish seedlings to a static magnetic field from a small permanent magnet. The roots grew in a magnetic field gradient of 1.8 - 14.7 T m^{-1}, away from the magnet. The response to the south pole of the magnet was significant, while that to the north pole was not.

Table 8. Magneto-mechanical effects

Authors	Cells	Endpoint	Exposure	Results	Comments
Static magnetic field effects					
(Murayama, 1965)	Erythrocytes	Orientation	0.35 T	Sickle erythrocytes orient perpendicular to the magnetic lines of force.	Number of independent experiments not described. No statistical analysis.
(Brody et al., 1985)	Erythrocytes	Orientation	0.38 T (flowing system: < 0.1 h)	Deoxygenated sickle erythrocytes in flowing suspension align perpendicular to a magnetic field.	SMF may affect capillary blood flow.
(Higashi et al., 1993)	Human erythrocytes	Orientation	1 - 8 T 0.5 - 2 h	Erythrocytes oriented with disk plane parallel to SMF direction. Influenced by a 1 T field and almost 100% oriented when exposed to 4 T.	

(Higashi et al., 1995)	Human erythrocytes	Orientation	0.5 - 8 T 1 h	Intact erythrocytes oriented within 5 s with disk planes parallel to SMF. Glutaraldehyde-fixed erythrocytes oriented perpendicular to SMF. State of haemoglobin had no effect on degree of orientation.	
(Higashi et al., 1996)	Glutaralde-hyde-fixed erythrocytes	Orientation	1 - 8 T 1 hour	Orientation of glutaraldehyde-fixed erythrocytes with disk plane perpendicular to SMF. Effect depends on field intensity.	
(Emura et al., 2001)	Glutaralde-hyde-fixed bull sperm	Orientation	1.7 T 10 min	Very strong orientation in comparison with erythrocytes or platelets. Orientation increased sigmoidally as function of SMF intensity and reached 100% at just below 1 T.	No statistical analysis, but effect very obvious. Number of experiments not indicated.
(Hirose et al., 2003a)	Human glioblastoma cells	Orientation, cell viability	10 T 1 h or 7 d	Cells embedded in collagen gel oriented perpendicular to direction of the SMF, due to arrangement of microtubules under influence of magnetically oriented collagen fibres. No specific orientation in cells not exposed or cultured in absence of collagen.	Number of experiments not described. No quantitative data nor statistical analysis. Descriptive study.

(Eguchi et al., 2003)	Rat Schwann cells	Orientation	8 T 2 or 60 h	Orientation parallel to 8 T SMF after 60 h. In collagen: after 2 h SMF exposure alignment perpendicular, along aligned collagen fibres.	
(Kotani et al., 2000)	Mouse osteoblasts	Cell orientation	8 T 60 min, 14 d	Collagen from osteoblasts aligns parallel to SMF; incubation of osteoblasts + collagen results in perpendicular orientation.	
(Iwasaka et al., 2003)	A7r5 rat smooth muscle cells	Orientation	8, 12, 14 T 60 h	Circular spots of proliferated cells became elliptical in presence of SMF. Ellipticity significant for fields > 8 T.	
(Iwasaka & Ueno, 2003)	Rat smooth muscle cells	Orientation of intracellular components	14 T 2 - 3 h	SMF induces change in polarized light intensity through lamellar cell assembly; corresponds to behavioural changes in cell components.	Descriptive study of limited value: only a single experiment with one Petri dish.
(Okazaki et al., 1988)	Human erythrocytes	Flow of erythrocyte suspension	110 - 300 mT	Inhomogeneous SMF redistributed flow of erythrocytes dependent on magnetic properties of erythrocytes and haematocrit concentration.	

(Okazaki et al., 1991)	Human erythrocytes	Sedimentation rate	110 - 300 mT up to 3 h	Higher sedimentation rate of paramagnetic erythrocytes with inhomogeneous SMF.	Number of independent experiments not described. No statistical analysis, but rate differences calculated
(Iino, 1997)	Human erythrocytes	Erythrocyte sedimentation rate (ESR) and aggregation	6.3 T vertical, exposures up to 1 h	SMF enhances ESR. Effect in plasma (> 20 min), not in saline solution. Increase in size of aggregates.	No statistical analysis for increase in size of aggregates.
(Iino & Okuda, 2001)	Human erythrocytes	Erythrocyte sedimentation rate (ESR) and aggregation	6.3 T up to 3 h	ESR only enhanced in anisotropic erythrocytes.	No statistical analysis for increase in size of aggregates.
(Pacini et al., 1999b)	Normal human neuronal cell culture (FNC-B4); mouse leukaemia; human breast carcinoma cells	Morphology, cell proliferation, production of endothelin-1, genome instability	0.2 T 5 - 15 min	No alterations in genome instability; dramatic changes of morphology only in neuronal cells. Significant decrease in cell proliferation, changes in production of endothelin-1.	
(Short et al., 1992)	Human melanoma cells; normal fibroblasts	Cell number, adhesion, and viability	0.5, 2, 4.7 T 12 - 72 h	Adhesion of melanoma cells diminished. No effect on normal fibroblasts.	No statistical analysis. Number of experiments not specified.
(Danielyan et al., 1999)	Human breast cancer and normal glandular tissues	Water content in tissues, ouabain ^{3}H binding	0.2 T 1 h	Decrease or increase of ouabain binding at low or high concentrations, respectively. Decrease in hydration of cancer tissues.	

(Papadopul os et al., 1992)	Rat osteoblasts	Activity	178 mT 21 d	No effect.	
(Testorf et al., 2002)	Fish melano-phores	Aggregation	8, 14 T up to 5 h	No effect on aggregation except for statistically significant irregularity in the speed of aggregation under exposure to 8 T.	8 T and 14 T experiments performed in different seasons. Significant difference between control groups for 8 T and 14 T.
(Yano et al., 2001)	Primary roots of radish (*Raphanus sativus*) seedlings	Tropism	13 - 68 mT 24 h	Roots responded tropically to SMF field gradient of 1.8 - 14.7 Tm^{-1}; significant response to south pole of magnet.	

Studies considered to be uninformative

(Hong et al., 1971)

(Malinin et al., 1976)

(Pate et al., 2003)

7.1.3 Cellular metabolic activity

Effects on enzyme activity may well lead to changes in cellular metabolic activity. Lysozymal degranulation and cell migration in response to static magnetic field exposure at 0.1 T for 30 min were studied in human polymorphonuclear leucocytes (PMNs) (Papatheofanis, 1990). Time dependent effects on enzymatic activity, such as increased release of lysozyme and lactate dehydrogenase (degranulation), were observed. Static magnetic fields inhibited cell migration. The calcium channel antagonists diltiazem, nifedipine, and verapamil protected PMNs exposed to static magnetic fields. The results indicated that calcium channels might be involved in the effects of static magnetic fields on enzymatic activity.

Human peripheral blood mononuclear cells (PBMC) and Jurkat cells were exposed to 4.75 T for 1 h by Aldinucci et al. (2003b). Concentrations of interleukins (IL-1β, -2, -6), interferon (IFN-γ), and tumour necrosis factor α (TNFα) in PBMC were not affected. On the other hand, static magnetic fields led to very low concentrations of IL-2 and Ca^{2+} in Jurkat cells. The data suggested that static magnetic fields might affect calcium transport in Jurkat cells, but not in normal PBMC. In contrast to this, Salerno et al. (1999) detected increased release of IFN-γ in normal PBMC after exposure to 0.5 T. They observed reduced expression of CD69 and increased release of IFN-γ and IL-4. A decrease in metabolic activity of human HL-60 promyelocytic cells in response to exposure for 72 h to 1 T was seen in a later study (Sabo et al., 2002). This decrease was also seen in the presence of the antineoplastic drugs 5-fluorouracil, cisplatin, doxorubicin, and vincristine. The data from these independent studies (Sabo et al., 2002; Aldinucci et al., 2003b) may indicate that normal and transformed cells might have different sensitivity to static magnetic fields.

Chignell and Sik (1995a; 1998a) studied effects of static magnetic fields on the photohaemolysis of human erythrocytes by ketoprofen and protoporphyrin IX. In these studies, application of a static magnetic field during UV-irradiation of ketoprofen and erythrocytes decreased the time required for photohaemolysis. This observation might be explained by increased concentration and/or lifetime of free radicals generated by the reduction of ketoprofen in its triplet excited state by erythrocyte membrane constituents, probably lipids. In contrast, no effects were observed on the protoporphyrin IX-induced photohaemolysis, which is initiated by singlet oxygen (Chignell & Sik, 1995b).

Heine et al. (1999) investigated the influence of magnetic fields emitted from a 1.5 T MRI device on human neutrophil function. Blood samples were obtained from 12 patients immediately before and after exposure, and then subjected to flow cytometric analysis of the induced respiratory burst by the intracellular oxidative transformation of dihydrorhodamine 123 to the fluorescent dye rhodamine 123. No significant differences were found between the percentage of superoxide-anion-producing neutrophils before and after MRI, suggesting short time exposure during MRI does not induce the respiratory burst of neutrophils in patients. Aldinucci et al. (2003a) exposed human lymphocytes and Jurkat cells using an NMR apparatus. They found an increase in intracellular free Ca^{2+} in lymphocytes, without changes in proliferation and cytokines. Ca^{2+} and proliferation decreased in Jurkat cells, also without cytokine activation. The effect in Jurkat cells is similar with or without RF (Aldinucci et al., 2003b), but combined exposure affected intracellular free Ca^{2+} in human lymphocytes.

71

Table 9. Cell metabolic activity

Authors	Cells	Endpoint	Exposure	Results	Comments
Static magnetic field effects					
(Papatheofanis, 1990)	Human polymorpho-nuclear leucocytes (PMNs)	Lysozymal degranulation and cell migration	0.1 T 30 min	Increased release of lysozyme and lactate dehydrogenase; inhibition of cell migration; channel antagonists protected cells exposed to SMF.	Blood samples pooled from three donors. No significance levels provided for the reported effects. The electromagnet could have produced alternating magnetic fields that were not controlled and might have produced the effects.
(Aldinucci et al., 2003b)	Human lymphocytes, Jurkat cells	Ca^{2+} movement, cell proliferation, production of pro-inflammatory cytokines	4.75 T 1 h	No effects on human lymphocytes. In Jurkat cells, changed properties of cell membranes lead to decreased Ca^{2+} transport and concentrate-ions, and to decreased cell proliferation.	

(Salerno et al., 1999)	Human peripheral blood mononuclear cells (PBMC)	Expression of activation markers and interleukin release	0.5 T 2 h	Reduced expression of CD69; increased release of IFN-γ and IL-4; release of TNF-α, IL-6 and IL-10 not modified.	
(Sabo et al., 2002)	Human HL-60 promyelo-cytic cell line	Metabolic activity	1 T 72 h	Retardation of metabolic activity, including in the presence of antineoplastic drugs.	The custom-made DC power supply could have produced alternating magnetic fields, which were not controlled and might have produced the effects.
(Chignell & Sik, 1995d)	Human erythrocytes	UV-induced photohaemolys is by the phototoxic drug ketoprofen and the photodynamic agent protoporphyrin IX	335 mT 20 min or up to 150 min	Reduced time for 50% ketoprofen-induced haemolysis. Possibly by increased concentration and/or lifetime of free radicals. No effects on proto-porphyrin IX - induced photohaemo-lysis. No difference between short and long exposure times.	The electromagn et could have producedalte rnating magnetic fields, which were not controlled and might have contributed to the observed effects.

(Chignell & Sik, 1998b)	Human erythrocytes	UV-induced photohaemolysis by the phototoxic drug ketoprofen	10 - 150 mT 20 min	SMF decreased the time required for UV-photo-haemolysis through increasing the concentration of radicals released during photolysis.	Unspecified source of SMF. Significance levels of effects and number of independent experiments not provided.	
MRI or Combined Exposure Studies						
(Heine et al., 1999)	Human neutrophils	Intracellular oxidative transformation of dihydro-rhodamine 123 to the fluorescent dye rhodamine 123	1.5 T 27.6 (±11.4) min	No influence on the production of radical species in living neutrophils.		MRI exposure.
(Aldinucci et al., 2003a)	Human lymphocytes, Jurkat cells	Intracellular Ca^{2+} concentration, cell proliferation, production of pro-inflammatory cytokines	4.75 T + pulse modulated RF 1 h	Increase in intracellular free Ca^{2+} without changes in proliferation and cytokines.		
Studies considered to be uninformative						
(Jajte et al., 2003)						

7.1.4 Cell membrane physiology

The cell membrane represents an interface between the cellular components inside the cell and the extracellular environment. As such, it regulates the intracellular environment, maintains the negative (approximately 70 mV) potential of the interior to that of the exterior (the 'resting' potential), and regulates the flow of molecules (for example, through voltage-gated or ligand-gated ion channels and carrier proteins such as the Na-K-ATPases).

Most studies on the effects of static magnetic fields on membranes concern exposures of short duration and low flux densities.

Rodent nerve preparations and hippocampal slices are frequently used, but snail ganglia and single snail neurons also serve as models because the relatively large size of molluscan neurons makes them easy to manipulate.

Rosen performed studies with mouse phrenic nerve preparations. In his 1992 paper, nerve-diaphragm preparations were exposed to 120 mT for 50 seconds (Rosen, 1992). No change in postsynaptic membrane resting potential was observed. There was a modest increase in action potential firing frequency at ambient temperatures < 35 °C, but a prominent decrease appeared at temperatures > 35 °C. Since the effect did not appear in the absence of Ca^{2+}, it was suggested that static magnetic fields may influence the release of neurotransmitter by stimulating calcium influx into the nerve terminal. Using murine neuromuscular junction preparations, Rosen observed increased inhibition of miniature endplate potentials between 50 and 150 seconds of exposure to 123 mT (Rosen, 1993). Discontinuation of the field resulted in full recovery.

In cultured neuroblastoma cells, Sonnier et al. (2000) found no effect on the resting potential after 5 seconds of exposure to 0.1, 0.5, 5 or 7.5 mT. Santini et al. (1994) did not see any response of membrane conductivity in primary chick embryo myoblasts after exposure to 1, 3 or 5 mT for 1 h. Carson et al. (1990) exposed HL-60 cells to 150 mT for 23 min and observed no effect on cytosolic free Ca^{2+}. In contrast, Rosen (1996) saw small reversible effects on the activation of time constant of calcium ion channels in GH3 cells after 150 seconds of exposure to 120 mT. He suggested that this was probably due to conformational changes in the plasma membrane resulting from membrane deformation.

Yost and Liburdy (1992) investigated calcium signal transduction after mitogenic stimulation in lymphocytes following exposure to static and time-varying magnetic fields. The presence of static fields alone resulted in no change.

Exposures of human neuroblastoma cells to static magnetic fields of up to 7.5 mT did not result in changes in any of the studied parameters of the action potential (Sonnier et al., 2003). Results suggested that the cellular mechanism responsible for the action potential is not affected under the employed conditions. Opposite results were reported by Rosen (2003a), who saw a transient increase in the activation time-constant of the sodium channel component of the action potential. However, Rosen (2003) observed this effect only at temperatures above 35 °C, greater than the 25 °C temperature used by Sonnier et al. (2003).

Miyamoto et al. (1996) did not observe any alterations in active and passive influxes of K^+ ions in human HeLaS3 cells exposed to static magnetic fields of different flux densities (0.5, 1, 1.6 T). Increasing the temperature from 37.4 to 45.0 °C did not change the outcome of the experiment.

McLean et al. (1995) exposed mouse dorsal root ganglion neurons to approximately 11 mT for 200 seconds. They observed a temporary reduction in the number of stimuli that elicited an action potential. The effect was maximal at 200 - 250 seconds after the start of exposure and returned to normal at 400 - 600 seconds. The effect was only found with magnet stacks of alternating polarity, not with single magnets. They speculated that there was a direct or indirect effect on action potential generating sodium channels.

Trabulsi et al. (1996) exposed mouse hippocampal slices to 2 - 3 or 8 - 10 mT for 20 min and measured excitatory postsynaptic potentials (EPSPs). They observed a biphasic effect of exposure in the 2 - 3 mT range (a small depression followed by a longer amplification) and a depression of EPSP in the 8 - 10 mT range. They suggested that changes in intracellular Ca^{2+} concentration were responsible for the effects.

The effect of exposure of isolated snail neurons to static magnetic fields was the object of three studies. Azanza (1989) exposed the cells to flux densities of 116 or 260 mT for 1 min and measured action potentials. She observed a Ca^{2+}-dependent effect, where 86% of the cells were excited and 14% were inhibited. Balaban et al. (1990) measured resting potential and input resistance of snail neurons during exposure to 23, 120 or 200 mT for 20 min. They observed a stimulus-dependent decrease in input resistance in normally silent cells, but an increase in resistance in spontaneously active cells. Exposure also resulted in changes in EPSPs. No effects were found after removal of glial cells surrounding the neuronal perikarya. The authors suggested that the observed effects were mediated by metabolic processes and that glial cells played a mediating role in these. Ayrapetyan et al. (1994) found that exposure to 2.3 - 350 mT for 3 - 5 min increased the firing of Ca^{2+}-dependent action potentials. They also exposed physiological solutions to static magnetic fields and found that the conduction of Ca^{2+}-containing solutions was altered. The activity of exposed neurons was further diminished when they were incubated in previously exposed Ca^{2+}-containing physiological solutions. The authors speculated that static magnetic field exposure might alter the hydration state of the Ca^{2+} ions and that this might have effects on their functionality.

Raybourn (1983) investigated the effect of exposure to 1 - 10 mT fields for up to 3 minutes on isolated turtle retinas by measuring the electroretinographic b-wave. The functional capacity of the retinas was assessed by using changes in sensitivity resulting from altered illumination conditions. A reduction of the response by static magnetic fields was found only at the transition from light to dark. No effect of dose was observed, which indicates a saturation effect occurred already at 1 mT. The sensitivity of the retinas was not altered.

Aoki et al. (1990) exposed human acute leukaemia-derived TALL-1 cells to 0.4 T for 15 minute, and observed an increased efflux of the drug adriamycin. They concluded that this was caused by alterations in the plasma membrane.

In the only study using plant material, Reina and Pascual (2001; 2001) studied water uptake through lettuce seed cell membranes. They exposed seeds to 0 - 10 mT for 10 minutes and observed a dose-dependent increase in water uptake. They explained the observations by (unspecified) alterations in cell membrane properties.

Höjevik et al. (1995) studied cyclotron resonance effects in rat insulin-producing RINm5F cells. They exposed the cells to 20.9 µT static fields in combination with 20.9 μT_{peak} ELF fields, with frequency varying from 12 - 60 Hz. No cyclotron resonance effects were observed.

Table 10. Cell membrane physiology

Authors	Cells	Endpoint	Exposure	Results	Comments
Static magnetic field effects					
(Rosen, 1992)	Murine phrenic nerve-diaphragm preparation	Miniature end-plate potentials	120 mT 50 s	No change in postsynaptic membrane resting potential. Modest frequency increase < 35 °C; prominent decrease > 35 °C; no effect in absence of Ca^{2+}.	
(Rosen, 1993)	Isolated murine neuro-muscular junction preparation	Miniature end-plate potentials. Reversible alteration in presynaptic membrane function	123 mT 150 s	Increasing inhibition between 50 and 150 s; recovery time constant at 135 s.	

(Sonnier et al., 2000)	Human neuro-blastoma cells	Resting potential	0.1, 0.5, 5, 7.5 mT 5 s	No effect.	
(Santini et al., 1994)	Primary chick embryo myoblasts	Membrane conductivity and permittivity	1, 3, 5 mT 1 h	No effect.	Lack of statistical methods (only means and SD given), but absence of changes was clear.
(Carson et al., 1990)	Human HL-60 promyelo-cytic cell line	Ca^{2+} concentration	0.15 T 23 min	No effect.	Number of independent experiments not reported.
(Rosen, 1996)	GH3 cells	Calcium channel activation	120 mT 150 s	Small reversible changes in calcium channels, probably due to membrane deformation of the intra-membrane part.	
(Yost & Liburdy, 1992)	Rat thymic lymphocytes	Calcium signal transduction	23.5 µT 1 h	No effect of SMF alone, only in combination with ELF field.	
(Sonnier et al., 2003)	Human SH-SY5Y neuroblastoma cell	Action potentials	0.1, 0.5, 7.5 mT	No detectable change in any of the studied parameters of the action potential.	
(Miyamoto et al., 1996)	Human HeLa S3 cells	Active and passive influx of K^+	0 - 2 T 15 min	No effect of SMF on total K^+ channels and different channel subtypes.	

(Rosen, 2003a)	GH3 cells	Kinetics of voltage activated Na^+ channels	125 mT 150 s	Slight shift in current-voltage relationship; < 5% reduction in peak current. Increase in activation time constant during and following exposure > 35 °C.	
(McLean et al., 1995)	Adult mouse dorsal root ganglion neurons	Action potentials (AP)	approx. 11 mT 200 sec	Reduction in number of stimuli that elicit AP; maximal at 200 - 250 s, returned to normal at 400 - 600 s; effect only seen with stacks of alternating polarity, not with single magnet.	
(Trabulsi et al., 1996)	Mouse hippocampal slices	Excitatory postsynaptic potential (EPSP)	2 - 3, 8 - 10 mT 20 min	Biphasic effect in 2 - 3 mT range; depression of EPSP in 8 - 10 mT range.	No statistics, only examples.
(Azanza, 1989)	Isolated snail neurons	Action potentials	116 or 260 mT 1 min	Ca^{2+} dependent inhibition or excitement; 86% of cells excited, 14% inhibited.	No statistics, no effect of flux density described.

(Balaban et al., 1990)	Snail neurons	Resting potential, input resistance	23, 120, 200 mT 20 min	Strength-dependent decreased input resistance in normally silent cells, increased in spontaneously active cells; changes in excitatory postsynaptic potentials; no effect after glia removal.	
(Ayrapetyan et al., 1994)	Land snail neurons	Action potentials (AP)	2.3 - 350 mT 3 - 5 min	Increase of firing of Ca^{2+}-dependent AP. Exposure of physiological solutions alters their properties, which leads to changes in neuron activity.	
(Raybourn, 1983)	Turtle retinas	Electroretino-graphic b-wave response	1 - 10 mT up to 3 min	Short-term reduction; only shortly, after lights off; no dose effect. No reduction in retinal sensitivity. Brief suppressive effect on extracellularly monitored light-elicited ionic current fluxes.	
(Aoki et al., 1990)	Human acute leukaemia-derived TALL-1 cell line	Accumulation and efflux of adriamycin	0.4 T 15 min	Increased efflux of adriamycin.	

(Reina & Pascual, 2001)	Lettuce seed cell membrane	Water uptake	0 - 10 mT (1 mT steps) 10 min	Dose-dependent increase in water uptake, induced by alterations in cell membranes.	Strong point is the backup by theoretical explanation.
MRI or combined exposure studies					
(Höjevik et al., 1995)	Rat insulin-producing RINm5F cells	Ca^{2+} transmembrane transport	20.9 µT SMF, 20.9 $µT_{peak}$ ELF fields, f = 12 - 60 Hz 100, 500 ms	No cyclotron resonance effects observed.	
Studies considered to be uninformative					
(Bellossi, 1986b)					
(Rosen, 1994)					
(Cavopol et al., 1995)					
(Osuga & Tatsuoka, 1999)					
(Wieraszko, 2000)					

7.1.5 Gene expression

The cell membrane is also a prime site for receiving external physical or biochemical 'signals', and can, through a signal transduction process acting via specialized receptor molecules, activate intracellular metabolic signalling pathways that result in the expression of specific genes. These in turn lead to the expression of specific proteins that initiate appropriate cellular responses.

One study focused on protein expression in cultured rat primary cortical and hippocampal cells in response to short, 15 min, exposure to 100 mT (Hirai et al., 2002). This study analysed DNA binding activator protein-1 (AP1), neuronal marker protein MAP2, neuronal differentiation marker proteins GAP-43, Fos-family proteins c-Fos, Fos-B, Fra-2 and Jun-family proteins c-Jun, Jun-B, and Jun-D, along with cytoplasmic Ca^{2+} and LDH activity. The authors found increased AP1 DNA binding through expression of Fra-2, c-Jun, and Jun-D proteins in immature hippocampal neurons. The results suggested that the short exposure to weak static magnetic fields may have lead to desensitisation of N-methyl-d-aspartate (NMDA) receptor channels through modulation of *de novo* synthesis of particular inducible target proteins at the level of gene transcription by the AP1 complex in immune hippocampal neurons. The effects were not observed in mature hippocampal neurons or in cortical neurons.

Hirose et al. (2003b) explored the effects of static magnetic fields on the expression of proto-oncogenes, including c-Jun, c-Myc, and c-Fos proteins, by exposing HL-60 cells to spatially homogeneous 10 T or inhomogeneous 6 T static magnetic field (with a 41.7 T m^{-1} gradient) for up to 72 h. The data revealed that c-Jun was expressed after exposure to the inhomogeneous 6 T for 24, 36, 48, and 72 h with increased protein amount and phosphorylation level, but that no response was found with shorter exposure duration and after exposure to a homogeneous 10 T field. C-Myc and c-Fos did not respond to either field. The authors concluded that a static magnetic field gradient has significant biological effects and needs to be taken into consideration.

Human L-132 cells were exposed to 1.5 T for 240 min (Guisasola et al., 2002a). Heat shock proteins hsp70, hsp27, and corresponding mRNAs, were measured, along with cAMP and Ca^{2+} ions. No effects of static magnetic fields were observed.

Table 11. Gene expression

Authors	Cells	Endpoint	Exposure	Results	Comments
Static magnetic field effects					
(Hirai et al., 2002)	Rat neuronal cells: primary cortical and hippocampal cell cultures.	DNA binding activator protein-1 AP1; neuronal marker protein MAP2; neuronal differentiation marker protein GAP-43; c-Fos, Fos-B, Fra-2; c-Jun, Jun-B, Jun-D. Cytoplasmic Ca^{2+}. LDH activity	100 mT 15 min	Increased AP1 DNA binding through expression of Fra-2, c-Jun, and Jun-D proteins in immature hippocampal neurons. Suggestive of desensitization of NMDA receptor channels at the level of gene transcription by the AP1 complex.	

(Hirose et al., 2003b)	Human HL-60 cells	c-Myc, c-Fos, c-Jun expression	6 or 10 T 1 - 72 h	No effect on c-Myc, c-Fos and c-Jun by homogeneous 10 T SMF. SMF gradient field induced c-Jun expression.	6 T field included exposure to gradient field.
(Guisasola et al., 2002b)	Human L-132 cells	hsp70, hsp27, and corresponding mRNAs; cAMP, Ca^{2+}	1.5 T 240 min	No effect of SMF. SMF exposure during MRI procedures does not induce any cellular stress response.	Number of independent experiments not reported.

Studies considered to be uninformative
(Cohly et al., 2003)
(Mnaimneh et al., 1996)
(Hiraoka et al., 1992)
(Richardson et al., 1992)
(Schneeweiss et al., 1995)

7.1.6 Cell growth, proliferation and apoptosis

Both proliferative and apoptotic responses, often the result of the activation of appropriate signalling pathways and the consequent expression of relevant genes, may be involved in carcinogenic processes, if activated inappropriately. A proliferative stimulus to a cell carrying an oncogene or having lost a tumour suppressor gene through mutation, or inhibition of apoptosis in damaged cells, may initiate the clonal expansion of a colony of such cells, thereby paving the way for the growth of a tumour.

A number of investigators have studied the effect of static magnetic fields exposure on *in vitro* cell growth and proliferation. Most studies have been designed to determine the effects of long-lasting, continuous exposure.

No effects were observed in a number of different cell types using a variety of exposure conditions. Rockwell (1977) did not find any effects after exposure of EMT6 mouse mammary tumour cells to 0.148 T for 48 h. Chinese hamster V79 cells were not influenced by several hours of exposure to 0.75 T (Ngo et al., 1987). Considerably higher flux densities of 1.5 T applied for 1 h or 7.05 T for 4 or 24 h did not influence the cell cycle progression of human HL60 and EA2 tumour cells. Exposure for 48 and 96 h to 1.5 T did not alter the growth rate of human HeLa and Gin-1 (gingival fibroblast) cells (Sato et al., 1992). Yamaguchi et al. (1993) also exposed Gin-1 cells, but to 0.2 T and for 6 - 8 months without an effect on cell growth. In yeast cells, 1.5 T applied for 15 h did not result in growth changes (Malko et al., 1994). No effect was observed of exposure to fields as high as 7 T for up to 8 days in P388 mouse leukaemia cells and V79 Chinese hamster fibroblasts (Sakurai et al., 1999), nor of 10-T fields applied for 4 days to Chinese hamster CHO-K1 cells (Nakahara et al., 2002). Finally, repetitive exposure to 1.5 T (3 times 1 h per week for 3 weeks) did not result in alterations of proliferation and clonogenicity of human fetal lung fibroblasts (Wiskirchen et al., 1999). Aldinucci et al. exposed human peripheral blood mononuclear cells (PBMC) and Jurkat cells to 4.75 T for 1 h (Aldinucci et al., 2003b). No proliferative effects of static magnetic fields were observed in the human lymphocytes, either quiescent or activated by phytohaemagglutinin (PHA).

In contrast, a number of studies with a variety of mammalian cells of different origin did find effects. Buemi et al. (2001) exposed rat renal VERO cells and cortical astrocytes to 0.2 T for up to 6 days. They observed an influence of exposure on the balance between cell proliferation and death. Linder-Aronson and Lindskog (1995) observed impaired attachment and growth of human periodontal fibroblasts during exposure to 0.1 - 0.2 T for up to 5 weeks. Exposure to 0.2 T for up to 3 hours led to decreased ^{3}H thymidine incorporation in the human MCF-7 breast cancer and NC-B4 neurons cell lines (Pacini et al., 1999a). No effect was found in murine leukaemia WEHI-3 cells, nor was there an effect on colony formation in any of the three cells lines.

Pacini et al. (1999b) also investigated cell proliferation and signalling following the exposure of human neurons (FNC-B4) to a 0.2 T static field. Cell proliferation, assessed by ^{3}H thymidine incorporation was inhibited in the neurons but not in the controls. Further tests indicated that the field did not affect twelve DNA microsatellites, indicating that no genomic instability was induced by static magnetic field exposure.

The viability of lymphocyte cells was followed after exposure to a 10 T field (Onodera et al., 2003). Without lymphocyte stimulation, there were no significant differences in the viability of exposed and unexposed T cells (CD4+ and CD8+), B cells and NK cells. Stimulated T cells had reduced viability following exposure. A 10 T static magnetic field had acute effects on immune cells during cell division, but a minimal effect on cells in a nondividing phase.

Raylman applied flux densities of 7 T to human lymphoma (Raji) cells for 18 hours and observed an 11% reduction in the number of viable cells and a reduced growth rate (Raylman et al., 1997). Exposure to 7 T for 64 hours reduced the viable cell number in human melanoma (HTB 63) cells, human ovarian carcinoma (HTB 77 IP3) cells and human lymphoma (Raji; CCL 86) cells (Raylman et al., 1996). The authors attributed the effect to growth retardation, although the cell cycle was unaltered. No increased number of DNA breaks was found, which is in agreement with the lack of effect on viability.

Norimura et al. (1993) exposed human T-lymphocytes to 2 - 6.3 T for up to 3 days. They observed inhibition of growth by field strengths of 4 - 6.3 T in cells stimulated by phytohaemagglutinin, but not in unstimulated cells. The radiosensitivity of the cells increased and the repair capacity decreased after exposure to 6.3 T. The authors concluded that temporary physiological alterations were induced by exposure to static magnetic fields of 4 T and higher. Apparently, these alterations are only observed when the cells are challenged.

Human and mammalian cells in culture were used in a few studies devoted to functional activity in response to long static magnetic field exposure. Flipo et al. (1998) analysed the mitogen response to concanavalin A, phagocytosis, Ca^{2+} influx, and apoptosis in C57Bl/6 murine macrophages, spleen lymphocytes, and thymic cells exposed to static magnetic fields at 2.5 - 150 mT for 24 h. Static magnetic fields altered several functional parameters in all cell types. No intensity threshold was observed in this study. Exposure of murine immune cells to static magnetic field decreased macrophage phagocytosis, enhanced apoptosis of thymocytes, and inhibited the response of lymphocytes to the mitogen concavalin A in association with an increased Ca^{2+} influx. Fanelli et al. (1999) analysed apoptosis and Ca^{2+} influx in human U937 and CEM cells. Exposure to 0.6 - 6 mT for 4 h increased cell survival by inhibiting apoptosis induced by several agents in an intensity-dependent fashion. Protective effects on apoptosis could be attributed to increased Ca^{2+} influx. However, this effect was not seen in rat cells where apoptosis was induced by Ca^{2+} influx.

Teodori et al. (2002) followed the occurrence of apoptosis in human HL60 cells exposed to a 6 mT static magnetic alone (18 hours) or in combination with the known apoptosis-inducer camptothecin (5 hours). They used two approaches (flow cytometry and laser scanning cytometry) and found no effect of static magnetic fields, alone or in combined treatment, on overall apoptosis. However, the authors observed a different distribution of early versus late apoptotic cell populations in the co-exposure treatment, suggesting a premature shift of cells into late apoptosis. It is unclear whether this could lead to inflammatory events.

Several authors used bacterial strains and plant cells to study the effects of static magnetic field exposure. Stansell et al. (2001) exposed *E. coli* to 8 - 60 mT for 19.5 h and studied the effect of the antibiotic piperacillin. Exposure increased the resistance against the antibiotic. In contrast, Benson et al. (1994) observed enhancement of the effect of the antibiotic gentamicin to *Pseudomonas aeruginosa* exposed to 0.5 - 2 mT for 20 min. It cannot be excluded that the decreased growth might have been influenced by different light conditions.

When grown in a mixed culture in stationary phase, the *E. coli* strains ZK126Nalr and ZK126Smr have different death rates, which lead to a growth advantage for ZK126Smr. When grown under continuous exposure to inhomogeneous 5.2 - 6.1 T fields, or 7 T homogeneous fields, the death rate of the ZK126Nalr cells decreases and the growth advantage of the other strain disappears (Okuno et al., 2001). The effect is stronger with the inhomogeneous fields.

Stasiuk (1974) exposed *Mycobacterium tuberculosis* to static magnetic fields (180 mT) and found that exposures of up to 1 h did not change the bacterial growth, but that longer exposure (2 h and more) resulted in significant inhibition. No changes were observed in sensitivity to antibiotics or growth in tissues of infected animals. Khar'kova et al. (1976) studied the effect of long exposure of *Staphylococcus* to a 5 mT field. Permanent changes in colour of colonies (after 16 days), and changes in morphology and in fermentation of proteins and hydrocarbons, were observed by 18 months. By 8 months, the sensitivity to antibiotics increased significantly. The lethality increased in mice upon infection with static magnetic field-exposed *Staphylococcus*. These results could have implications for human health, but they must first be independently replicated.

The growth and viability of the plant-growing bacteria *Serratia marcescens* and of callus cells of *Hordeum vulgare* (barley) and *Rubus fructiosus* (blackberry) was investigated after exposure to an inhomogeneous field varying between 6 and 10 mT for 24 or 48 h (Piatti et al., 2002). The number of bacterial cells was reduced, while both the number and viability of *H. vulgare* cells were lower after exposure. *R. fructiosus* cells were not influenced.

Several studies looked at the effects of MRI exposures on *in vitro* cell growth. Schiffer et al. (2003) used a clinical MR scanner to investigate the effects of signals relevant to MRI exposure on the cell cycle of two human cell lines. Appropriate controls were included (positive control for cell cycle alteration, as well as temperature and vibration controls). Combining static magnetic fields (1.5 or 7.05 T) with either a time-varying bipolar gradient field for 1, 2 or 24 hours or a pulsed radiofrequency field did not alter the cell cycle distribution, nor did a one-hour exposure to the MRI signal.

To elucidate the effect of MRI exposure on early murine embryo development, two-cell embryos were treated for various lengths of time by MRI using pulse sequences employed in current clinical imaging (Chew et al., 2001). There were no significant differences detected in the rate of blastocyst formation between control and exposed groups.

Tofani et al. (2001) exposed human colon adenocarcinoma (WiDr), breast adenocarcinoma (MCF-7), and embryonal lung fibroblasts (MRC-5) cells to either a static magnetic fields alone (1 - 30 mT) or in combination with ELF (3 mT at 16, 50 or 100 Hz). They observed apoptosis in WiDr and MCF-7 cells after exposure to static magnetic fields only with flux densities > 1 mT. The effect increased with simultaneous 50 Hz ELF exposure, but only for latency times up to 24 h.

Table 12. Cell growth, proliferation and apoptosis

Authors	Cells	Endpoint	Exposure	Results	Comments
Static magnetic field effects					
(Rockwell, 1977)	Mouse mammary tumour cells (EMT6)	Viability or growth	140 mT 48 h	No effect.	Lack of statistical information, but absence of effect was clear.
(Ngo et al., 1987)	Chinese hamster fibroblast cells (V79)	DNA synthesis, survival	0.75 T several h or 1 h following neutrons	No effect. Data indicated that SMF exposure alone does not exert any changes in survival and DNA synthesis in comparison with the effects from neutron radiation.	Results clear cut and experiments seem well-performed; however, no information on statistical analysis.
(Sato et al., 1992)	Human HeLa cells, human gingival fibroblast cells (Gin-1)	Growth, DNA content, DNA synthesis, labelling index	> 1.5 T 48, 96 h	No effect.	

(Yamaguchi et al., 1993)	Human gingival fibroblast cells (Gin-1)	Growth, DNA content, rate of lactate production, glucose consumption, ATP content and cell morphology	0.2 T 6, 8 mo + 1 or 2 wk; Sm-Co magnets	No influence on growth, morphology and glycolytic activity.	
(Malko et al., 1994)	Yeast cells	Growth	1.5 T 15 h	No effect.	
(Sakurai et al., 1999)	Mouse leukaemia cells (P388), Chinese hamster fibroblast cells (V79)	Growth pattern of cells, DNA distribution and sensitivity to bleomycin	7 T 3 h - 8 d	No effect.	Only one experiment per endpoint.
(Nakahara et al., 2002)	Chinese hamster ovary cells (CHO-K1)	Growth, cycle distribution, micronucleus (MN) formation	10 T 4 d	No effects of SMF alone, but enhancement of 4-Gy-induced MN-formation. SMF exposure may have been a co-factor.	
(Wiskirche n et al., 1999)	Human fetal lung fibroblast	Proliferation, clonogenic assay	1.5 T 1 h, 3x/wk, 3 wk	No significant effects.	
(Aldinucci et al., 2003b)	Human lymphocytes, Jurkat cells	Ca^{2+} movement, cell proliferation, production of pro-inflammatory cytokines	4.75 T 1 h	No effects on lymphocytes. In Jurkat cells, changed properties of cell membranes lead to decreased Ca^{2+} transport and concentrations, and to decreased cell proliferation.	

(Buemi et al., 2001)	Rat renal cells (VERO); cortical astrocytes	Cell proliferation, cell death balance	0.2 T 2, 4, 6 d	Influence of SMF on cell proliferation / death balance; differs between cell lines. This could have been partly due to astrocytes being primary cells and renal cells being immortalized. SMF exposure may have interacted with apoptosis.	
(Linder-Aronson & Lindskog, 1995)	Human periodontal fibroblasts	Attachment and growth	107 - 230 mT (intradisk variation) 1 - 5 wk	Impaired attachment and growth.	With increasing passage number, there was also decrease in attachment & growth in controls, but difference with exposed cells was clearly significant.
(Pacini et al., 1999a)	Human breast cancer cell line (MCF-7); neurons (NC-B4); murine leukaemia cells (WEHI-3)	Cell damage and proliferation	0.2 T 5 min - 3 h	Decreased ^{3}H thymidine incorporation in human cells, not in murine; no effect on formation of cell colonies. Effect of vitamin D permanent, that of SMF temporary.	

(Pacini et al., 1999b)	Normal human neuronal cells (FNC-B4); mouse leukaemia cells; human breast carcinoma cells	Morphology, cell proliferation, production of endothelin-1, genome instability	0.2 T 5 - 15 min	No alterations in genome instability; dramatic changes of morphology in neuronal cells only. Significant decrease in cell proliferation, changes in production of endothelin-1.	
(Onodera et al., 2003)	Human peripheral blood mononuclear cells (PBMC)	Viability, apoptosis, lymphocyte subpopulations	field increase 0 - 10 T over 0.5 h, constant for 3 h, decrease to 0 T over 0.5 h	Without lymphocyte stimulation, no significant differences in viability of exposed and unexposed T cells (CD4$^+$ and CD8$^+$), B cells and NK cells. Stimulated T cells had reduced viability following exposure.	
(Raylman et al., 1997)	Human lymphoma cells (Raji)	Viable cell number	7 T 18 h	11% reduction of number of viable cells due to exposure; growth rate retarded.	
(Raylman et al., 1996)	Human melanoma cells (HTB 63), ovarian carcinoma cells (HTB 77 IP3), and lymphoma cells (CCL 86, Raji)	Cell viability; flow cytometry	7 T 64 h	Reduction in viable cell number – HTB63 19%, HTB77 22%, Raji 41%; cell cycle unaltered; no increase in DNA breaks, growth after exposure slowed for 1 d. Cell growth recovered when SMF exposure was halted.	Sensitive testing method (cell cycle analysis).

(Norimura et al., 1993)	Human T-lymphocytes	Cell growth and radiation response	2 - 6.3 T up to 3 d	No effect in normal cells; growth inhibition in stimulated cells only at >4 T; radiosensitivity up, repair decreased after 6.3 T. Stimulated or stressed cells possibly more susceptible to SMF than normal growing cells.	Peculiar way of determining cloning efficiency.
(Flipo et al., 1998)	Murine macrophages (C57Bl/6), spleen lymphocytes, and thymic cells	Mitogen response to concanavalin A, phagocytosis, Ca^{2+} influx, apoptosis	2.5 - 150 mT 24 h	Decreased macrophage phagocytosis, enhanced apoptosis of thymocytes, and inhibited response of lymphocytes to Con A in association with an increased Ca^{2+} influx.	Data support conclusion about non-linear dependence of effects.
(Fanelli et al., 1999)	Human U937 and CEM cells; human peripheral blood leucocytes; rat thymocytes	Apoptosis, Ca^{2+} influx	0.6 - 6 mT 4 h	Protective effect on apoptosis was due to increase of Ca^{2+} influx. Effect not seen in rat cells where apoptosis was induced by Ca^{2+} influx.	
(Teodori et al., 2002)	Human HL-60 cells	Apoptosis	6 mT 18 h	No effect of SMF alone, slight acceleration of apoptosis in camptothecin-treated cells.	
(Stansell et al., 2001)	Bacteria (E. coli)	Number of cells with piperacillin treatment	8 - 60 mT 19.5 h	Increased number of cells.	

(Benson et al., 1994)	Bacteria (*Pseudomonas aeruginosa*)	Number of cells with gentamicin treatment; autoradiograms from ^{111}In uptake	0.5 - 2 mT 20 min	Decreased number of cells due to SMF enhancement of antibiotic activity.	No sham controls; growth difference may have been influenced by different light conditions.
(Okuno et al., 2001)	Bacteria (*E. coli* ZK126Nalr and ZK126Smr)	Differential cell growth	5.2 - 6.1 T, inhomogeneous (maximum gradient 23 T/m) 7 T homog.	Growth advantage in stationary phase disappears; effect stronger with inhomogeneous field.	
(Stasiuk, 1974)	*Mycobacterium tuberculosis*	Cell growth in culture, resistance to antibiotics, growth of bacteria from infected guinea pigs	180 mT 1, 5, 30, 60, 120 min and 24 h	No effects at 1, 5, 30 and 60 min exposures. Significant inhibition of cell growth at 120 min and almost complete blockage at 24 h exposure. No changes in sensitivity to antibiotics. No effects on growth in tissues from exposed animals.	Amount of independent exposures not reported.

(Khar'kova et al., 1976)	Haemolytic Staphylococcus, strain 209-P	Colour and morphology of colonies, fermentation of proteins and hydro-carbons sensitivity to antibiotics. Pathogenic properties upon infection of mice.	5 mT up to 18 months	Permanent changes in colour of colonies by 16 d exposure, changes in morphology and fermentation of proteins and hydrocarbons by 18 months. Sensitivity to antibiotics increased after 8 months. Increased lethality of mice after infection with SMF-exposed Staphylococcus.	Amount of independent exposures and number of measurements not reported.
(Okuno et al., 2001)	Bacteria (E. coli ZK126Nalr and ZK126Smr)	Differential cell growth	5.2 - 6.1 T, inhomo-geneous, 7 T homo-geneous	Growth advantage in stationary phase disappears; effect stronger with inhomogeneous field.	
(Piatti et al., 2002)	Bacteria, plant cell cultures	Growth, viability	6 - 10 mT 24 or 48 h; magnetic disks	Reduction in number of bacterial cells; reduction in number and viability of H. vulgare cells; no effect on R. fucticosus.	
MRI or combined exposure studies					
(Schiffer et al., 2003)	Human HL60 and EA2 tumour cells	Cell cycle distribution	1.5 T, 2 h 7.05 T, 4 or 24 h 7.05 T + gradient field, 2 or 24 h 1.5 T + RF, 1 h 1.5 T + gradient + RF, 1 h	No effect.	

(Chew et al., 2001)	Two-cell murine embryos	Rate of blastocyst formation	8 pulse sequences employed in current clinical imaging 1.5 T 2.27 - 6.11 min	No effect; development rates 70 - 75%. MR imaging sequences did not exert harmful effects to blastocyst formation.	Used standard MRI imaging sequences.
(Tofani et al., 2001)	Human colon adenocarci-noma cells (WiDr), breast adenocarci-noma cells (MCF-7), embryonal lung fibroblasts (MRC-5)	Growth, apoptosis	1, 3, 10, 30 mT SMF, 3 mT ELF at 16, 50 100Hz 20 min	Apoptosis observed in WiDr and MCF-7 cells only after > 1 mT SMF; increased with simultaneous 50 Hz ELF. Only for latency times up to 24 h.	

Studies considered to be uninformative
(Esformes et al., 1981)
(McDonald, 1993)
(Tsuchiya et al., 1999)
(Stepanian et al., 2000)
(Horiuchi et al., 2001)
(Ishizaki et al., 2001)
(Mariani et al., 2001)
(Horiuchi et al., 2002)
(Jajte et al., 2002)
(Zhang et al., 2002)

7.1.7 Genotoxic effects

The genotoxicity of an agent is an indication of its potential to damage DNA, and is therefore implicated in the process of mutagenesis. As a result of this, stable and heritable genetic mutations are generated, often through misrepair. Mutations leading to the activation of oncogenes, or the inactivation of tumour suppressor genes, are early events in the formation of cancers.

Tests of genotoxicity typically include chromosomal aberrations, sister chromatid exchange, micronucleus formation, different assays for mutagenesis, and measures of DNA damage (such as the comet assay).

Cooke and Morris (1981) analysed chromosomal aberrations and sister chromatid exchanges following 1-h exposure of human lymphocytes to static magnetic fields. Even while there was a trend for an increase in number of chromosome lesions and proportion of cells with lesions (50 - 80%) at both employed field intensities, (0.5 and 1 T), these increases were not statistically significant. The authors concluded that static magnetic fields had no significant effect on any of the measured parameters.

Effects of static magnetic fields on conformation of chromatin/nucleoids were studied in human and bacterial cells (Matronchik et al., 1996; Belyaev et al., 1997; Binhi et al., 2001). In these studies, transient condensation or decondensation of chromatin was observed at specific 'intensity windows' in the range of 0 - 110 μT. The authors attributed these transient changes to adaptation of cells to the changes in the static magnetic field. A possible interplay of these changes in chromatin conformation with genotoxic effects was suggested. The observed effects were explained on the basis of phase modulation of hypothetical natural high-frequency oscillations.

A number of studies have been designed to determine effects of long lasting continuous exposure in mammalian cells. Okonogi et al. (1996) did not find effects of a 6 h exposure to 4.7 T on the background level of micronuclei in Chinese hamster CHL/IU cells. On the other hand, a decrease in the formation of micronuclei induced by concomitant exposure to mitomycin C was observed. The authors suggested that static magnetic field exposure might have a protective effect on DNA damage produced by mitomycin C.

Exposure of rat lymphocytes to the much lower flux density of 7 mT for 3 h did not increase the number of cells with DNA damage, as measured with the comet assay (Zmyslony et al., 2000). The amount of damage was significantly increased when the $FeCl_2$-incubated cells were simultaneously exposed to static magnetic fields. However, the same exposure to static magnetic fields did not modify H_2O_2-induced DNA damage. According to the authors, the low level of $FeCl_2$ did not induce any noxious effects on lymphocytes. They hypothesized that the static magnetic field might have had an effect on radical pairs, leading to an increased number of free radicals generated in the cells by iron cations, but they also felt that reasonable explanations for their results were lacking. Nakahara et al. (2002) investigated the formation of micronuclei in Chinese hamster ovary CHO-K1 cells. Exposure to 1 or 10 T alone for 4 days did not result in induction of micronuclei. No synergistic effects were observed in combined treatments with X-irradiation, except for exposure to 10 T and 4 Gy. In those cases, static magnetic field exposure increased the formation of X-ray-induced micronuclei by 10%.

A similar variability in results was seen in studies with bacterial cells. Ikehata et al. used the Ames test to study effects of exposure to 2 - 5 T for 20 minutes up to 48 h (Ikehata et al., 1999). They observed no direct effect of static magnetic field exposure on mutagenicity or growth rate. Mutation rate in the static magnetic field-exposed groups was significantly higher than in the non-exposed groups when cells were treated with several (but not all tested) chemical mutagens. No dose-response for mutagenic effects was observed in this study. Mutagenic effects were also not detected with the Ames test at the higher magnetic fields of 5 and 7.2 T (Teichmann et al., 2000).

Zhang et al. analysed mutagenic effects of 24-h exposure to 5 or 9 T in *Escherichia coli* cells (Zhang et al., 2003). They observed no effects on survival and mutation rate in wild type, or in strains defective in DNA repair enzymes or redox-regulating enzymes. Mutation frequency increased in soxR and sodAsodB mutants (which are defective in defence mechanisms against oxidative stress). The expression of superoxide-inducible genes was stimulated. The data suggested that static magnetic fields above 5 T induce mutations through elevated production of intracellular superoxide radicals in *E. coli* (Zhang et al., 2003).

Baum and Nauman used plant cells to study mutagenic effects of static magnetic field exposure (Baum & Nauman, 1984). They analysed micronuclei and pink mutations in *Tradescantia*. Magnetic field at intensities of about 0.16 to 0.78 T applied continuously over 6 or 7 days did not induce genotoxic effects in *Tradescantia* cells.

Wolff et al. (1985) exposed human lymphocytes and Chinese Ovary cells to a 2.35 T static magnetic field combined with radiofrequency fields for 12.5 h. Sister chromatide exchange and chromosomal aberrations were assessed. No effects on these cytogenetic endpoints were found.

Table 13. Genotoxic effects

Authors	Cells	Endpoint	Exposure	Results	Comments
Static magnetic field effects					
(Cooke & Morris, 1981)	Human lymphocytes	Frequency of gross chromosome lesions, sister chromatid exchanges and proportion of amodal cells.	0.5 T, 1.0 T 1 h	No effect.	Trend for increased chromo-somal lesions and increased proportion of cells with lesions.
(Matronchik et al., 1996)	Bacterial *E. coli* cells	Conformation of nucleoids	0 - 110 µT 15 min	Changes on conformation of nucleoids dependent on SMF in specific 'intensity windows'. Condensation or decondensation of nucleoids was observed in specific windows.	
(Belyaev et al., 1997)	Normal human fibroblasts and lymphocytes	Conformation of chromatin	zeroed natural magnetic field 10 - 120 min	Time-dependent transient condensation of chromatin characteristic of stress response with maximum at 40 - 80 min. Effects reproduced in experiments with lymphocytes from the same donor.	

(Binhi et al., 2001)	Bacterial *E. coli* cells	Conformation of nucleoids	0 - 110 µT 15 min	Changes in conformation of nucleoids dependent on 'SMF intensity windows' with extrema at 0, 26, 43, 61, 72, 83 and 105 µT. Explained by phase modulation of ion interference in rotations of DNA-protein complexes.	
(Okonogi et al., 1996)	Chinese hamster cells (CHL/IU)	Micronuclei (MN) formation	4.7 T 6 h	No effects of SMF on the background level of MN. Decrease in formation of MN induced by Mitomycin C. Possibly influence on cell cycle.	
(Zmyslony et al., 2000)	Rat lymphocytes	DNA damage including single strand breaks and alkali labile sites	7 mT 3 h	No effect of SMF only. Enhancement of $FeCl_2$-induced DNA-damage by SMF. No effects on H_2O_2-induced damage.	
(Nakahara et al., 2002)	Chinese hamster ovary cells (CHO-K1)	Growth, cell cycle distribution, micronucleus (MN) formation	1, 10 T 4 d	No effects of SMF alone, but enhancement of 4-Gy-induced MN-formation. SMF exposure may have been a co-factor.	Enhance-ment was at the border of statistical significance

(Ikehata et al., 1999)	Bacterial strains from the Ames test	Mutagenicity and co-mutagenecity (Ames test), cytotoxicity	2, 5 T 20 min, 1.5, 3, 6, 15, 24, 48 h	Mutagenicity of several (but not all) tested compounds increased; no dose-response; no direct effect of SMF on mutagenicity or growth rate. Possibly influence of SMF on reaction intermediates.	
(Teichmann et al., 2000)	Bacteria from the Ames test	Mutagenicity (Ames test)	0.5, 7.2 T 1 h, 24 h	No effect.	Although statistics are lacking, it was clear from comparison of the means ± SD that there was no effect of SMF.

(Zhang et al., 2003)	*Escherichia coli* wildtype, soxR, sodAsodB mutants	Induction of mutations, clonogenic survival	5 or 9 T 24 h	No effects on survival and mutation rate in wild-type, or strains defective in DNA repair enzymes or redox-regulating enzymes. Mutation frequency increased in soxR and sodAsodB mutants (defective in defence mechanisms against oxidative stress). Expression of superoxide inducible gene was stimulated.	Changes larger than SD, however, statistical analysis was not performed.
(Baum & Nauman, 1984)	*Tradescantia* clones 4430 and 02	Micronuclei, pink mutations	0.16, 0.76 - 0.78 T 6 - 11 d	No effect of SMF applied continuously over 6 or 7 days on *Tradescantia* pollen mother cells.	Field variations of ± 25%.
MRI or combined exposure studies					
(Wolff et al., 1985)	Chinese hamster ovary cells; human lymphocytes	Chromosomal aberrations (CA), sister chromatid exchanges (SCE).	2.35 T + RF 12.5 h	MR imaging conditions did not cause cytogenetic damage.	

Studies considered to be uninformative
(Rossner & Matejka, 1977)
(Wolff et al., 1980)
(Geard et al., 1984)
(Takatsuji et al., 1989)
(Yamazaki et al., 1993)
(Mahdi et al., 1994)
(Schreiber et al., 2001)

7.1.8 Conclusions

The results of *in vitro* studies are useful for elucidating interaction mechanisms and for indicating the sorts of effects that might be investigated *in vivo*, but are not sufficient to identify health effects without corroborating evidence from *in vivo* studies.

A number of different biological effects of static magnetic fields have been studied *in vitro*. The observed effects are rather diverse and were found after exposure to a wide range of magnetic flux densities.

Despite some inconsistencies, the studies on cell free systems show that biologically relevant biochemical reactions can be affected by static magnetic fields in the millitesla to tesla range.

The body of reviewed data on magneto-mechanical effects showed that static magnetic fields can affect orientation of cells. These effects were observed under relatively high field intensities of more than 1 T, and for different exposure times that ranged from minutes to hours.

The studies on metabolic activity suggest that it may be affected by static magnetic fields, dependent on cell type or whether or not the cells are transformed. The data obtained from the 'cell-free system' studies indicated that radicals and calcium metabolism might be primary targets for effects of static magnetic fields. This is also the case for combined exposures to static magnetic fields and RF fields. It should be mentioned that most of the *in vitro* studies involved electromagnets that might create alternating fields, which were usually not measured.

The studies on membrane effects show that exposure to static magnetic fields in the millitesla range is able to change membrane properties in isolated systems and cultured cells, possibly through changes in (calcium) ion channel structure and/or activity. These changes may lead to changes in neuronal functioning, such as changes in action potential generation and, consequently, neurotransmitter release. However, most of the effects seem to be reversible.

Few studies have been performed on gene expression. The data show that static magnetic fields can affect the expression of specific genes in human and mammalian cells. These effects may depend on exposure duration and field gradients.

There are many studies on cell growth, with contrasting results. The occurrence of effects in mammalian cells appears highly cell-type dependent, since n several cell lines showed no effects on growth from fields up to 10 T. When an effect was found, it was generally growth retardation. The extent of any effect was usually dependent on exposure time and field strength (in the millitesla to tesla range). However, the dependence on field strength was addressed only in two studies and non-linear responses have been observed.

The few studies dealing with apoptosis in mammalian cells and those on growth of bacteria also show contrasting results. The effects in bacteria appear strongly strain-dependent.

Only a few studies on genotoxicity have been performed. No genotoxic effects of static magnetic fields up to 9 T have been shown, except for one study with repair-deficient bacterial strains. The studies with combined exposure to mutagens and static magnetic fields indicated modification of the effects of some of the tested mutagens. The effects may be strain/cell type dependent, but there are no indications for dose-dependence.

There are positive and negative findings regarding *in vitro* effects. There is evidence that static magnetic fields can affect several endpoints at intensities lower than 1 T, in the millitesla range. However, most data, both negative and positive, have not been replicated. Biological variables such as cell type, cell activation, and other physiological conditions during exposure were shown to be of importance. Thresholds for some of the effects were reported, but other studies indicated non-linear response without clear threshold values and even 'flux-density' windows were reported. The mechanisms for these effects are not known, but effects on radicals and ions may be involved. So far, dosimetric issues have not been studied and it is not clear whether the equivalent of 'dose' equals 'time of exposure' times 'intensity' is applicable for quantification of those effects and use in health risk assessments. In addition, there is no consistent knowledge regarding how prolonged or interrupted exposure would affect biological systems *in vitro*. Besides possible complicated dependence on physical parameters such as intensity, duration, recurrence and gradients of exposure, biological variables appear to be important for the effects of static magnetic fields. Finally, combined effects of static magnetic fields with other agents, such as genotoxic chemicals, seem to produce synergistic effects, both protective and stimulating. Further studies should clarify these issues.

7.2 Static field effects *in vivo*

This section discusses static field effects on *in vivo* biological systems, which are based on animal studies, in relation to possible health effects in humans. These kinds of investigation elucidate some *in vivo* mechanisms that cannot be investigated directly in humans, but are very important for understanding the mechanisms of static field interactions with complex living organisms. These investigations thus enable a more precise estimation of the Environmental Health Criteria and their applications.

Static electric fields induce a surface charge on animals and humans (see chapter 5). These can be perceived via surface charge effects such as hair movement. A few studies, mostly relating to perceptual effects, have been carried out and are briefly reviewed below. Most of the reviewed studies concern the effects of static magnetic fields; these can interact with living organisms in a number of different ways (see chapter 5 for a full discussion). This includes possible interactions with certain types of metabolic reactions and physiological processes, particularly those that involve the exchange of charged particles (ion fluxes) across cell membranes and the consequent generation of transmembrane electrical potentials (gradients of ion concentration).

7.2.1 Static electric fields

A review by Kowalczuk et al. (1991) concluded that the few published animal studies of static electric field effects provided no evidence of any adverse health effect. There have been few subsequent studies, and these have mostly examined surface charge effects. Rats showed aversive behaviour in an electric field of 55 kV m^{-1} and above, but not to fields of 42.5 kV m^{-1} or less (Creim et al., 1993). Exposure to 75 kV m^{-1} did, however, not induce taste aversion learning (Creim et al., 1995). The results of an earlier study suggested that locomotor and rearing activity was not significantly modified by exposure to up to 12 kV m^{-1} (Bailey & Charry, 1986).

103

Table 13. Static electric field effects

Authors	Animal	Endpoint	Exposure	Results	Comments
Static electric field effects					
(Creim et al., 1993)	Rats	Avoidance behaviour using a shuttle-box	Up to 80 kV m^{-1} for 1 h with constant or varied air ion concentration	Exposure to fields of 55 or 80 kV m^{-1} resulted in significant avoidance compared to sham exposed controls.	Air ion concentration, which simulates conditions under HVDC overhead lines, had no effect on avoidance behaviour.
(Creim et al., 1995)	Rats	Taste-aversion learning using a saccharin-flavoured drink	75 kV m^{-1} for 4 h at a constant air ion concentration	Exposure to 75 kV m^{-1} did not induce taste aversion.	Experimental procedure validated using a positive control.
(Bailey & Charry, 1986)	Rats	Locomotor and rearing activity; food and water intake	3 kV m^{-1} for 2, 18 or 66 h; 12 kV m^{-1} for 18 h.	Exposure even at 12 kV m^{-1} did not affect activity, or food and water intake.	
Studies considered to be uninformative					
(Möse & Fischer, 1970)					
(Fam, 1981)					

7.2.2 Static magnetic fields

Throughout life, all living organisms interact with geomagnetic fields in different ways. Some are thought to have developed specific sense organs with high magnetic sensitivity for the purposes of spatial orientation and directional cues during migration. Others, including humans, are not only constantly exposed to the action of geomagnetic fields, but are also occasionally exposed to much larger static fields produced by artificial sources.

To investigate the complex nature of static magnetic field effects on biological systems *in vivo*, a detailed analysis of the effects at different levels of organization is necessary. Animals, particularly in animal models of specific conditions, are very useful for investigating and interpreting the effects of static magnetic field exposure that are often difficult, or impossible, to investigate in humans. They provide qualitative information about possible human responses, but are unlikely to provide quantitative information (since there are many differences in metabolism, physiology, lifetime etc.).

This review has been structured according to basic principles of anatomical and physiological organization, with the objective of identifying probable static magnetic field effects in animals that could also occur in humans. The principal areas covered include neurobehavioural studies, the musculo-skeletal system, the cardiovascular system and haematology, the endocrine system, reproduction and development, and genotoxicity and cancer.

7.2.2.1 Neurobehavioural studies

The nervous system enables animals and humans to respond to their environment and communicate with each other, as well as to maintain their internal physiological state. It comprises the brain and spinal cord of the central nervous system, the motor and sensory nerves of the peripheral nervous system, and the sympathetic and parasympathetic nerves and ganglia of the autonomic nervous system. Individual nerve cells receive and transmit information along their axons by the propagation of electrical impulses (action potentials). Information transmission at synapses (junctions) with other nerve cells takes place via the release of specialized neurotransmitter substances. In addition, specialized neurosecretory cells in the hypothalamus, pituitary gland and pineal organ of the brain release hormones that exert control over more peripheral endocrine organs, such as the thyroid and gonads.

7.2.2.1.1 Neurophysiological studies

The Lorenz force that acts on moving charge carriers, such as ionic currents, might be expected to affect ion channel conduction properties, thereby affecting nervous system function. However, calculation by Wikswo and Barach (1980) suggested that a field of $\sim$ 24 T would be required to produce a 10% change in Na^+ or K^+ ion channel conductivity, with larger fields required for heavier ions.

Support for this view comes from the work of three groups. Schwartz (1978; 1979) found no effect of a 1.2 T field on action potential conduction velocity and ion channel currents in lobster giant axons. Similarly, Tenforde and colleagues found no effect of a 2 T field on conduction velocity, refractory period and excitation threshold in excised frog sciatic nerve preparations (Gaffey & Tenforde, 1983). Hong et al. (1986) and Hong (1987) found no effect of exposure to a static field of up to 1.2 T or to 1 T on nerve conduction velocity in anaesthetised rats nor in (awake) human subjects, respectively. In addition, a 1.5 T field had no effect on the amplitude or latency of somatosensory evoked potentials in volunteers (Hong & Shellock, 1990). (See chapter 8.8.1).

Rosen and colleagues have carried out a number of electrophysiological studies over the past 10-20 years, including both *in vitro* (previous chapter) as well as *in vivo* studies (see Rosen, 2003b for a review). With regard to the *in vivo* studies, Rosen and Lubowsky (1987) studied the effects of a pure static magnetic field of 120 mT on the excitability of striate cortex in three adult cats. To avoid effects from the anaesthesia, the animals were decerebrated (immobilised through surgical transection of the mid-brain). All animals subjected to a 120 mT field showed a gradual decrease in the maximum amplitude of the visual evoked potential, as well as a reduction in its variability. This change began 50 to 95 seconds after the field was turned on and persisted for 200 to 285 seconds after the field was turned off, with maximum effect evident at 100 to 175 seconds. At 80 mT, an effect was found in only one animal but not in the two others. Because the effects developed slowly and persisted for some time after the field was turned off, the authors suggested that the field alters the ionic environment or neurotransmitter availability at synapses, rather than having an effect on axonal conduction.

The same conclusion was drawn based on the results of the second study (Rosen & Lubowsky, 1990). The effects of 123 mT on spontaneous discharge frequency and discharge pattern of principle cells in the lateral geniculate body of five adult cats were examined. Effects on the lateral geniculate body would result in altered visual evoked potential, as was observed earlier. This experiment revealed that 45% of studied cells showed a decrease in frequency after the field was turned on. Once more, the effect developed slowly (75 seconds after field activation) and returned to baseline 250 seconds after the field was turned off.

These results appear consistent with other studies by Rosen (1996; 2003a) on cultured neuroblastoma cells, in which patch-clamp techniques revealed slow, long-lasting increases in the activation time-constants of the voltage-gated Na^+ and Ca^{2+}ion channels. These results are also consistent with studies by Wieraszko and colleagues (Trabulsi et al., 1996; Wieraszko, 2000) on the modulation of synaptic excitability by static fields of 2 - 3 mT (see Table 10).

Two Russian studies investigated the effect of a 10 to 30 min static field exposure on evoked potentials in rats (Klimovskaia & Smirnova, 1976; Smirnova et al., 1982). The first study found increased amplitudes and additional waves in the evoked potentials after 0.4 T exposure. The effects were reversible. In the second study, different exposure levels between 0.1 and 1.6 T had been applied. An intensity-dependent increase in the amplitude of the potentials as well as modified shapes were observed. Effects were stronger in the hippocampus than in the cortex.

Cordeiro et al. (1989) exposed rats that had been subjected to sciatic nerve transection to a static magnetic field of 1 T for 12 h per day for 4 weeks. Exposure, when compared to sham exposure, had no effect on the speed of nerve regeneration.

Several animal species use geomagnetic fields for their orientation and navigation. This means that these animals are very sensitive to static magnetic field changes. Lohmann et al. (1991) subjected the marine mollusc *Tritonia diomedea* to alterations in geomagnetic field orientation at a 1 minute-on, 1 minute-off schedule for 26 min, and observed increased action potential firing in two specific brain neurons.

It is known that the electro-fish *Apteronotus* emits weak sinusoidal electric signals. Stojan et al. (1990) observed a changed in the amplitude of the electric signal if a fish was exposed to a static magnetic field up to 10 T during 20 h. This effect was observed above a threshold of 1 T. The change in the amplitude was 8 to 10 mV for field strengths between 2 and 10 T. The effect was observed immediately after the field was turned on. The effect in the 2 T condition disappeared after 5 to 10 h, whereas the effect persisted almost unchanged until the field was turned off in the 10 T condition.

Table 14. Neurophysiological studies					
Authors	Animal	Endpoint	Exposure	Results	Comments
Static Magnetic Field Effects					
(Schwartz, 1978)	Lobster	Nerve conduction velocity in giant axon.	1.2 T SMF parallel or perpendicular to axon 20 - 30 min	No effect on nerve conduction velocity	

(Schwartz, 1979)	Lobster	Resting potential, membrane action potential and transmembrane currents in giant axon.	1.2 T SMF parallel or perpendicular to axon < 5 min or 20 - 30 min	No effects on membrane potential or transmembrane currents	The preparation viability declined after about 10 - 15 min.
(Gaffey & Tenforde, 1983)	Frog	Action potential amplitude, conduction velocity, absolute and relative refractory periods in sciatic nerve	Up to 2.0 T field parallel to or perpendicular to nerve 4 - 17 h	No significant effect of 2 T field on action potential amplitude, conduction velocity, absolute and relative refractory periods. No effect of 1 T field on threshold	
(Hong et al., 1986)	Adult Sprague-Dawley albino rat	Motor nerve conduction and excitability	0.3 - 1.2 T 15, 30 or 60 sec	No effect on nerve conduction. Increased motor nerve excitability at > 0.5 T and t>30 sec. Effect disappeared 1 minute after termination of the field exposure. Effects were dose related.	Anaesthetized with intraperitoneal chloral hydrate.
(Rosen & Lubowsky, 1987)	Cat	Visual evoked response	120 mT + 80 mT 100 sec	At 120 mT decrease in amplitude, variability of a visual evoked response; starts 50 sec after start of exposure, lasts 285 sec after termination.	Increased amplitude of the visual evoked response at 80 mT in one of three animals (no effect in the others).

(Rosen & Lubowsky, 1990)	Cat	Principle cells in the lateral geniculate body	123 mT 100 sec	Decrease of discharge frequency in 45% of the cells studied, starting 75 sec after field activation and returning to baseline 250 sec after field was turned off.	Decerebration before the experiment instead of anaesthesia. This paper documents a spontaneous change of discharge frequency in the same order as the magnetic field-induced ones.
(Klimovskaia & Smirnova, 1976)	Albino rats	Cerebral and cerebellar cortex potentials evoked by sciatic stimulation	0.05 - 0.4 T 10 - 20 min	SMF at 0.4 T increased the amplitude of evoked potentials. Appearance of additional waves in evoked potentials. Effects of SMF were reversible.	
(Smirnova et al., 1982)	White rats	Somatosensory potentials in brain cortex and hypo-thalamus	0.1 - 1.6 T 15, 30 min	Intensity-dependent changes in potential in both cortex and hippocampus, with stronger response in hippocampus. Effects of 1.6 T were the same for different electromagnets. One of those magnets had a weak component, 1.8%, of alternating field, 100 Hz.	
(Cordeiro et al., 1989)	Rat	Nerve regeneration	1 T 12 h/d, 4 wk	No effect on nerve regeneration.	

(Lohmann et al., 1991)	Marine mollusc (*Tritonia diomedea*)	Action potentials	Alterations in geomagnetic field orientation, 1min on, 1 min off, for 26 min	Increased action potential firing in response to changes in ambient earth-strength SMF.	
(Stojan et al., 1990)	Electric fish Aptero-notus	Natural electrical activity	0.5, 1, 1.5 2, 4 and 10 T 20 h	Prompt increase in amplitude of electric signals when field was turned on; threshold was 1 T. Amplitude decreased, but only marginally, after 2 - 5 h in a 10 T field.	
Studies considered to be uninformative					
(Tkach et al., 1987) (Kloiber et al., 1990)					

7.2.2.1.2 Sensory receptors: the eye and the ear

The eye and the ear are both very closely associated with the central nervous system. In fact the retina comprises, in addition to the photoreceptors, complex neural circuitry that is derived embryologically as an outgrowth of the forebrain. The hair cell receptors of the inner ear project via sensory nerve fibres to parts of the brain, and receive neural input projected from these brain nuclei.

Specialized nerve cells in the retina relay diurnal day/night information to the pineal, thereby affecting the release and production of melatonin and so affecting diurnal behaviour (see section 7.2.2.4.1). The retina is also thought to play a key role in orientation and migratory behaviour through detection of changes in the natural geomagnetic field. Although the mechanism for this is unknown, the participation of radical pairs from light sensitive molecules, e.g. cryptochromes, in magnetic field perception has been recently suggested (Mouritsen et al., 2004). Olcese et al. published two studies of the effect of artificial changes in the geomagnetic field on catecholamines in the neuroretina (Olcese et al., 1988; Olcese & Hurlbut, 1989). They observed a reduction in retinal nocturnal dopamine and norepinephrine levels in rats with no effect on melatonin synthesis in the retina itself. Further study with both nocturnal and diurnal animals revealed different reactions for cone-dominant and rod-dominant retina. An intact retina was essential for any effect to be detected. The mechanism and implications are unknown, although the authors speculated that the effect might influence diurnal rhythms.

Only one study has investigated the effects of exposure to static magnetic fields on hearing. Tausch-Treml et al. (1989) studied the acoustic action potentials of the cochlea in guinea pigs after exposure for up to 3 h to 8.5 T SMF. No effects were observed. Possible effects on the vestibular system of the inner ear are described in section 7.2.2.1.4 on animal behaviour.

Table 15. Sensory receptors: the eye and the ear

Authors	Animal	Endpoint	Exposure	Results	Comments
Static magnetic field effects					
(Olcese et al., 1988)	Rat	Retinal melatonin synthesis and catecholamine contents	Artificial geomagnetic field strength Duration?	Alteration of ambient SMF reduced retinal nocturnal dopamine and norepinephrine levels; no effect on melatonin synthesis.	Exact mechanism and implications not known.
(Olcese & Hurlbut, 1989)	Rat, hamster, ground squirrel	Retinal catecholamine contents	Artificial geomagnetic field strength SMF < 60 mT Duration?	Retinal dopaminergic system differentially responsive to SMF. Dopamine levels can be reduced by SMF. Different reaction for cone-dominant retina as compared to rod-dominant retina.	Exact mechanism and implications not known.
(Tausch-Treml et al., 1989)	Guinea pig	Acoustic action potential	8.5 T 3 h	No effect.	Non-quantitative analysis of ECGs.
Studies considered to be uninformative					
(Sacks et al., 1986)					

111

The effect of a hypogeomagnetic field on stress-induced analgesia in mice was investigated in two studies. The experimental procedure in the first study (Del Seppia et al., 2000) consisted of firstly maintaining the mice under various magnetic exposure conditions for 90 minutes, secondly immobilising the animals in a tube for 30 minutes and thirdly recording the nociceptive responses of the restraint-stressed mice as the latency of front paw lifting to an aversive thermal stimulus. Two experiments were conducted with 3 and 5 groups of mice. One group was exposed to a hypogeomagnetic field with a flux density of 4 µT and another group was exposed to an ambient geomagnetic field of 46 µT. The latency of foot-lifting responses in both experiments was significantly reduced in the animal group exposed to a hypogeomagnetic field compared to the group exposed to a normal geomagnetic field. The observed effect strength was comparable with the effect of an injection of 1.0 mg kg^{-1} of the specific opiate antagonist naloxone hydrochloride. Those effects were more systematically investigated in the second study (Choleris et al., 2002). A pre-stress exposure was necessary for the anti-analgesic effects to occur. An anti-analgesic effect was observed if the ambient field was strongly reduced by shielding during 2 h, but no effect was observed in two near-zero magnetic conditions. The authors suggested that the elimination of the extremely weak time-varying component of the magnetic environment, which was only achieved by shielding, may have been responsible for the observed effects.

Exposure to MRI fields where the static field component was 0.15 T was reported to alter morphine-induced analgesia to a heat stimulus in mice (Ossenkopp et al., 1985). The authors suggested that exposure resulted in alterations in neuronal calcium binding and/or alterations in nocturnal pineal gland activity. It is not possible, however, to determine whether exposure to the static magnetic field affected this response.

Table 16. Analgesia

Authors	Animal	Endpoint	Exposure	Results	Comments
Static magnetic field effects					
(Del Seppia et al., 2000)	Male C57 mice	Analgesia	Hypogeo-magnetic field using magnetic shield; SMF = 4 µT. Oscillating field: f < 0.1 Hz: 20-70 µT; 40 Hz: 80 µT 2 h	Reduction of the response latency, if Earths' natural field was shielded. This effect was similar with oscillating magnetic field (f < 0.1 Hz).	Effects are comparable with the effect of an injection of 1.0 mg kg^{-1} of the specific opiate antagonist naloxone hydrochloride.
(Choleris et al., 2002)	Female CD1 mice	Analgesia	< 0.1 µT 2 h	Reduction of analgesia by strong reduction of ambient magnetic field. However, no effect with zeroed field.	Zeroed field contained time-varying components (f < 0.1 Hz). Shielded field did not contain time varying components
MRI or combined exposure studies					
(Ossenkopp et al., 1985)	Mice	Analgesia	0.15 T 2x22.5 min	Alterations in day- and night-time responses to morphine.	Well-designed experiment. Exposure to SMF and RF fields (simulation of diagnostic procedure).

7.2.2.1.4 Behaviour

Behaviour is chiefly controlled by the central nervous system acting on the body's musculature via the peripheral nervous system and may be either spontaneous or a response to an environmental stimulus. Behaviour may be either innate or learned.

A number of studies have investigated the effects of static magnetic fields on the behaviour of animals. A majority of the papers have involved rodents (mice, rats, and mole rats), but studies of paramecium, turtles and mosquitoes have also been reported.

Davis et al. (1984) studied the behaviour of adult mice continuously exposed for up to 72 hours to 1.5 T. Three types of behavioural tests were employed, namely memory of electroshock, general locomotor activity and sensitivity to a seizure-inducing neuropharmacological agent (pentylenetetrazole or PTZ). No behavioural alterations were found in the exposed mice when compared to the controls in any of the experiments. Hong et al. (1988) exposed infant rats to 0.5 T for 14 postnatal days. Following a one-month rest period, there was no significant difference in learning ability (escape avoidance of a mild foot shock) between the control and exposed groups.

Nakagawa and Matsuda (1988) also exposed rats, but for a longer period. Rats were trained and observed for Sidman avoidance (SA) and for discriminative avoidance (DA) for 7 and 14 weeks, respectively. Prior to the completion of avoidance conditioning, rats in the SA group were exposed for 0.6 T for 16 hours/day for 4 days and rats in the DA group were exposed for 0.6 T for 6 hours/day for 4 days. Both exposed groups showed a diminished performance of avoidance responses. Trzeciak et al. (1993) exposed male, as well as pregnant and non-pregnant female, rats to 0.49 T for 2 hours per day for 20 consecutive days. Exposure had no effect on open-field behaviour and locomotor activity for either the male or female rats. However, a decrease in the 'irritability' of the rats, i.e. their responsiveness to being touched, was noted.

Weiss et al. (1992) investigated the aversive response of rats at static magnetic field levels of 0, 1.5 and 4 T using a simple T-maze with one arm extended into the bore of the magnet. No behavioural differences were found for 0 and 1.5 T. However, at 4 T it was found that the rats would not enter the exposed arm of the maze in 97% of the trials, and that this effect persisted for a short while when the exposed and sham exposed arms were reversed. The authors proposed that the aversive response was due to magnetic induction effects caused by motion in the strong magnetic field gradient. A similar experiment by Nolte et al. (1998), in which rats were given a conditioned stimulus (a taste solution) followed by exposure for 30 min to a 9.4 T magnetic field, showed a conditioned taste aversion that lasted for up to 8 days after the cessation of field exposure.

These behavioural effects of exposure to intense static fields were further explored in a series of recent studies by Houpt and co-workers (Lockwood et al., 2003; Houpt et al., 2003), who exposed restrained rats, and unrestrained and restrained mice, to static magnetic fields of up to 14 T. Exposure to a 9.4 T magnetic field for the same duration used by Nolte et al. (1998) resulted in increased c-Fos expression, taken as an index of neural activity, in the vestibular and visceral nuclei of the brain, suggesting activation of the vestibular and visceral neural pathways

(Snyder et al., 2000). These authors noted that such effects were consistent with the suggestion by Schenck (2000; 2005) that small head movements in a strong static field could induce vestibular stimulation through the action of magnetohydrodynamic forces on the fluid within the semicircular canals. Further study by these authors (Lockwood et al., 2003; Houpt et al., 2003) found that exposure of rats to either 7 or 14 T suppressed rearing as well as inducing tight circling, the direction of which was related to orientation within the field. Conditioned taste aversion was induced after exposure to either field strengths. Very similar results were obtained with mice following exposure to a 14.1 T static field. All mice developed a conditioned taste aversion and a significant number displayed tight circling and a suppression of rearing. Unrestrained mice exhibited larger effects than those that were restrained, supporting the view that these responses are consistent with vestibular stimulation as well as the reports of vertigo and nausea in people during movement in very strong static magnetic fields.

Tsuji et al. (1996) reported decreased food and water intake in mice exposed in a 5 T magnetic field for 24 or 48 h. The authors raise a number of possible explanations, including the suggestion that this was caused by discomfort experienced in the 5 T field.

A number of investigators have studied magnetic fields as navigational markers and their effects on spatial discrimination. Kimchi and Terkel (2001) used the blind mole rat in an eight-arm maze under natural and artificial magnetic fields to show that the rodent was able to perceive and use the Earth's magnetic field to orient in space. Lohmann et al. (2001) found that hatchling loggerhead sea turtles, when exposed to magnetic fields found in widely separated oceanic regions, swam in the direction that would keep them within the currents that facilitate their migratory pathway.

Strickman et al. (2000) found that mosquitoes placed in a 0.1 mT magnetic field moved until they were orientated parallel to the field. Mosquitoes were tested for the presence of a remnant ferromagnetic material indicative of a biological compass, but it was found that the external surface appeared to have an affinity for ferromagnetic particles.

Rosen and Rosen (1990) studied the motility of Paramecium following exposure to a 126 mT magnetic field. They observed a reduction in swimming velocity and a disorganization of movement pattern. The authors speculated that a realignment of anisotropic molecules within the membrane could have been responsible for the observation. This work was supported by a more recent study by Nakaoka et al. (2002), in which they found that the Paramecium swam perpendicular to 0.78 T.

Levine and Bluni (1994) and Levine et al. (1995) investigated whether a decrement in spatial discrimination learning in mice following exposure to a static magnetic field was due to an interaction between the field and physiological ferromagnetic material (magnetite) or instead to an effect on circulating melatonin levels. These authors exposed mice to static magnetic fields of up to 2 T for up to 100 min. The data partially supported learning interference following magnetic field exposure, but no consistent effect on levels of circulating melatonin was found. However, the exposure was reported as having duplicated a 'spin-echo' MRI sequence, and so the possibility that pulsed gradient fields were also present cannot be ruled out.

Two studies by Ossenkop and colleagues (Innis et al., 1986; Ossenkopp et al., 1986) examined the effects of exposure of rats to MRI fields for about 23 min upon the performance of several behavioural tests (namely spatial memory, open field behaviour and passive avoidance learning). The MRI exposure had no effect on task performance by exposed animals compared to those that were sham exposed. Similarly, Messmer et al. (1987) found that the exposure of rats for 30 min to MRI fields where the static field component was 1.9 T did not induce taste aversion. In this test, taste aversion to e.g. saccharin is induced by an associated exposure to a stimulus that was perceived as unpleasant.

Table 17. Behaviour					
Authors	**Animal**	**Endpoint**	**Exposure**	**Results**	**Comments**
Static magnetic field effects					
(Davis et al., 1984)	Mouse	Behaviour: passive avoidance trials, locomotor activity, PTZ seizure threshold	1.5 T 72 h	No effect on behaviour.	
(Hong et al., 1988)	Rat	Learning ability (escape-avoidance of mild foot shock)	0.5 T 14 d, 3x5 min d^{-1} (postnatal)	No effect of SMF on learning.	

(Nakagawa & Matsuda, 1988)	Rat	Behaviour	0.6 T 6 or 16 h d^{-1}, 4 d	Performance of avoidance responses inhibited, staying low for 2 - 3 wk after exposure.	
(Trzeciak et al., 1993)	Rat	Behaviour	0.49 T 2 h d^{-1}, 20 d	Decrease in irritability; no effect on open-field behaviour, locomotor activity.	
(Weiss et al., 1992)	Rat	Behaviour: walking into or avoiding magnetic field	0, 1.5, 4 T 4 min	Behaviour disruption at 4 T: initially 4 T is avoided; trained animals abruptly stop upon encountering a 4 T field.	Consistency with other high field experiments affecting vestibular region. Not clear if it is induced field or a direct effect of SMF exposure.
(Nolte et al., 1998)	Rat	Aversion to a conditioned taste stimulus	9.4 T 30 min	With one SMF conditioning day, approximately half of the rats showed conditioned taste aversion; with three conditioning days, 7/8 rats showed taste aversion lasting up to 8 days.	Consistent with other high field experiments affecting vestibular region. Not clear if it is induced fields or a direct effect of SMF exposure.

(Snyder et al., 2000)	Rat	c-Fos induction in visceral and vestibular nuclei of the rat brain stem	9.4 T 30 min	More c-Fos-positive cells in brainstem: neural activation in visceral and vestibular nuclei. Counterclockwise turning behaviour after exposure in 4/6 rats.	Consistency with other high field experiments affecting vestibular region. Not clear if it is induced fields or a direct effect of SMF exposure.
(Lockwood et al., 2003)	Mice	Behaviour: locomotor activity, conditioned taste aversion (CTA)	14 T 30 min	All restrained and unrestrained mice developed CTA; a significant number displayed tight circling and suppression of rearing. Effects larger in unrestrained mice.	Restraint stress might suppress effect somewhat, or effect might be enlarged due to movement of unrestrained animals
(Houpt et al., 2003)	Rat	Behaviour: locomotor activity, conditioned taste aversion (CTA)	7 or 14 T > 30 min	Exposure suppressed rearing and induced tight circling and CTA acquisition; strongest effect with 14 T.	Follow up of experiments of Nolte et al. 1998. Influence of restraint stress unknown.
(Tsuji et al., 1996)	Mouse	Food and water intake	5 T 24, 48 h	Exposure-dependent decreased food, water intake, body weight; no effect on organ weight.	

(Kimchi & Terkel, 2001)	Mole rat	Eight-armed maze test	Artificial geomagnetic field strength 2 d	Significant directional preference shown independent of light stimulation; decrease in performance under shifted SMF.	Relevance to human health unclear.
(Lohmann et al., 2001)	Sea turtles (hatchling)	Appropriate migratory direction	Artificial geomagnetic field strength Duration not reported	Significant directional preference shown.	Relevance to human health unclear.
(Strickman et al., 2000)	Mosquito	Blood-sucking	0.1 mT 5 min	Oriented parallel to SF; two of 3 species took fewer blood meals in a rotating MF (90° each 15 sec) than in the Earth's normal MF.	Advantage of orientation not clear; disrupted feeding possibly because of unnatural field conditions.
(Rosen & Rosen, 1990)	Paramecium	Motility	126 mT 48 h	Reduction in velocity, disorganization of movement.	Low numbers of organisms.
(Nakaoka et al., 2002)	Paramecium	Swimming orientation	0.68 T 0.5 - 1 sec	*Paramecium* swam perpendicular to SMF; no effect in AC MF (60 Hz, 0.65 T).	Lack of statistics, but effect clear. A result of diamagnetic anisotropy of cilia and trichocysts?

MRI or combined exposure studies

(Levine & Bluni, 1994)	Mouse	Left-right discrimination learning ability and serum melatonin levels	0.3 T 30 min	Significant interference with spatial discrimination learning; variable melatonin levels.	MRI fields present. Animals transported 12 miles between MRI unit and laboratory.
(Levine et al., 1995)	Mouse	Left-right discrimination learning ability and serum melatonin levels	2.0 T 100 min	Significant interference with spatial discrimination learning; no changes in serum melatonin levels.	Possible confounding with other MRI magnetic fields.
(Innis et al., 1986)	Rat	Spatial memory test	0.15 T 23 min	No effect on spatial memory.	
(Ossenkopp et al., 1986)	Rat	Open field behaviour and passive avoidance test	0.15 T 22.5, 23.3 min, 5 d	No effect.	
(Messmer et al., 1987)	Rat	Taste aversion paradigm	1.89 T 30 min	No effect.	Positive control group (injected with 0.15 M lithium chloride) developed taste aversion.

Studies considered to be uninformative

(Grzesik et al., 1988)
(Nikolskaia et al., 1999)
(Nikol'skaia et al., 2000)
(Phillips et al., 2001)
(Nikolskaia & Echenko, 2002)
(Wiltschko et al., 2002)

7.2.2.2 Musculoskeletal system

The body musculature is, by and large, an effector organ of the nervous system. The skeletal system of animals provides an articulated frame against which the muscles of the body act to produce movement. In most animals, muscle contraction can be rapid, and results from the inherent excitability of muscle fibres. Muscles of the gastrointestinal tract and cardiovascular system are also under nervous system control, but have more of a 'housekeeping' regulatory role.

The bones of the skeletal system are relatively stable, but undergo constant remodelling in response to mechanical stresses. Piezoelectric effects within the bone are thought to have a role in this remodelling process, through the generation of electric fields.

7.2.2.2.1 Muscles

The biomechanical activity of muscle results from its chemical, electrical and mechanical excitability. The release of neurotransmitter from a motor nerve terminal results in an action potential in the muscle fibre that is transmitted along the cell membrane, activating a contractile mechanism. *In vivo* regulation of the biomechanical activity of the muscles is a complicated and integrated process. Animal models are very useful for investigation of the processes of *in vivo* effects of static magnetic field action on the processes of regulation of muscle activity.

The effects of chronic application of 0.02 T on specific ATPase activities, and bioelectrical and biomechanical responses, in isolated rat diaphragm muscle have been reported by Itegin et al. (1995). The mean activities of Na^+-K^+ ATPase and Ca^{2+} ATPase determined from diaphragm homogenates were significantly higher in the magnetic field exposed group, but that of Mg^{2+} ATPase was not significantly lower compared to the control group.

Static magnetic field effects on motor nerve conduction and resting membrane potential on muscle have been reported by Hong et al. (1986) and Itegin et al. (1995). The resting membrane potential, amplitude of muscle action potential, and overshoot values have been investigated. The latency was found to increase in the experimental group, and all the above-mentioned bioelectrical differences between the groups were statistically significant. Force of muscle twitch was found to decrease significantly in the magnetic field-exposed group. This finding was attributed to the augmenting effect of magnetic field on Ca^{2+} ATPase activity. According to Itegin et al. (1995), these results suggest that static magnetic field exposure changes specific ATPase activities and, hence, bioelectrical and biomechanical properties in the rat diaphragm muscle. Hong et al. (1986) described measurements of motor nerve conduction and excitability on the tail nerve of anaesthetized rats before and after nerve exposure to a static magnetic field of various intensities and durations. No significant change was found in either the distal latencies or the amplitudes of the compound muscle action potential (CMAP) measured from stimulating the tail nerve after it was exposed to 1.2 T for 60 seconds. However, the nerve excitability expressed as changes of the amplitudes of the submaximally evoked CMAP increased significantly when the tail nerve was exposed to a static magnetic field with a magnetic flux density higher than 0.5 T for more than 30 seconds.

Table 18. Muscles

Authors	Animal	Endpoint	Exposure	Results	Comments
Static magnetic field effects					
(Itegin et al., 1995)	Rat diaphragm muscle	ATPase activities and bioelectrical and biomechanical responses.	0.2 mT 4 h d^{-1}, 19 wk	Na$^+$-K$^+$ ATPase and Ca^{2+} ATPase activity increased; Mg^{2+} ATPase not increased; resting membrane potential, amplitude of muscle action potential, and overshoot values lowered.	
(Hong et al., 1986)	Adult Sprague-Dawley albino rat	Motor nerve conduction and excitability	0.3 - 1.2 T 15, 30 or 60 sec	No effect on nerve conduction. Increased motor nerve excitability at > 0.5 T and t > 30 sec. Effect disappeared 1 min after termination of exposure. Effects dose related.	Anaesthetized with intraperitoneal chloral hydrate.
Studies considered to be uninformative					
(Gorczynska & Wegrzynowicz, 1986b)					
(Tamaki et al., 1987)					
(Takeshige & Sato, 1996)					
(Satow et al., 2001)					

7.2.2.2.2 Bone growth

Osteoblasts and osteoclasts cells are dynamic components in this stable and slow-changing system. Environmental factors that have direct or indirect action on these two types of cells in bone tissue can play a very important role in processes of remodelling and re-shaping of the bones, as well as bone healing processes. The long bones are first modelled in cartilage and transformed into bone by ossification that begins in the shaft of the bone (enchondral bone formation). Osteoblast precursors secrete factors that affect osteoclast development, an observation that is not surprising given the necessity of maintaining a balance between resorption and formation. The influence of static magnetic fields on the growth of rodent bones has been studied using various methods. In general, low field strengths and long exposure times were employed.

Yan et al. (1998) implanted magnetic rods in rat femurs. The flux density close to the magnet was approximately 180 mT at most, while at 5 mm from the rod it was practically zero. The authors claimed to have observed a decrease in bone mineral density and calcium content in femurs implanted with non-magnetized rods at 12 weeks after the procedure. The authors concluded that normal bone mineral density and calcium levels were observed when the rods were magnetized. However, no significant differences seemed to be present in the data. It is likely that the statistical analysis of the data was incorrect. A further indication for this might be that the authors also claimed to observe changes in bone mineral density and calcium in the areas of the femur where the flux density was zero.

The same group also studied the effect of the same procedure in rat femurs that were made ischaemic (Xu et al. (2001). In this case, exposure lasted for 3 weeks. The authors observed significant differences between magnetized and unmagnetized rods only in the parts of the bone where the flux density was zero. Again, the statistical analysis of the data seems problematic. The authors speculated that exposure to the static magnetic field from magnetized rods resulted in an improvement in the blood circulation, leading to an improvement of bone growth. It is difficult to envisage that this would have an effect only in the unexposed areas. These experiments seem well-performed, but the analysis of the data is flawed. There is no effect of the implanted magnetic rods on bone growth.

Camilleri and McDonald (1993) used permanent magnets to apply 100 mT for 1 to 10 days to the sagittal sutures of rats. They observed a transient reduction in thymidine uptake at 3 days after the start of exposure, but no difference in tetracycline-incorporation. No effect on bone growth and inhibition of cell division could be demonstrated.

Fracture healing in a rabbit radius was studied by Bruce et al. (1987). They applied 22 - 26 mT for 4 weeks, using permanent magnets, and determined the force needed to break bone units consisting of ulna and radius, which could not be separated without damaging the healing callus. Greater forces were needed to break the static magnetic field-exposed units. The authors suggested that static magnetic fields might accelerate the maturation of tissues, leading to thicker trabecular bone and thereby increasing the strength of a callus. However, no histological differences were detected.

The presumed effect of static magnetic field exposure on bone remodelling has led to the exploration of the use of permanent magnets in orthodontics to accelerate the repositioning of teeth. Tengku et al. (2000) studied the effect of such orthodontic magnets on the movement of the rat tooth. The magnets resulted in maximum flux densities of 10 - 17 mT and remained in position for 1 - 14 days. Tooth movement was identical in the animals treated with magnets and those treated with equal seized unmagnetized weights. However, a transient greater root resorption, an increased width of the periodontal ligament space and greater activity of clastic cells that are needed for bone remodelling were observed at 7 days in the animals with magnets. The force exerted by the device was reduced to zero by day 7 and remained so until day 14. It is possible that only force-induced alterations are influenced by the static magnetic field, but the overall effect on tooth movement is nil.

The influence of much higher fields on bone formation has also been studied. Kotani et al. (2002) implanted mice with pellets containing bone morphogenetic protein (BMP) 2 and exposed them for 60 hours to an 8-T field. Bone growth in and around the pellets was significantly higher in the exposed animals compared to the unexposed controls. The orientation of bone formation was parallel to the static magnetic field. The authors speculated upon several mechanisms, varying from alterations in membrane phospholipids to static magnetic field-induced mechanical stress, both leading to osteoblast differentiation. Exposure to a strong static magnetic field in combination with bone morphogenetic protein might be a clinically viable option for improving bone healing.

Kwong-Hing et al. (1989) used autoradiography and liquid scintillation to examine acute exposure effects of MRI on dentin and bone formation in mice. They found that exposure to a standard 23.2 min clinical multislice MRI (0.05 T) procedure caused a significant increase in the synthesis of the collageneous matrix of dentin in the incisors. The results suggest that the magnetic fields associated with MRI can affect cell activity. The mechanisms that may alter the incorporation of ^{3}H-proline into the predentin layer remain largely speculative. The relative role of the three magnetic fields (static, radiofrequency, and time-varying) associated with MRI on the increase in the incorporation of ^{3}H-proline still need to be examined.

Table 19. Bone growth

Authors	Animal	Endpoint	Exposure	Results	Comments
Static magnetic field effects					
(Yan et al., 1998)	Rat	Bone formation	Implanted magnetic rods ~ 180 mT 12 wk	Authors reported a decrease in bone mineral density (BMD) and Ca content in femurs implanted with non-magnetized rods and normal levels in femurs implanted with magnetized ones.	No effect was observed.
(Xu et al., 2001)	Rat with ischaemic bone model	Bone formation	Implanted magnetic rods ~ 50 mT 3 wk	Bone mineral density lower in ligated + unmagnetized rods at 3 wk ; strongest in proximal and distal parts. Enhancement of femoral bone formation.	Stated flux density of 180 mT not in bone; 50 mT max, but at 5 mm from rod practically zero (i.e. in proximal and distal parts).
(Camilleri & McDonald, 1993)	Rat	Bone growth	100 mT 1 - 10 d	Transient reduction in thymidine uptake at 3 d. No difference in tetracycline-incorporation. No effect on bone growth.	
(Bruce et al., 1987)	Rabbit	Fracture healing	22 - 26 mT 4 wk	Greater forces needed for breaking bone units exposed to SMF; no difference in histopathologic comparison.	Change in breaking force not supported by histology.

126

(Tengku et al., 2000)	Rat	Orthodontic tooth movement	10 - 17 mT 1 - 14 d	Greater root resorption, increased width of periodontal ligament space and greater tartrate-resistant acid phosphatase activity at 7 d. SMF did not enhance tooth movement.	No description of magnetic material.
(Kotani et al., 2002)	Mouse	Bone formation (induced by implanted bone morpho-genetic protein [BMP-2] – containing pellets).	8 T 60 h	Increase of ectopic bone formation in and around BMP-2-containing pellets, with orientation of bone formation parallel to SMF.	Orientation of bone formation parallel to SMF possibly due to diamagnetic anisotropy of membrane phospholipid in osteoblastic cells.
MRI or combined exposure studies					
(Kwong-Hing et al., 1989)	Mouse	Formation of dentin and bone	0.15 T 23.2 min	Increase in the synthesis of the collagenous matrix of dentin in the incisors.	
Studies considered to be uninformative					
(Linder-Aronson & Lindskog, 1991)					
(Linder-Aronson et al., 1992)					
(Darendeliler et al., 1995)					
(Linder-Aronson et al., 1995)					
(Linder-Aronson et al., 1996)					
(Darendeliler et al., 1997)					

7.2.2.3 Circulatory system

The circulatory system is the transport system of the organism that supplies O_2 and substances absorbed from the gastrointestinal tract to the tissues, and returns CO_2 to the lungs and other products of metabolism to the liver and kidneys. It also has a central role in the regulation of body temperature, and the distribution of the hormones and other agents that regulate tissue and cell function.

Blood, the carrier of these substances, is pumped through a closed system of blood vessels. The circulation is controlled by multiple regulatory systems, from blood pressure and heart rate controlling systems to those maintaining adequate capillary blood flow in all organs (but particularly in the heart and brain). The main components of the circulatory system are blood cells (erythrocytes, leucocytes and platelets), blood plasma (protein and non-protein component) and lymph. This section is concerned with static magnetic field effects on the circulatory system and on pharmacologically-induced changes to this system.

7.2.2.3.1 Cardiac function

The rhythmic beating of the heart, which maintains blood circulation, is driven by periodic waves of electrical excitation These begin in the pacemaking region of the right atrium, spread through the right and left atria, triggering atrial contraction, then move through the atrio-ventricular node and conducting system of the bundle of His to the ventricular septum and walls, triggering ventricular contraction. This electro-mechanical process of wave propagation through the heart causes the pumping action of the heart and the circulation of blood.

Electrical potentials (flow potentials), generated across a blood vessel by the flow of blood in static magnetic field, have been recorded in a number of animal species exposed to magnetic fields greater than about 100 mT. While the physiological significance of these flow potentials remains unclear, they are of great importance in the light of the strong static fields used by MRI systems for clinical diagnostic analysis. They result from Lorenz forces acting on moving charges (see chapter 5) which are generally associated with ventricular contraction and the ejection of blood into the aorta. They appear superimposed on the T-wave of the ECG, which indicates the repolarisation of the ventricular heart muscle as electrical excitability gradually recovers following contraction.

Studies have been performed on a number of animal species. Briefly, flow potentials have been recorded in rats (Gaffey & Tenforde, 1981), rabbits (Togawa et al., 1967), dogs (Gaffey & Tenforde, 1979), monkeys (Beischer & Knepton, Jr., 1964; Beischer, 1969; Tenforde et al., 1983; Gorczynska & Wegrzynowicz, 1989) and baboons (Gaffey et al., 1980). These and other studies are reviewed by Tenforde (2005). In large animal species, the flow potential can be detected in the ECG at magnetic field levels above approximately 0.1 T. The flow potential is a linear function of field strength up to 1.0 T. At higher field levels, the total electrical potential at the T-wave locus in the ECG increases more rapidly as a function of magnetic field strength, possibly as a result of the superposition of additional, weaker flow potentials. Total electrical potential also increases with body size; for example, the average increase in the T-wave signal amplitude in a 1.0 T field in rats is ~ 75 µV, whereas it is ~ 175 µV in juvenile baboons. Similar alterations in the ECG have been observed in humans exposed to strong magnetic fields (see section 8.1.2.2.1).

Three studies have been performed on large mammals. Tenforde et al. (1983) exposed Macaca monkeys to 0.5 - 1.5 T fields. The authors observed an increase in the ECG signal amplitude with fields > 0.1 T but no magnetohydrodynamic effect on blood flow and no effect on blood pressure. They concluded that there was little or no cardiovascular stress. Kangarlu et al. (1999) performed cardiac and physiological safety studies in relation to magnetic resonance imaging in pigs. The animals were exposed in an MRI machine for 3 h to a field that had a flux density of 8 T at the location of the heart. This did not result in effects on heart rate, blood pressure, cardiac output or several other vital parameters. Finally, Bourland et al. (1999) reported that exposure to a static magnetic field of 1.5 T had no effect on the cardiac ectopic beat threshold of anaesthetized dogs in which a temporary and reversible cardiac arrest had been induced by vagus nerve stimulation. The ectopic beat was induced by eddy currents resulting from rapidly switched gradient magnetic fields. A lack of effect on ectopic beat threshold was also seen in two dogs in which the heart was beating normally during stimulation.

As part of a study on potentially hazardous effects of magnetic field produced by MRI on cardiac function in the rat and guinea pig, Willis and Brooks (1984) exposed the animals to 0.16 T static magnetic fields only (5 min on, 5 min off, repeated four times). No changes were observed in blood pressure, heart rate, or ECG. No sham exposures were performed, but a comparison was instead made between the field on and field off periods.

Other studies have been more equivocal. Nakagawa (1984) reported that 600 mT fields for 33 min had no effects of various rabbit heart rate parameters, but that a transient effect was seen immediately after exposure to the field. A previous study by Nakagawa (1978) revealed that reserpine-treated rabbits exposed to 60 mT for 5 weeks had an increased in heart rate and blood flow when compared with the sham exposed animals.

Klimovskaia and Smirnova (1975) exposed rabbits to 0.45 T for 30 min or 3 h. They observed a transient hypotension, a decrease in respiratory rate and a trend towards brachycardia. They also subjected the animals to accelerations of 6 and 10 G. The compensatory reactions of the cardiovascular and respiratory system induced by such treatments were not influenced by SMF exposure.

In two papers, Gmitrov and Ohkubo (2002a; 2002b) reported the effects on cardiovascular regulation of exposure to an artificial SMF in relation to geomagnetic field disturbances. The baroreflex sensitivity (BRS), arterial pressure and heart rate were determined in rabbits before and after 40 min of local 0.35 T SMF exposure applied at the position of the sinocarotid baroreceptor. Increased geomagnetic field disturbances decreased baroreflex sensitivity, which lead to deregulated blood pressure. Administration of nitroprusside interrupted the baroreceptor reflex, and the static magnetic field antagonized this effect. Verapamil, a Ca^{2+} channel-blocking agent, antagonized the effects of applied static magnetic field and geomagnetic field disturbances. The authors speculated that exposure of the sinocarotid baroreceptor to static magnetic field, along with modification of the pharmacotherapy for hypertension, should be effective on days with intense geomagnetic disturbance, perhaps through modulation of Ca^{2+} channel permeability.

Table 20. Cardiac function

Authors	Animal	Endpoint	Exposure	Results	Comments
Static magnetic field effects					
(Gaffey & Tenforde, 1981)	Rat	ECG, heart rate, breathing rate	up to 2.1 T 2 - 3 min (ECG, heart rate, breathing rate); 1.5 T 5 h (post-exposure ECG)	If SMF > 0.3 T, T-wave amplitude increased in a field strength-dependent manner; no changes in heart rate or breathing rate. No short-term or long-term effects of 5-h exposure.	Effect might be caused by field gradient.
(Tenforde et al., 1983)	Monkey	ECG, blood pressure	0.5 - 1.5 T	Increase in ECG signal amplitude in fields > 0.1 T; no effect on blood pressure; magnetohydro-dynamic effect on blood flow. Little or no cardiovascular stress.	

(Kangarlu et al., 1999)	Swine	Cardiac function	8 T 3 h	No effect on body temperature, heart rate, ventricular pressure, and cardiac output	
(Bourland et al., 1999)	Dogs	Ectopic beat threshold in temporarily arrested and beating hearts	1.5 T Ectopic beats stimulated by rapidly changing gradient magnetic field	No difference in ectopic beat threshold in exposed and unexposed animals.	Dogs anaesthe-tised with pentobarbital
(Willis & Brooks, 1984)	Rat, guinea pig	ECG, blood pressure	0.16 T 5 min on, 5 min off, x 4	No effect on ECG and blood pressure.	
(Nakagawa, 1984)	Rabbit	Electrophysio logical responses	600 mT 33 min	Transient decrease in heart rate after exposure.	No description of methods for statistical analysis.
(Nakagawa, 1978)	Rabbit	Cardiovascul ar system	60 mT 5 wk	Increase in heart rate (at 3 and 5 weeks) and blood volume of a central artery of an ear lobe (2 - 5 weeks) as compared with reserpine treated animals.	
(Klimovskaia & Smirnova, 1975)	Rabbit	EEG, arterial pressure, heart rate, respiratory rate, reactions to adrenalin, and electrical stimulation of brain	0.45 T 30 min and 3 h	Transient hypotension; decrease in respiratory rate; bradycardia. No decrease of compensatory reactions in response to accelerations of 6 and 10 G.	

(Gmitrov & Ohkubo, 2002a)	Rabbit	Baroreflex sensitivity (BRS), arterial pressure, heart rate	0.35 T 40 min	Increase in BRS by SMF for nitroprusside depressor test; SMF antagonized decrease in BRS by geomagnetic disturbance.	
(Gmitrov & Ohkubo, 2002b)	Rabbit	Baroreflex sensitivity (BRS), arterial pressure and heart rate	0.35 T 40 min	SMF and geomagnetic effect on BRS antagonized by Ca^{2+} channel blocker.	
Studies considered to be uninformative					
(Reno & Beischer, 1966)					
(Behari & Mathur, 1997)					

7.2.2.3.2 Blood pressure

The regulation of blood pressure by the cardiovascular system during circulatory changes faced normally in everyday life and abnormally in disease illustrates the integrated operation of the cardiovascular regulatory mechanisms.

Hypertension is sustained elevation of the systemic arterial pressure. The arterial pressure is determined by the cardiac output and the peripheral resistance (pressure = flow × resistance). The peripheral resistance is determined by the viscosity of the blood and, more importantly, by the calibre of the resistance vessels. Hypertension can be produced by elevating the cardiac output, but sustained hypertension is usually due to increased peripheral resistance.

Meszaros (1991) investigated effects of 40 mT and platelet activating factor on blood pressure in rats. Transient hypotension (lasting 1 - 2 hours) was induced by injection of iron beads and 5-min exposure to the static magnetic field, but this was only seen when the middle part of the body was exposed and when there were short intervals between bead injections and static magnetic field exposure. Hypotension was prevented or reverted by a platelet activating factor antagonist.

Okano and Ohkubo (2001) examined the effects of static magnetic fields on blood pressure in conscious rabbits. Blood pressure was pharmacologically altered and a flux density of 1 mT was applied locally to the ear for 30 min. Blood pressure was decreased by nicardipine, a Ca^{2+}

channel blocker, or increased by the nitric oxide synthase inhibitor N(omega)-nitro-L-arginine methyl ester (L-NAME). Static magnetic field exposure counteracted the effects of both drugs. However, the field was only locally applied to part of the ear. The exposed area is probably too small to alter blood pressure in the entire animal, especially in the presence of the pharmacological agents. The effect might possibly have been mediated by the autonomic nervous system.

The study by Okano and Ohkubo (2003a) is a continuation of the above-mentioned paper (Okano & Ohkubo, 2001). In this case, they investigate anti-pressor effects of whole-body exposure to a static magnetic field (5.5 mT for 30 min) on pharmacologically-induced hypertension in conscious rabbits. A suppression of both noradrenaline-induced and L-NAME-induced vasoconstriction and hypertension was observed, but there was no effect on microcirculation and blood pressure without pharmacological treatment. The mechanisms of the reduction of artificial hypertension are unknown.

Okano and Ohkubo (2003b) investigated the effects of static magnetic fields on the development of hypertension using young male, stroke resistant, spontaneously hypertensive rats (SHRs) beginning at 7 weeks of age. The animals were exposed to static magnetic fields of 3.0 - 10.0 mT or 8.0 - 25.0 mT for 12 weeks. Static magnetic fields suppressed and retarded the development of hypertension for several weeks in both exposed groups to a statistically significant extent when compared with an unexposed group. A recent paper by Okano et al. (2005a) indicated that a static magnetic field at 5 mT, but not at 1 mT, suppressed and retarded hypertension, and also reduced plasma concentrations of NO metabolites, angiotensin II and aldosterone, in rats. The antipressor effects are probably related to the extent of reduction in plasma levels of angiotensin II and aldosterone in the SHRs. Okano et al. (2005b) also reported that static magnetic fields in the range of 7.5 - 25.0 mT applied for 2 - 12 wks reversed reserpine-induced hypotension and bradykinesia in rats.

Table 21. Blood pressure

Authors	Animal	Endpoint	Exposure	Results	Comments
Static magnetic field effects					
(Meszaros, 1991)	Rat	Blood pressure	40 mT 5 min	No effect after saline+ SMF. Rapid decrease in arterial blood pressure, lasting 1 - 2 h after iron+SMF; only seen when middle part of body was exposed and with short interval between iron and SMF; hypotension prevented or reverted by PAF antagonist.	
(Okano & Ohkubo, 2001)	Rabbit	Blood pressure (BP) and cutaneous micro-circulation	1 mT 30 min	Reduced vasodilatation, enhanced vasomotion; antagonized reduction of BP; attenuation of vasoconstriction, suppression of elevation of BP.	
(Okano & Ohkubo, 2003a)	Rabbit	Pharma-cologically induced hypertension	5.5 mT 30 min	No effects in normal animals. Hypertension suppressed by SMF.	
(Okano & Ohkubo, 2003b)	Rat	Blood pressure	3 - 10 or 8 - 25 mT 12 wk	SMF suppressed and retarded hypertension. Also reduction in angiotensin II and aldosterone. No dose effect.	

(Okano et al., 2005b)	Rat	Reserpine-induced hypotension	3.0 - 10.0, 7.5 - 25.0 mT 12 wk	SMF in the range of 7.5 –2 5.0 mT for 2 - 12 wk reversed reserpine-induced hypotension and bradykinesia compared with sham-exposed reserpine-treated rats.	
(Okano et al., 2005a)	Rat	Blood pressure	0.3 - 1 or 1 - 5 mT 12 wk	SMF at 1 - 5 mT suppressed and retarded hypertension. Also reduction in NO, angiotensin II and aldosterone.	

7.2.2.3.3 Blood flow

One possible site of the action of static magnetic fields is on blood flow. As a dynamic system of movable charges, this system is one that is at a susceptible point for static magnetic field action on the level of organism. Ohkubo and co-workers in Japan have performed a series of experiments in rodents. Most studies concerned acute effects of short exposures to low flux densities.

Ohkubo and Xu (1997) studied cutaneous microcirculation in conscious rabbits using an ear chamber, a device that allows direct observation of cutaneous capillaries. A flux density of 1, 5 or 10 mT was applied for 10 min. Static magnetic field exposure induced non-dose-dependent changes in vasomotion in a biphasic manner. With high amplitude of vasomotion, static magnetic fields induced vasoconstriction; with low amplitude of vasomotion static magnetic fields induced vasodilation. The physiology of this effect is still unclear. It could be the result of autonomic nervous system regulation mechanisms, or stimulation and suppression of normal metabolism in tissues that is related to changes in oxygen consumption. Immobilization stress cannot, however, be excluded.

In another study from this group, Okano et al. (1999) performed a more extensive investigation of the biphasic effect. They exposed conscious rabbits to 1 mT for 10 min while either increasing the vascular tone by noradrenaline administration, or decreasing it using acetylcholine. Static magnetic fields resulted in vasodilatation and increased vasomotion under high vascular tone and in vasoconstriction and decreased vasomotion under low vascular tone. Thus, static magnetic fields counteract the effects of noradrenaline and acetylcholine.

Gmitrov et al. (2002) studies the effect of exposure to 0.2 and 0.35 T static magnetic fields on haemodynamics in anaesthetized rabbits. They found an increased blood flow during and after exposure, when compared with pre-exposure baseline and sham exposed controls. The authors postulated that long exposure to high level non-uniform static magnetic fields modifies microcirculatory homeostasis through modulation of the local release of endothelial neurohumoral and paracrine factors that act directly on the smooth muscle cells of the vascular wall, presumably by affecting ion channels or a second messenger system. However, data analysis in this paper is not completely clear. In the controls, anaesthesia resulted in a decrease in blood flow. A similar mechanism might be the cause of the observed trend for a decrease in blood flow after cessation of static magnetic field exposure.

In a study by Xu et al. (1998), subchronic effects of a locally applied static magnetic field on cutaneous microcirculation in rabbits were observed. The microcirculation was studied using ear chambers in conscious animals after exposure, by Sm-Co permanent magnets attached to the ear chamber, to 180 mT for 24 hours to 4 weeks. Exposures for 1 - 3 weeks significantly increased the amplitude of long-lasting vasodilatation and enhanced the vasomotion. The increased vasomotion in the exposed group decreased again to the initial values after exposure. It is peculiar that a short 1-mT exposure still has a measurable effect after prolonged 180 mT exposure. Xu et al. (2001) studied acute microhaemodynamic effects of whole-body exposure in anaesthetized mice to static magnetic fields. Exposure was to 0.3, 1 and 10 mT for 10 min. An increased peak blood velocity was observed for flux densities of 1 mT or higher. The effect remained for up to 35 hour after exposure.

The effects of short exposures to very high flux densities of 8 T on blood flow were investigated in three studies by Ichioka. Such a strong magnetic field could evoke induction of electrical potentials and magnetomechanical forces. Ichioka et al. (1998) exposed anaesthetized rats for 20 min and measured microcirculatory blood flow. Following exposure, blood flow initially increased for about 5 min, and gradually decreased and returned to control level thereafter. The effect is probably a rebound of the reactive hyperaemia and the action of magneto-hydrodynamic forces that induced a reduction of blood flow during exposure.

In a more elaborate study that followed this preliminary one, Ichioka et al. (2000) observed that a high-intensity static magnetic field (again 8 T applied for 20 min) can simultaneously modulate skin microcirculation and body temperature in anaesthetized rats. A decrease of the skin blood flow and temperature during exposure were observed, both of which tended to recover after cessation of exposure. It is possible, however, that the anaesthesia reduced the temperature-controlling mechanisms. In a subsequent study, Ichioka et al. (2003) demonstrated that an 8-T field induced water vapour movement over the body of the animals, thereby decreasing the humidity in the air around the animals. This may well explain the decrease in skin temperature observed in the earlier experiments. In a study with both mice and rats exposed to a uniform 1.5 T field and to a 60 T m^{-1} gradient field, Tenforde (1986b) found no effects on core body temperature of exposures up to 3 h in duration.

Table 22. Blood flow

Authors	Animal	Endpoint	Exposure	Results	Comments
Static magnetic field effects					
(Ohkubo & Xu, 1997)	Rabbit	Cutaneous micro-circulation in rabbit ear chamber	1, 5, 10 mT 10 min	Non-dose-dependent variation of vasomotion;10 sec. latency	
(Okano et al., 1999)	Rabbit	Cutaneous micro-circulation in rabbit ear chamber	1 mT 10 min	Vasodilatation, vasomotion under noradrenaline-induced high vascular tone; vasoconstriction, reduced vasomotion under acetylcholine-induced low vascular tone.	
(Gmitrov et al., 2002)	Rabbit	Micro-circulation	0.25 T 80 min	Increased blood flow during and after exposure when compared with pre-exposure baseline and control experiments.	Data analysis not fully clear.

(Xu et al., 1998)	Rabbit	Cutaneous micro-circulation in rabbit ear chamber	180 mT 24 h - 4 wk	Vasodilation, enhanced vasomotion at 1 - 3 wk, disappears thereafter.	
(Xu et al., 2001)	Mouse	Muscle capillary micro-circulation	0.3, 1, 10 mT 10 min	Peak blood velocity increased at 1 and 10 mT.	
(Ichioka et al., 1998)	Rat	Cutaneous micro-circulation in dorsal skinfold chamber	8 T 20 min	After exposure, 5 min increase in blood flow, then return to control values.	
(Ichioka et al., 2000)	Rat	Cutaneous micro-circulation in dorsal skin pocket	8 T 20 min	Decreased skin blood flow and temperature during exposure; rectal temperature tended to decrease.	
(Ichioka et al., 2003)	Rat	Skin temperature changes	8 T 5 min	Skin temperature decrease related to SMF-induced decrease in humidity around the body.	
MRI or combined exposure studies					
(Tenforde, 1986b)	Rat, mouse	Temperature changes	1.5 T + 60 T m^{-1} up to 3 h	No effects on core temperature.	
Studies considered to be uninformative					
(Lud & Demeckiy, 1990) (Steyn et al., 2000)					

7.2.2.3.4 Blood brain barrier

The tight junctions between capillary endothelium in the brain and between the epithelial cells in choroid plexus effectively prevent proteins from entering the adult brain and slow the penetration of smaller molecules. The rate of passage of molecules is inversely proportionate to their size and directly proportionate to their lipid solubility. This barrier to the exchange of substances between the brain and the blood and cerebrospinal fluid is referred to as the blood-brain barrier.

Shivers et al. (1987) reported that exposure to a short clinical MRI procedure (0.15 T) elicited a temporary dysfunction of the blood-brain barrier in rats. Recovery of normal blood-brain barrier function was completed 15 - 30 min following cessation of the MRI exposure.

Prato et al. (1990) exposed adult rats to a clinical MRI procedure at 0.15 T. They measured the concentration of a radioactive tracer, [153]Gd-DTPA, in whole-brain homogenates and in blood samples. A significant increase in the blood-brain barrier permeability was observed in the MRI exposed group compared to a sham exposed group. Prato et al. (1994) also exposed adult rats to various exposure scenarios. An MRI examination was simulated in two animal groups. A third group was exposed to a pure static field of 1.5 T and a fourth group to 1.89 T. A significant increase in the blood-brain barrier permeability was observed in one of the MRI exposed groups, whereas a decrease was found, compared to a sham exposed group, in the other MRI exposed group. Both groups exposed to static magnetic fields showed significant increased blood-brain barrier permeability only when compared to their respective sham controls. However, the extent of increase in permeability was small and within the range of diurnal variation. In addition and as the authors noted, interpretation is complicated by the fact that the increased tracer concentration in brain tissue could also have resulted from an increase in cerebral blood volume, without any change in the permeability of the blood-brain barrier.

Table 23. Blood Brain Barrier

Authors	Animal	Endpoint	Exposure	Results	Comments
MRI or combined exposure studies					
(Shivers et al., 1987)	Rat	Blood brain barrier (BBB)	0.15 T (MRI) 23.2 min	Temporary opening of BBB, recovered 15 - 30 mins after exposure.	
(Prato et al., 1990)	Rat	Blood brain barrier permeability (BBBP)	0.15 T (MRI) 2 x 23.2 min	BBBP significantly increased.	

(Prato et al., 1994)	Adult male Sprague-Dawley rat	Blood brain barrier permeability (BBBP)	1.5 T (MRI); 1.5 T (MRI with reduced RF and increased gradient field); 1.5 T (SMF only); 1.89 T (SMF only) 2 x 22.5 min	BBBP increased after regular MRI, but decreased after modified MRI. Both SMF only levels increased BBBP.	

7.2.2.3.5 Blood cells

The results from several researchers are quite contradictory. This may be due to different testing systems, as well as to different magnetic field exposures (static magnetic fields alone, static magnetic fields in combination with RF exposure, etc.).

Atef et al. (1995) reported effects on haemoglobin structure and function of 10 min exposures to magnetic fields of 0.4 T. No changes in dimensions and shape of haemoglobin molecules were observed, but a decrease in auto-oxidation reaction rate was found. It was suggested that auto-oxidation might be reduced by static magnetic field exposure through a stabilizing effect on the tertiary conformation of haemoglobin. Bhatia (1999) detected an increased phagocytic activity at 37 °C and a decreased activity at 27 °C after exposing mice to 1.4 T for 60 min. However, the changes involved a maximum of 25% and the clinical relevance of this observation is questionable.

Feinendegen and Muhlensiepen (1987) reported an increase in thymidine kinase activity in mouse bone marrow cells after static magnetic field exposures from 0.2 to 1.4 T for 5 to 30 minutes. The mice were anaesthetised and body temperature was manipulated using a thermostatically controlled chamber. Thymidine kinase activity was increased at a body temperature of 27 °C and decreased at 37 °C. The effects were not lasting. The measured values returned to baseline within several minutes after completion of static magnetic field exposures. The differences in the size of the experimental groups (with a range from 9 to 45 mice) and the lack of information concerning the controls are weaknesses of the study. Stegemann et al. (1993) reported about the effects on the activity of acetylcholinesterase in mouse bone marrow cells, which was inhibited by about 20% after a static magnetic field exposure of 30 min to a 1.4 T field. However, they did not mention the number of the control animals nor the conditions that they were kept in. As the experiments were obviously not blinded, it is unclear whether or not there was bias in the reporting of static magnetic field-associated effects.

The viability of bone marrow cells *in vivo* can be tested by isolating these cells, injecting them in recipient animals, and counting the number of spleen colonies formed. In a follow-up experiment to the one cited above, Peterson et al. (1992) used this technique to study the effect of variations in field strength (0.5 - 1.4 T), exposure time (15 - 60 min) and body temperature (20 - 37 °C) on murine bone marrow cells. An increase in cell viability was observed after a 30 min exposure to 1.4 T only with a body temperature of 27 °C, but not with lower or higher temperatures. No effect was seen with lower field strengths. When the body temperature was kept constant at 27 °C and the field strength at 1.4 T, an effect of exposure duration was found: that is, longer exposure resulted in higher cell viability. The authors speculated that the specificity of the effect might be membrane related.

Several other studies reported on the effects of long-term continuous or intermittent static magnetic field exposure. Tenforde and Shifrine (1984) examined the effects of long continuous magnetic field exposure (6 d at 1.5 T) on the immune system of mice being exposed to a static magnetic field. No effects were detected.

Gorczynska and Wegrzynowicz (1983) and Gorczynska (1987b) published several studies regarding long intermittent magnetic field exposure (maximum 0.3 T, 1 h d⁻¹, 7 weeks maximum). Gorczynska described alterations in the coagulation system, in blood cell numbers, and in the haematopoietic organs of guinea pigs. In nearly every study published by this group, effects were described which were more or less linked to static magnetic field exposure. Unfortunately, only limited information is given about the experimental and environmental conditions. The data reported in the publications appear to be incomplete and the statistical analysis, if mentioned, seems to be questionable.

Table 24. Blood cells

Authors	Animal	Endpoint	Exposure	Results	Comments
Static magnetic field effects					
(Atef et al., 1995)	Mouse	Haemoglobin structure and function	0.1 - 0.4 T 10 min	No changes in dimensions or shape of Hb molecule; decrease in auto-oxidation reaction rate.	
(Bhatia, 1999)	Mouse	Membrane and receptors of the reticulo-endothelial cells of bone marrow	1.4 T 60 min	Increased phagocytic activity at 37 °C and decreased activity at 27 °C	The increase or decrease of phagocyte activity is a max of ~ 25 %. Relevance is unclear.
(Feinendegen & Muhlensiepen, 1987)	Mouse	Thymidine kinase acitivity	0.2 - 1.4 T 5 - 30 min	Dose-dependent increase at body temperatures of 27 °C and 29 °C, decrease at 37 °C. Max effect in 30 min, return to baseline in 5 - 10 min. Membrane effect?	Effects were only measurable for minutes, not lasting. Relevance is unclear.
(Peterson et al., 1992)	Mouse spleen colonies (CFU-S7d)	Numbers of spleen colonies at different body temperatures	> 1.4 T > 15 min 20 - 37 °C	Increase in number of spleen colonies if SMF exposure was at least for 30 min at 1.4 T at a body temperature of 27 °C. Specificity of effect may be membrane effect.	
(Stegemann et al., 1993)	Mouse	Acetylcholin-esterase activity	1.4 T 30 min	Max inhibition at 3.5 (27 °C) or 2 h (37 °C); incomplete recovery at 15 h.	Reduction of approximately 20%. Relevance is unclear.

(Tenforde & Shifrine, 1984)	Mouse	Humoral and cell-mediated immune responses	1.5 T 6 d	No effects.	
(Gorczynska & Wegrzynowicz 1983)	Guinea pig	Platelet count; platelet aggregation; prothrombin and partial thromboplastin times; fibrinogen and fibrinolysis	5, 300 mT 1 h d^{-1}, 7 wk	Decreased platelet count; increased platelet aggregation; increased prothrombin and partial thromboplastin times; decreased fibrinogen, increased fibrinolysis.	No statistical test specified.
(Gorczynska 1987b)	Guinea pig	Myelopoiesis	0.05, 0.3 T 1 h d^{-1}, 7 wk	Alterations in numbers of various blood cells, independent of exposure time.	
(Gorczynska 1987a)	Guinea pig	Ceruloplasmin activity and iron content in serum; liver and spleen morphology	5, 300 mT 1 h d^{-1}, 7 wk	Drop in ceruloplasmin activity; unchanged serum iron content; morphological changes of spleen; functional disturbances of liver.	
Studies considered to be uninformative					
(Barnothy & Barnothy, 1970)					
(Battocletti et al., 1981)					
(Turieva-Dzodzikova et al., 1995)					
(Zhernovoi et al., 2001)					

7.2.2.3.6 Blood serum enzymes

Blood serum is a colloid system with proteins and an inorganic component. Some of the proteins have a transport function, some have an immune defence function and some are enzymes. The accent in this section is especially on static magnetic field effects on enzyme activity in blood plasma. Most of the studies reviewed below were judged to be scientifically weak.

Gorczynska and Wegrzynowicz (1984; 1985; 1986a; 1986b; 1989) and Gorczynska (1986; 1987a; 1988) have published a series of experiments on the effects of static magnetic field exposure on various outcomes. Guinea pigs were used in the majority of experiments, but use was also made of rabbits and rats. The exposures were homogenous static magnetic fields created by a 'resistive electromagnet', with exposure levels varying between 0.005 T and 0.3 T. Animals were exposed for one hour per day, 1 - 7 weeks. Control animals were placed for one hour per day in glass vessels similar to the ones used with the exposed animals. For almost all of the studied outcomes, an effect of the exposure was found that was independent of exposure level, but that generally increased with the duration of exposure. The findings included an indication of decreased concentration of serum protein, an increase in acid phosphatase activity, increased Na^+ concentration, indications of increased K^+ concentration, decreased chloride concentration, decreased glutamic pyruvic transaminase (GPT) activity, an increased level of fibrinogen degradation products (FDP) and a corresponding decrease in the concentration of fibrinogen in plasma. No morphological changes in the cardiac or skeletal muscles, kidneys, cerebellum, and lung tissue were observed. In one experiment using Wistar rats (Gorczynska & Wegrzynowicz, 1989), effects were independent of both magnetic field level and duration of exposure, showing increased GPT activity, increased glutamic oxaloacetic transaminase (GOT) activity, increased lactic dehydrogenase activity, increased alkaline phosphatase activity, and reduced cholinesterase activity for all exposure levels regardless of exposure duration (1 - 7 weeks). However, experimental setup was only briefly described, and there was no description of animal pre-experimental conditions or of their conditions during the experiment. The statistical methods used were also not described.

Watanabe et al. (1997) studied lipid peroxidation in the liver, kidneys, heart, lungs, and brain of mice exposed to 3.0 T or 4.7 T for 1, 3, 6, 24, or 48 hours, or to a sham control. No effect was found at 3.0 T exposures, whereas lipid peroxidation in liver, but no other organ, was increased after 3 hours or longer of exposure to 4.7 T. Increased lipid peroxidation in liver and GOT and GPT activities, were found after administration of CCL$_4$ combined with exposure to 4.7 T, exceeding the effect of each exposure alone.

Osbakken et al. (1986) studied effects of exposure to a 1.89 T superconductive magnet on adult and offspring mice. The study design included cage-control groups, control groups housed in the magnet room 20 feet from the magnet, and exposed groups housed in the magnet room.

Animals were exposed during a certain part of the day, for one to three months, for a total of 360 - 624 h. Animal populations and their living conditions were clearly described. No consistent differences were found in gross and microscopic morphology, haematocrit and white blood cell counts, or in plasma creatine phosphokinase, lactic dehydrogenase, cholesterol, triglyceride, or protein concentrations.

Papatheofanis and Papatheofanis (1989a; 1989b) studied acid and alkaline phosphatase activity in bone and blood, and calcium and phosphate ion concentrations, in serum from exposed, sham-exposed, and cage controlled groups of mice. Animals were exposed for 30 minutes per day during 10 consecutive days to a 1 T homogenous static magnetic field generated by an electromagnet. No effects were found on ion concentrations or any of the other studied endpoints.

Table 25. Blood serum, enzymes

Authors	Animal	Endpoint	Exposure	Results	Comments
Static magnetic field effects					
(Gorczynska & Wegrzynowicz, 1984)	Guinea pig	Serum protein concentration	0.005 - 0.3 T 1h d^{-1}, 6 wk	Indication of decrease in serum protein concentration dependent on duration of exposure, but not on magnetic field level.	Weak methodology.
(Gorczynska & Wegrzynowicz, 1985)	Guinea pig	Acid and alkali phosphatase	0.005, 0.3 T 1 h d^{-1}, 1 - 7 wk	Increase of acid, but not alkali phosphatase regardless of exposure level.	Weak methodology.
(Gorczynska & Wegrzynowicz, 1986a)	Guinea pig	K$^+$, Na$^+$ and chloride concentrations in serum	0.005 - 0.3 T 1 h d^{-1}, 6 wk	Increasing Na$^+$, decreasing Cl$^-$ in serum; no statistically significant effect on K$^+$. No differences were found 14 days after exposure cessation.	Weak methodology.

(Gorczynska & Wegrzynowicz, 1986b)	Guinea pig	Glutamic pyruvic transaminase (GPT) activity and morphological changes in the cardiac or skeletal muscles, kidneys, cerebellum, and lung	0.005, 0.05, 0.1, 0.3 T 1 h d⁻¹, 7 wk	Changes in enzyme activity related to exposure duration; no morphological changes. Decrease of GPT in guinea pig, but increase in rat (see 1989 paper below).	Weak methodology.
(Gorczynska & Wegrzynowicz, 1989)	Rat	Cytoplasmatic enzymes, cholinesterase activity, alkaline phosphatase activity	0.008, 0.15 T 1 h d⁻¹, 1 - 7 wk	Increased activity of cytoplasmatic enzymes (GPT, GOT, LDH), decreased cholinesterase activity, increased alkaline phosphatase activity; independent of exposure intensity or duration; reversible, return to normal 2 months after experiment.	Weak methodology.
(Gorczynska, 1986)	Rabbit	Fibrinogen degradation products	0.005, 0.12, 0.3 T 1 h d⁻¹, 2 - 4 wk	Increased fibrinogen degradation product related to duration of exposure, not to dose.	Weak methodology.
(Gorczynska, 1988)	Rabbit	Fibrinolysis	0.005, 0.1, 0.3 T 1 h d⁻¹, 4 wk	Duration-dependent increase in rate of fibrinolysis.	Weak methodology.

(Watanabe et al., 1997)	Mouse	Lipid peroxidation, GOT and GPT activity	3.0, 4.7 T 1, 3, 6, 24, or 48 h	Increase of lipid peroxidation in the liver after exposure to 4.7 T, but not 3.0 T. The increase did not vary with duration of exposure. Effect of exposure to 4.7 T on GOT or GPT, only after treatment with CCL_4. No effect on lipid peroxidation in kidney, heart, lung, or brain.	
(Osbakken et al., 1986)	Mouse	Gross and microscopic morphology; haematocrit and white blood cell counts; plasma creatine phosphokinase, LDH, cholesterol, triglyceride and protein concentrations	1.89 T 360 h over 1 month - 624 h over 3 months	No effects.	Weak methodology.
(Papatheofanis & Papatheofanis, 1989a)	Mouse	Bone acid and alkaline phosphatase activity	1 T 30 min d^{-1}, 10 d	No effects.	Weak methodology.
(Papatheofanis & Papatheofanis, 1989b)	Mouse	Ionic and enzymatic constituents of the circulatory system, e.g. blood alkaline phosphatase, acid phosphatase, calcium ion concentration and phosphate ion concentration	1 T 30 min d^{-1}, 10 d	No effects.	Weak methodology.

7.2.2.4 Endocrine system

The endocrine system, like the nervous system, adjusts and correlates the activities of the various bodily systems to the changing demands of the external and internal environment of the body.

The pineal and pituitary neuroendocrine glands, both situated in the brain and under neural control, release hormones into the blood stream that exert a profound influence on body metabolism and physiology, partly via their influence on the release of hormones from other endocrine glands situated elsewhere in the body. For example, hormones from both the pineal and pituitary glands play a central role in the control of reproduction.

7.2.2.4.1 Pineal gland

The pineal gland, or epiphysis, secretes melatonin, which functions as a timing device to keep internal physiological processes synchronized with the light-dark cycle in the environment. Melatonin is produced and released by the pineal gland only during the dark. Changes in day length can be taken as a marker of season, and melatonin has an important role in controlling the onset of reproduction in seasonally breeding animals.

A series of experiments from the University of Mainz, Germany, have focused on the effects of static magnetic field exposure on pineal gland melatonin synthesis and cell activity. An artificial magnetic field was generated by a pair of Helmholtz coils, of either 1.5 m or 3.0 m in diameter, creating an inversion of the horizontal component of the Earth's magnetic field. The response of pineal cells from guinea pigs and rats to a direct stimulation of a static magnetic field was investigated in two experiments (Semm et al., 1980; Reuss et al., 1983). The majority of cells (80% of cells from guinea pigs and 67% from rats), did not respond at all, while the remaining cells elicited different types of responses, e.g. inhibition in the guinea pig (Semm et al., 1980) or excitation of activity in the rat (Reuss et al., 1983). A decrease in pineal serotonin-N-acetyltransferase (NAT) activity and melatonin content (measured per gland) in rats was found after exposure during 15 minutes or 2 hours before midnight in an initial experiment (Welker et al., 1983).

An additional series of experiments were performed to elucidate the mechanism(s) through which magnetic fields affect NAT activity and melatonin content. NAT activity and melatonin content in acutely blinded rats were not affected by 30 minutes exposure to a magnetic field, in contrast to the decrease that was found in intact animals (Olcese et al., 1985). In another experiment, the effect was found to be species dependent, but independent of ocular pigmentation. That is, a reduction of

NAT activity and melatonin content was found both in albino Sprague Dawley rats and in Long-Evans hooded rats, but no effect was found in golden hamsters (Olcese & Reuss, 1986). However, a later study showed that pigmentation was important; no effect was seen in pigmented gerbils, whereas NAT activity was decreased by exposure in male albino gerbils (Stehle et al., 1988). Another study demonstrated that the effect was found only in the presence of dim red light (Reuss & Olcese, 1986). The number of animals in most of the above-described experiments was small, it is unclear whether animals were randomized into experimental groups, the ages of animals were not clearly reported, and levels of NAT activity varied considerably between control groups of the same species in different experiments.

A Swiss research group exposed rats to a one hour inversion of the horizontal component of the Earth's magnetic field, and compared pineal cyclic adenosine monophosphate (cAMP) content to that in unexposed siblings (Rudolph et al., 1988). A 38% reduction of cAMP was found in exposed rats. In another rat experiment, no effect on NAT activity or melatonin content was found after exposure to an artificial magnetic field that compensated for the Earth's natural magnetic field (Khoory, 1987).

Kroeker et al. (1996) exposed rats to a static magnetic field that could vary between $5x10^{-5}$ T and 0.08 T. One daytime and one nighttime control group was used. The magnetic field was created by placing a disk magnet on the bottom of each animal cage. No effects of the magnetic field exposure on melatonin content were found in any of the experimental groups. The only group with lower melatonin content was the daytime control group.

Jankovic and collaborators studied aspects of the immune system and melatonin in rats. In one study (Jankovic et al., 1991), they implanted small magnets, or same size iron beads, a number of days before or after immunization or challenge with various biochemical agents. Several immune response markers showed significantly elevated levels with the various static magnetic field treatments, while they were not visible in sham exposed or sham operated subjects. It is difficult to determine any localization information from this study (while the magnets are small, so are rat brains). Following suggestions from other research in magnetosensitivity, the authors studied the influence of magnetic fields in combination with pinealectomy, with appropriate controls (Jankovic et al., 1993; 1994). Magnetic fields again increased the immune response, and the absence of the pineal reduced the same markers, but the papers failed to make a strong case for linking the two.

Lerchl et al. (1990; 1991) reported an influence of intermittent exposure to a 40 μT static magnetic field on serotonin and melatonin metabolism in laboratory animals. The results were supported by Yaga et al. (1993), who reported changes in diurnal melatonin rhythm from pulsed static magnetic fields (40 μT) that resulted in a net reduction of melatonin secretion. In contrast, Levine et al. (1995) exposed mice to a 2 T pulsed magnetic field without an effect on melatonin secretion. In all these studies, the exposure contained time varying components due to rapid field switching or pulsing. Thus, firm conclusions on static magnetic field effects cannot be drawn from the results.

Table 26. Pineal gland

Authors	Animal	Endpoint	Exposure	Results	Comments
Static magnetic field effects					
(Semm et al., 1980)	Guinea pig	Electrical activity of pineal cells	Artificial geomagnetic field strength	Depression of pineal activity by an induced SMF; restoration by the inverted SMF.	
(Reuss et al., 1983)	Rat	Electrical activity of pineal cells	Artificial geomagnetic field strength 4 - 5 min	Activation of pineal cells continued after switching off the magnetic stimuli.	Variable responses.
(Welker et al., 1983)	Rat	Pineal serotonin-N-acetyl-transferase (NAT) activity; melatonin content	Artificial geomagnetic field strength 2 h	Reduction of nocturnal pineal NAT activity and melatonin content by changing the inclination of the ambient SMF, 63 - 58°, 68° or 78°.	Seem to report selected results. Weak methodology.
(Olcese et al., 1985)	Rat	Pineal serotonin-N-acetyl-transferase (NAT) activity; melatonin content	Artificial geomagnetic field strength 30 min	Reduction of nocturnal pineal NAT activity and melatonin content in intact rats; no effects in blinded rats.	Incomplete description of methodology.

(Olcese & Reuss, 1986)	Rat, hamster	Pineal serotonin-N-acetyl-transferase (NAT) activity and melatonin content	Artificial geomagnetic field strength 30 min	Reduction of nocturnal pineal NAT activity and melatonin content by 50° rotation of the horizontal component of the ambient SMF in rats; no effect in hamsters.	Incomplete description of methodology. NAT activity in unexposed rats was considerably lower than in their previous study (1985).
(Stehle et al., 1988)	Mongo-lian gerbil, rat	Pineal serotonin-N-acetyl-transferase (NAT) activity and melatonin content	Artificial geomagnetic field strength 30 min	Decreases in nocturnal pineal NAT activity and melatonin content in albino gerbils and rats regardless of sex; no effect in pigmented gerbils.	Results not fully reported. Incomplete description of methodology.
(Reuss & Olcese, 1986)	Rat	Pineal serotonin-N-acetyl-transferase (NAT) activity and hydroxyl-indole-O-methyl-transferase (HIOMT) activities	Artificial geomagnetic field strength 15 min	Magnetic field reduces nocturnal NAT and activity, and HIOMT activity, only under dim red light. No effect of the field alone.	Method-ological uncertainties; variable control data.
(Rudolph et al., 1988)	Rat	Pineal cAMP	Inverting of horizontal component of natural SMF 1 h	Decrease in pineal cAMP.	Methodology inadequately described.
(Khoory, 1987)	Rat	Pineal N-acetyl-transferase (NAT) activity, melatonin content	Artificial geomagnetic field strength 30 min	No effect on NAT activity or melatonin content.	Unclear if randomized. Experiment not blinded.

(Kroeker et al., 1996)	Rat	Neuro-chemistry	80 mT or 7 T 12 h and 8 d	No effect on melatonin, catecholamines, serotonin, or their metabolites.	Unclear if randomized. Experiment not blinded.
(Jankovic et al., 1991)	Rat	Weight change: spleen, thymus Immune response: plaque-forming cell (PFC) response, haemag-glutinin production, local hyper-sensitivity skin reactions, experi-mental allergic encephalo-myelitis (EAE), antibody production, peripheral blood CD4+ and CD8+ cells	60 mT 14, 24, 34 and 36 d	The highest immune response was observed with exposure of the occipital brain region for 24 d in the SMF group.	
(Jankovic et al., 1993)	Rat	Immune response: plaque-forming cell (PFC) response and hemag-glutination reaction	60 mT 21 d	Increased immune response in the presence of implanted magnets. Reduced immune response in the absence of the pineal gland.	

(Jankovic et al., 1994)	Rat	Weight change: spleen, thymus Immune response: plaque-forming cell (PFC) response, haemag-glutinin production, local hyper-sensitivity skin reactions,	60 mT 29, 39 d	Various immune responses were increased by SMF. SMF recovered decrease of immune reactions caused by pinealectomy.	Results are more supportive of interactions with some other structure than the pineal gland. No description of methods for statistical analysis.

MRI or combined exposure studies

(Lerchl et al., 1990)	Mouse, rat	Pineal serotonin metabolism	Inversion of horizontal component of Earth's magnetic field 5 min, 5 min off, 1 h; rapid on/off switching of field	Pineal serotonin increased; in rats: increase of pineal 5-hydroxyindole acetic acid, decrease of serotonin-N-acetyltransferase activity; pineal and serum melatonin levels not altered.	Age of animals not reported. Unclear if randomized. Experiment not blinded.
(Lerchl et al., 1991)	Rat	Serotonin-N-acetyl-transferase, melatonin, serotonin, 5-hydroxy-indole acetic acid	Inversion of horizontal component of Earth's magnetic field Rapid on/off switching of field	Reduced serotonin-N-acetyltransferase activity, lower melatonin; increased serotonin, 5-hydroxyindole acetic acid; effects not due to SF, but to on/off switching	Age of animals not reported (but little variation in body weight). Unclear if randomized. Experiment not blinded.

(Yaga et al., 1993)	Rat pineal glands	Pineal serotonin-N-acetyl-transferase (NAT) activity, melatonin content	40 μT, pulsed 45 min	Suppression of pineal NAT activity, and melatonin content by exposure during mid- or late dark phase; no changes after exposure early in the dark phase or during the day.	Age and sex of animals not reported, however, little variation in weight. Unclear if randomized.
(Levine et al., 1995)	Mouse	Serum melatonin levels	2 T 100 min	No effect on melatonin levels.	

7.2.2.4.2 Other endocrine gland effects

Other endocrine gland functions under static magnetic field action were reported by Gorczynska and Wegrzynowicz (1991a). They measured glucose homeostasis in rats after exposure to 1 mT and 10 mT fields for 10 days. They observed relatively small, but significant and consistent, changes, such as increased glucose levels, decreased insulin release. They interpreted the observed immune system changes as stress responses. Sutter et al. (1987) also studied effects on body weight and insulin release in rats after long, intermittent exposures to 0.4 T or 0.8 T fields. They saw no changes in organ or body weights. Although the two field levels affected glucose oxidation, the changes for the two field levels had different signs.

Teskey et al. (1987) exposed rats to MRI fields for 20 minutes per day for 5 or 21 days and evaluated survivability, hormone levels and weight parameters 13-22 months after the exposure. They found no differences from controls at this distant observation point.

Table 27. Other endocrine glands

Authors	Animal	Endpoint	Exposure	Results	Comments
Static magnetic field effects					
(Gorczynska & Wegrzynowicz 1991a)	Rat	Glucose homeostasis	1, 10 mT 1 h d^{-1}, 10 d	Slight increase in glucose, insulin release decreased, glucagons content increased as compared to controls.	Subtle but relatively solid effects.
(Sutter et al., 1987)	Rat	Pancreatic insulin content and *in vitro* insulin release of Langerhans islets; glucose and insulin plasma levels; body and pancreas weight	400, 800 mT 2h d^{-1}, 5d wk^{-1}	In adipocytes, 400 mT increased insulin-stimulated 1-^{14}C-glucose oxidation and 800 mT diminished it; no effect on body weight.	Opposite signs of the effects on glucose oxidation.
MRI of combined exposure studies					
(Teskey et al., 1987)	Rat	Survival, stress reactions	0.15 T 22.5 min d^{-1}, 5 d; 23.3 min d^{-1}, 21 d	No effect on hormone levels and weight parameters at 13 - 22 months after the exposure. No change in survivability.	.

7.2.2.5 Reproduction and development

Few studies have examined the effect of static magnetic fields on fertility. Most studies concern possible effects on the developing embryo and fetus (teratogenic effects). Key factors in the investigation of the potential teratogenic effects of any agent include an awareness of the potential sensitivity of the different developmental stages and the underlying developmental processes. Periods of cell proliferation and migration are particularly vulnerable to many teratogens. With regard to statistical analyses, those based on the numbers of affected fetuses (as used by some authors) will tend to overestimate the significance of any effect seen. This is because the assumption that individual fetuses within a litter are independent leads to an underestimate of the true variance.

7.2.2.5.1 Male fertility

Withers et al. (1985) did not detect any effect on spermatogenesis after exposing mice to a magnetic field of 0.3 T for 66 hours. Narra et al. (1996) reported slight changes in spermatogenesis and embryogenesis in mice exposed at 1.5 T for 30 min, but no abnormalities in sperm head shape (although the data were rather variable). Tablado et al. (1996; 1998; 2000) reported that maturation of sperm movement in mice, as well as postnatal testicular and epididymus development, was largely unaffected by either single, short-term exposure, or intermittent (1 h per day) or continuous, long-term exposure at 500 - 700 mT. In 1996, no effects on sperm motility, maturation and production were reported after exposing mice to a maximum of 0.7 T, 24 h d^{-1} for a maximum of 35 days. Tablado et al. (1998) used the same experimental set up two years later and reported sperm head abnormalities. However, developmental changes in the testes were not detected by the same authors in a subsequent experiment when dams were exposed, starting at the 7th day after gestation until birth (Tablado et al., 2000).

Table 28. Male fertility

Authors	Animal	Endpoint	Exposure	Results	Comments
Static magnetic field effects					
(Withers et al., 1985)	Mouse	Spermato-genesis	0.3 T 66 h	No effect on spermatogenesis.	
(Narra et al., 1996)	Mouse	Spermato-genesis, embryo-genesis	1.5 T 30 min	Reduction in testicular sperm; no increase in sperm head shape abnormalities; decreased survival of pre-implantation embryos.	
(Tablado et al., 1996)	Mouse	Sperm develop-ment	0.7 T 1 or 24 h d^{-1}, 10 or 35 d	No effect on sperm motility, maturation, production	
(Tablado et al., 1998)	Mouse	Sperm develop-ment	0.7 T 1 or 24 h d^{-1}, 35 d	More sperm head abnormalities with continuous exposure; no effect on tail.	
(Tablado et al., 2000)	Mouse	Testis develop-ment	0.5 - 0.7 T d 7 of gestation to day of birth	No effect up to 35 days of age.	

7.2.2.5.3 Mammalian development – static field exposure

Studies of possible teratogenic effects on mammalian species are more relevant to humans than are those on non-mammalian species. An early, rather comprehensive study by Sikov et al. (1979) did not find any effect of exposure to a static field of 1 T, either before implantation, during organogenesis or during fetal development, on the pre-natal and post-natal development of mice. A later study by Konermann and Monig (1986), which focused particularly on cortical development in mice, also found no developmental effect of exposure to fields of 1 T. Similarly, Zimmermann and Hentschel (1987) also reported a lack of effect on development in mice following exposure to a static magnetic field of 3.5 T over the whole period of gestation. More recent studies of mice exposed to fields of 4.7 T (Okazaki et al., 2001) and 6.3 T (Murakami et al., 1992) confirmed the lack of effect of exposure during organogenesis on *in utero* mouse development.

More variable results have been seen in two studies looking at possible developmental effects in rats. Mevissen et al. (1994) reported a significant decrease in the number of live fetuses per litter in rats exposed for the entire period of gestation to a 30 mT static field. The authors suggested that such exposure might be embryotoxic. A significant increase in the total number of resorptions and number of fetuses with common skeletal variants was also reported, although, as indicated above, the significance of findings based on individual fetuses may well be overestimated.

Table 29. Mammalian development - static field exposure

Authors	Animal	Endpoint	Exposure	Results	Comments
Static magnetic field effects					
(Sikov et al., 1979)	Mouse	Prenatal and postnatal development	1 T for varying periods for up to the whole of gestation	No consistent effects seen on prenatal or post-natal development.	Small litter numbers and large litter variability preclude firm conclusions
(Konermann & Monig, 1986)	Mouse	Prenatal development	1 T 1 h, 7, 10, 13 d post conception	No effect.	

157

(Zimmermann & Hentschel, 1987)	Mouse	Reproduction, development, haematology	3.5 T during mating and whole period of pregnancy (18 d)	With mating during 7-d period in field, reduced number of pregnancies (less mating); no teratology and pathology.	
(Okazaki et al., 2001)	Mouse	Fetal development	4.7 T 2 d	No effect on prenatal death and malformations but enchondral ossification enhanced and vascular endothelial growth factor reactivity altered.	
(Murakami et al., 1992)	Mouse	Fetal development	6.3 T 1 h d^{-1}, d 7-d 14 of gestation	No significant effects on litter size, fetal weight, intrauterine mortality rate, or skeletal abnormalities.	
(Mevissen et al., 1994)	Rat	Reproduction, fetal development	30 mT d 1-d 20 of pregnancy, or whole period of pregnancy	Decreased fetal survival; no malformations; increased skeletal ossification; postnatal growth enhanced after exposure during whole pregnancy.	
Studies considered to be uninformative					
(High et al., 2000)					

7.2.2.5.4 Mammalian development – MRI exposure

The exposures of pregnant mouse dams to all three magnetic field used in MRI (static, gradient and RF), have been examined by three research groups. While such exposures are more realistic (regarding MRI), any observed effects cannot be reliably attributed to any single field component. Significant heating, which can result from excessive RF magnetic field absorption, is a known teratogen (see Edwards et al., 2003). In addition, high levels of acoustic noise, resulting from rapid gradient field switching, may induce stress-related effects. A lack of effect, however, indicates that if the experimental model used was appropriate and the experimental design of sufficient power, none of the above conditions would have significantly affected the outcome.

Tyndall (1993) examined the effects of exposure for 36 min to a 1.5 T field (plus unspecified gradient and RF fields) on day 7 of gestation, during development of the anterior neural plate. An increased percentage of fetuses per litter with reduced craniofacial perimeter and crown-rump length was reported in the exposed groups compared to sham exposed animals. The author discussed RF-induced heating as a possible mechanism, although no rise in body temperature was recorded. Earlier studies (Tyndall, 1990; Tyndall & Sulik, 1991) reported that a similar exposure increased the incidence of eye abnormalities in the same strain of mouse (which is prone to this condition), but did not enhance the effect of x-ray-induced increases in this endpoint.

Heinrichs et al. (1988) carried out a comprehensive study of the effects of exposure of mice for 16 h around the same period (~ day 9 gestation) to MRI fields where the static magnetic field was 0.35 T. Pulsed gradient and RF magnetic fields were also present. There were no effects on the incidence of prenatal deaths, nor that of skeletal defects, but crown-rump length was significantly reduced in the MRI-exposed group. This effect may have been overestimated; however, since the analysis was based on the number of affected fetuses and appeared to neglect litter effects (see above). The authors noted that the noise generated within the magnet (by the switched gradient fields) may have been stressful. They further commented on the 10% reduction in body weight seen in both exposed and sham exposed groups due to dehydration over the 16 h treatment period.

An earlier study (Carnes & Magin, 1996) had reported significantly reduced fetal weight, which is strongly influenced by litter size, in mice exposed for 8 h on day 9 gestation to a 4.7 T static magnetic field, a switched gradient field and a 200 MHz RF field where the whole-body power absorption (specific energy absorption rate, or SAR) was estimated as 0.015 mW kg^{-1}. Sound levels were not provided. No effect was seen after exposure on day 12 of gestation, nor after exposure on day 9 and day 12 combined. In addition, no effect was seen on the number of fetal deaths in any MRI exposure group. Sperm production, which was not significantly affected in the study described above (Magin et al., 2000), was significantly reduced in mice exposed on day 12 gestation, but not on day 9, nor on day 9 and 12 combined. Overall, even ignoring the differences in experimental protocol, it is difficult to conclude that the effects described in the two studies are reproducible, either within or between the studies. A more likely explanation is of spurious differences introduced by small numbers, incomplete analysis, and variable data.

Later studies by Magin, Carnes and colleagues (Carnes & Magin, 1996; Magin et al., 2000) examined the effects of exposure of mice on days 9 and/or 12 gestation, i.e. during organogenesis, to static magnetic fields of around 4-5 T, combined with switched gradient and RF fields. In the study by Magin et al. (2000), mice were exposed to a static field of 4 T, a switched gradient field and a 170 MHz RF field, for which the average whole-body SAR was estimated to be 0.2 W kg^{-1}. Litter size was unaffected, but significantly increased numbers of resorptions and fetal deaths occurred in the group exposed on day 12 of gestation, but not on day 9, nor on days 9 and 12 combined. In addition, a significant increase in the rate of acquisition of motor skills was seen in the mice exposed on day 9 of gestation, whereas this was decreased in the group exposed on day 12. However, the numbers of pregnant dams per treatment group were rather small, the analyses often based on total numbers rather than numbers affected per litter, and the data were rather variable. Furthermore, only the exposed groups experienced the loud (90 - 100 dB) acoustic noise generated by the switched gradient fields.

Table 30. Mammalian development - MRI exposure

Authors	Animal	Endpoint	Exposure	Results	Comments
Static magnetic field effects					
(Tyndall, 1993)	Mouse	Crown-rump length and craniofacial perimeter	1.5 T 36 min	Decreased crown-rump length and craniofacial perimeter.	
(Tyndall, 1990)	Mouse	Eye developmental abnormalities induced by x-radiation at up to 30 cGy	1.5 T less than 1 h on d 7 of gestation	No effect on x-ray-induced eye abnormalities.	
(Tyndall & Sulik, 1991)	Mouse	Eye development	1.5 T 36 min, d 7 of gestation	Increased number of malformations.	
(Heinrichs et al., 1988)	Mouse	Placental resorptions, stillbirths, fetal weight at birth and crown-rump length	0.35 T 16 h, beginning on d 8 of gestation	Reduction of crown-rump length and fetal weight.	

(Carnes & Magin, 1996)	Mouse	Fetal growth, postnatal development, testicular development	4.7 T 8 h, d 9, d 12 of gestation	Reduction of sperm production in adults.	Small number, incomplete analysis, variable data.
(Magin et al., 2000)	Mouse	Fetal growth, postnatal development	4 T 1 or 2 x 9 h	No effect.	Small number, incomplete analysis, variable data.

7.2.2.5.2 Development in non-mammalian vertebrate embryos

In contrast to mammals, where development of the embryo and fetus occur *in utero*, amphibian and avian embryos develop in eggs, which are in some ways easier to experimentally manipulate. However, effects on such development may be less directly relevant to humans than studies on mammals.

An early, preliminary study by Brewer (1979) reported an inhibitory effect of static magnetic field exposure of 0.05 T on the reproduction of fish. However, the data were not analyzed. In contrast, Asahishima et al. (1991) reported that magnetic shielding (5 nT) induced early developmental abnormalities in the newt. The control data were, however, rather variable.

The possibility that strong magnetic field gradients may affect embryonic development in amphibia has been raised by IARC (2002). Early studies (Neurath, 1968; Ueno et al., 1984) had described abnormal growth and increased malformations in such embryos exposed to a static field of 1 T with field gradients of 10 - 1000 T m^{-1}. However, Mild et al. (1981) reported a lack of effect on the development of amphibian embryos of exposure to a spatially homogeneous static magnetic field of 0.25 T for up to 7 days. In addition, later studies by Ueno et al. (1990; 1994) briefly reported a lack of developmental effects following exposure during the early stages of development to 6.34 and 8 T fields, but it was not clear whether such exposure included strong field gradients.

More recently, Denegre et al. (1998) investigated the effect of exposure to static magnetic field of up to ~ 17 T on the first three cleavages of the fertilized egg of the African clawed toad *Xenopus laevis* used previously by Ueno et al. (1984; 1994). The authors found that the second and third cleavage oriented parallel to the plane of the magnetic field. The proportion of cleavages parallel to the field increased with field strength above around 2 T, to a maximum effect at around 17 T. The largest effects occurred in the homogeneous field rather than the gradient field, and the authors suggested that the effect resulted from the interaction with diamagnetically anisotropic molecules in the mitotic apparatus, possibly the microtubules of the spindle formation. These effect on the mitotic apparatus of cells exposed to high magnetic fields (up to 22 T) were confirmed in a further study by Valles et al. (2002). However, it is not clear whether the effects reported by Denegre et al. (1998) altered the proportion of eggs that developed into normal tadpoles.

Espinar et al. (1997) reported effects on cell migration and on differentiation of the cerebellar cortex in chickens after a long continuous exposure to 20 mT. The changes included cell degeneration and delay in the process of neuronal differentiation. Jové et al. (1999) found slight changes in the rate of development of chick embryos, including the pineal gland, in chicks exposed to static magnetic fields of 18 or 36 mT for up to 15 days incubation.

Behr et al. (1991) found no effects on embryonic development from exposure to a 4 T static magnetic field before and during incubation of chick embryos. MRI-specific exposure combinations with ELF and RF fields were also investigated in the study, but they are not relevant in this context.

Prasad et al. (1982; 1990) evaluated the effects of MRI exposure in an amphibian (frog) system. In one study (Prasad et al., 1982) frog spermatozoa, eggs and embryos were exposed to 0.7 T in combination with RF fields for 20 minutes. In another experiment fertilized frog eggs were exposed to a maximum of 4.5 T, again in combination with RF fields, for 60 minutes (Prasad et al., 1990). No deleterious effects were detected. Yip et al (1994a; 1994b; 1995) found no effect on the development of the central nervous system of exposed chickens in a total of three studies highlighting the effects of long continuous MRI field exposure (6 hours at 1.5 T in combination with RF and gradient fields). Kay et al. (1988) evaluated the exposure effects of MRI on frog embryogenesis. They found no abnormal morphology, function, or developmental delays of frog embryogenesis.

Table 31. Development in non-mammalian vertebrate embryos

Authors	Animal	Endpoint	Exposure	Results	Comments
Static magnetic field effects					
(Brewer, 1979)	Fish	Reproduction	0.05 T 3 generations	1st generation: reduced gestation time; 2nd: reduction spawn rate; 3rd: reproduction inhibited. Increase in size with exposure. Effects reversed after removal from field.	No statistics.
(Asashima et al., 1991)	Newt	Development	5 nT 5 d	Increased number of abnormalities.	Variable data
(Ueno et al., 1984)	Frog	Embryonic development	1.0 T; different gradients 8 - 12 h	No effect of 1 T field. Minor malformations with gradient field exposure.	
(Mild et al., 1981)	Frog	Embryonic development	0.25 T up to 7 d	No effect.	
(Ueno et al., 1990)	Frog	Embryonic development	4.5, 6.34 T up to 20 h	No effect of 6.34 T up to 7 h or 4.5 T up to 20 h on rapid cleavage and differentiation.	
(Ueno et al., 1994)	Frog	Embryonic development	40 nT, 8 T up to 20 h	No difference in development between control (Earth magnetic field), magnetic shielded (40 nT) and 8 T.	

(Denegre et al., 1998)	Frog	Development	1.74 - 16.7 T duration?	Alteration of cleavage planes (dose response). 50% abnormal embryos with parallel SMF (no dose effect), no abnormal embryos with perpendicular SMF.	
(Valles, Jr. et al., 2002)	Frog	Embryonic development	17 - 22 T duration?	Exposure during first two cell cycles induced third cycle mitotic apparatus and the third cleavage plane to align without changing cell shape.	
(Espinar et al., 1997)	Chicken	Brain development	20 mT 24 h at d 6, or from d 0- d 13	Exposure-dependent irreversible effects on cell migration and differentiation of cerebellar cortex.	
(Behr et al., 1991)	Chicken	Embryonic development	1, 4 T 18.8, 37.6, 56 or 75.1 min	No effect.	Includes SMF only group, but no statistics.
(Jové et al., 1999)	Chicken	Embryo pineal gland development	18, 36 mT from d 0 - d 5,10,15	Unequal promotion of embryo pineal gland development. Effect depended on exposure intensities and duration.	

MRI or combined exposure studies					
(Prasad et al., 1982)	Frog	Development after exposure of spermatozoa, eggs and embryos	0.7 T + RF 20 min	No effect.	
(Prasad et al., 1990)	Frog	Embryonic development	0.15, 4.5 T + RF + gradient 1 h	No effect.	.
(Yip et al., 1995)	Chicken	Axonal outgrowth	1.5 T + RF + gradient 6 h	No effect.	Controls not exposed to noise and vibration as in MRI.
(Yip et al., 1994a)	Chicken	Brain	1.5 T + RF + gradient 6 h	No effect.	
(Yip et al., 1994b)	Chicken	Embryonic development	1.5 T + RF + gradient 6 h	No immediate effects, but after 6 d higher abnormality and mortality rates.	More detailed studies should be performed, as the effect of noise and vibration cannot be ruled out.
(Kay et al., 1988)	Frog	Embryo-genesis	1.5 T + RF + gradient 2 x 1 h d^{-1}, prolonged exposure	No effect.	.

7.2.2.5.5 Developmental effects in non-vertebrate embryos

A few studies have been carried out with non-vertebrate species. These are phylogenetically distant from mammalian species, but may nevertheless (in principle) provide useful information. Levin and Ernst (1997) detected an effect of long continuous low field exposure (10 mT - 100 mT) in a sea urchin model. Ho et al. (1992) reported that static magnetic field exposure up to 9 mT during early embryogenesis of the fruit fly caused a dose-dependent increase in the number of abnormalities. Ramirez et al. (1983) evaluated the exposure effect of weak static magnetic field (4.5 mT) exposure on oviposition and development of the fruit fly. They found no effects on oviposition, but an increase in mortality of eggs and larvae.

These studies were regarded as relatively uninformative for health risk assessment.

Table 32. Other developmental effects

Authors	Animal	Endpoint	Exposure	Results	Comments
Static magnetic field effects					
(Levin & Ernst, 1997)	Sea urchin	Embryo development	10 mT - 0.1 T 26 h	Onset of mitosis delayed, species-dependent; exogastrulation by 30 mT, not 15 mT in one species, none in other.	Methodology weak.
(Ho et al., 1992)	Fruitfly larvae	Embryo-genesis	up to 7 mT 30 min 9 mT 24 h	Dose-dependent increase in abnormalities.	
(Ramirez et al., 1983)	Fruitfly	Oviposition, development	4.5 mT 14 d (oviposition) 48 h (development)	No difference in oviposition between control and SMF on d 1 - 7, avoidance of SMF on d 8 - 14. Mortality of eggs, larvae increased; adult viability decreased.	Variable data; inappropriate analysis.

7.2.2.6 Genotoxicity and cancer

Animal studies are often used in the evaluation of suspected human carcinogens, either screening for an increased incidence of spontaneous tumours or for the incidence of tumours induced by known carcinogens.

7.2.2.6.1 Genotoxicity and mutagenesis

Genotoxic effects of exposure to static magnetic fields have been mostly examined in cell cultures (see section 7.1.7). Few *in vivo* studies of genotoxicity or possible effects on other carcinogenic processes have been carried out.

Kale and Baum (1979) were unable to detect an enhanced mutation rate in the fruit fly *Drosophila melanogaster* exposed up to ten days to 1.3 T, and up to seven days to 3.7 T. In a subsequent study, Kale and Baum (1980) examined the effect of a long, continuous magnetic field exposure (166 h at 3.7 T) on chromosomal mutations in *D. melanogaster*, but were not able to detect any measurable magnetic field-induced changes. Koana et al. (1995; 1997) exposed *D. melanogaster* and their larvae to a 0.6 T magnetic field for 24 hours and observed a decrease of the surviving mutant genotype adults. The same group (Koana et al., 1997) also studied 5 T static magnetic fields for 24 hours and observed an enhancement of somatic recombination that was suppressed by vitamin E supplement. However, the genotoxicity equalled the effect of half to a quarter of the daily sunlight in Japan, thus making its clinical relevance questionable.

More recently, Suzuki et al. (2001) used a standard micronucleus assay and reported a significant, time-dependent and dose-dependent increase in micronucleus frequency in mice exposed to static magnetic fields of 2, 3 or 4.7 T for 24, 48 or 72 h. Micronucleus frequency was significantly increased following exposure to 4.7 T for all three time periods, and to 3 T after exposure for 48 or 72 h, whereas exposure to 2 T had no significant effect. The authors suggested that exposure to higher fields may have induced a stress reaction, or directly affected chromosome structure or separation during cell division.

With regard to combined exposures, Prasad and his co-workers (1984) examined the possible effects of exposure to RF and static magnetic fields on DNA in a study using mice. They did not find any chromosomal damage after exposing mice to 30 MHz in a magnetic field of 0.75 T for 60 minutes.

In 1995 Rofsky et al. reported the effects of MRI exposure (1.5 T static magnetic field with gradient and RF magnetic fields) with and without administration of the MRI contrast agent gadopentetate dimeglumine in a rat model (Rofsky et al., 1995). Neither magnetic fields alone nor the combination with contrast agent resulted in measurable chromosomal damage.

Table 33. Genotoxicity and mutation

Authors	Animal	Endpoint	Exposure	Results	Comments
Static magnetic field effects					
(Kale & Baum, 1979)	Fruitfly, egg, larva, pupa and adult	Lethal mutations	1.3 - 3.7 T 24 h, 10 d low field, 7 d high field	No effect.	
(Kale & Baum, 1980)	Fruitfly	Lethal mutations	3.7 T 166 h	No effect on production of induced sex-linked, recessive, lethal mutations.	
(Koana et al., 1995)	Fruitfly, 1st and 2nd instar larvae	Genotoxicity	0.6 T 24h	Decrease of surviving mutant genotype adults.	
(Koana et al., 1997)	Fruitfly, 3rd instar larvae	Genotoxicity and mutagenesis	5 T 24 h	Enhancement by SMF of somatic recombination, no effect on non-disjunction, terminal deletions, gene mutations. Effect suppressed by vitamin E supplement.	
(Suzuki et al., 2001)	Mouse	Micronucleus frequency	2, 3, 4.7 T 24, 48, 72 h	Increased number of micronuclei at higher exposure intensities and longer durations.	
MRI or combined exposure studies					
(Prasad et al., 1984)	Mouse	Chromo-somes in bone marrow	0.75 T 1 h	No effects, no chromosomal damage.	Exposure to SMF and RF.
(Rofsky et al., 1995)	Rat	Unstable chromosomal damage in regenerating liver cells	1.5 T + RF + gradient T1 (5.45 min) and T2 (10.45 min) imaging sequences	No effect of MRI alone or in combination with gadopentetate dimeglumine.	

7.2.2.6.2 Cancer

Few studies investigating the potential carcinogenicity of static magnetic fields have been carried out. With regard to possible effects on induced tumours, Bellossi (1984) reported a lack of effect on survival time in mice with chemically-induced epidermal tumours that were exposed to up to 800 mT for up to 1 h per day for 5 days per week until death was reported. In a later study, Mevissen et al. (1993) reported that exposure of rats to a magnetic field of 15 mT for 13 weeks did not significantly affect the incidence of chemically-induced mammary tumours, nor did it affect the number of tumours per animal compared with controls, although the weight per tumour was significantly increased. A complication is that the tumour multiplicity was reduced in rats treated with a static magnetic field as compared to the reference control, although the difference was not statistically significant. However, it is hard to draw any conclusions from this study because of the large range of tumour weights and the relatively small group size.

The growth of transplanted tumours were reported to be unaffected by exposure of mice to static fields of at least 1 T (Bellossi & Toujas, 1982; Bellossi, 1986c). Bellossi and colleagues studied the effect of static field exposure on the growth of tumours in mice injected with Lewis Lung tumour cells. Exposure to uniform static fields of up to ~ 1 T for up to 8 h per day for 5 days per week until death had no effect on the survival time (Bellossi & Toujas, 1982). Neither did exposure to non-uniform static magnetic fields of up to ~ 1 T, with gradients of up to 3 T m^{-1} (Bellossi, 1986c). The same group also studied the influence of static magnetic field exposure on spontaneous development of lymphoblastic leukaemia in mice (Bellossi, 1986b). Neither uniform nor non-uniform static magnetic fields had an effect. A somewhat longer lifespan was observed after intermittent exposure to 600 - 800 mT, but the number of animals in this group was quite small. The experimental procedures and analysis of the data in all these studies were rather briefly described, reducing the confidence that can be placed in them.

Table 34. Cancer

Authors	Animal	Endpoint	Exposure	Results	Comments
Static magnetic field effects					
(Bellossi, 1984)	Mouse	Methyl-cholanthren carcino-genesis	25 - 600 mT 2 h d^{-1}, 5d wk^{-1} 400 mT 5, 10, 15, 30 or 60 min d^{-1}, 5 d wk^{-1} 300, 600 or 800 mT 30 min d^{-1} for unspecified time	No effect on splenic index or survival.	Methods incomplete.
(Mevissen et al., 1994)	Rat	Develop-ment of mammary tumors induced by DMBA	15 mT 91 d	Increased tumour weight.	Small sample size and large range of tumour weights; source of increased tumour weight not stated. Histopathology showed no obvious peculiarities.
(Bellossi & Toujas, 1982)	Mouse	Tumour growth	13 - 900 mT 0.5, 1, 2, 3, or 4 h d^{-1}, 5 d wk^{-1}, from 2 months of age until death	No effect on survival after grafted Lewis Lung tumour.	Small group size. Also missing statistics, but there are no obvious differences.
(Bellossi, 1986c)	Mouse	Tumour growth	0.4 mT uniform SMF; non-uniform SMF: average gradient 3 T m^{-1}	No effect on life span, splenic weights or thymic weights.	

(Bellossi, 1986a)	Mouse	Spon- taneous carcino- genesis, survival	400 - 800 mT 2 h d⁻¹, 5 d wk⁻¹ 4.6 mT from age 9 wk up to death	Neither uniform nor non- uniform SMF had effects on development of viral lymphoblastic leukaemia. Longer lifespan after 600 - 800 mT (intermittent).	Small group size for 600 - 800 mT intermittent.

Studies considered to be uninformative
(Imajo et al., 1989)
(Gray et al., 2000)
(Tofani et al., 2003)

7.2.2.7 Other biological endpoints

This summary covers the category of studies that did not fit neatly into the other animal sub-categories. These studies are generally of a poor quality and were not considered informative for human health assessment.

Table 35. Other biological endpoints

Authors	Animal	Endpoint	Exposure	Results	Comments
Studies regarded as uninformative					
(Duda et al., 1991)	Rat	Liver and kidney concentration of copper, manganese, cobalt and iron	490 mT 0.5 - 4 h d⁻¹, total 8 - 64 h	SMF had no effect; 50 Hz MF changed metal concentration in kidneys of non-fertilized female rats.	Some differences observed, but these may well be due to multiple comparisons.
(Satoh et al., 1996)	Mouse	Metallothionein (MT) synthesis in liver, kidney, brain	3.0, 4.7 T 1, 3, 6, 24, or 48 h	MT synthesis induced in liver; CCl₄-induced hepatic MT synthesis enhanced. No effect in kidney or brain.	Quite long exposure needed to see the reported effects.

(Danielyan & Ayrapetyan, 1999)	Rat	Hydration of tissues and cell volume (number of ouabain binding receptors)	200 mT 0 - 5 h	Decrease of hydration in brain and liver tissue for 3.5 - 5 h; decrease of cell volume in brain, liver and spleen; increase of cell volume in kidney.	
(Barnothy & Sumegi, 1969)	Mouse	Histopathology of various organs	0.9 T, 2 T m^{-1} gradient 13 d	Disorganization in 40% of adrenal cortex slices. Increased mitotic index in liver cells.	Changes in bone marrow megakaryocytes decreased, the opposite of normal stress response. No description of methods for statistical analysis.
(Bellossi et al., 1984)	Rat, mouse	Body weight	400, 600, 800 mT 2 h d^{-1}, 5 d w^{-1} (4.6 mT in some mice), rats exposed for 4 wk and mice for ≥ 250 d	No effect on growth observed 4 weeks after exposure.	Varying physical parameters without any apparent rationale. Generally shorter exposures than the preceding studies. No description of methods for statistical analysis
(Bellossi et al., 1981)	Mouse	Water structure in brain: brain relaxation times (spin-lattice T1 and spin-spin T2), measured 1 - 5 d after exposure	600 mT 2 h	No effect on brain relaxation times T1/T2 five days after exposure.	Using a magnetic method to analyse these effects does not seem like a very good idea. Waiting 5 days is very long for structured water. Statistical analysis deficient.

(Bellossi, 1983)	Mouse	Trypano-somiasis	400 mT 10, 30, 60, 120 min, 5 d 200 - 600 mT 90 min	No effect.	No statistical analysis. Very consistent survival after injection suggestive of a very robust disease progression. This animal model may not be adequate to detect SMF effect.
(Gorczynska et al., 1986)	Rat	Cell respiration (liver mitochondria)	0.008, 0.15 T 1 h d^{-1}, 7 wk	Respiration through NADH dehydro-genase, succinic dehydrogenase and cytochrome oxidase influenced by duration, intensity (more at 0.008 T); reversible after 3 months.	
(Gorczynska & Wegrzynowicz, 1991b)	Rat	Structural changes in hepatocytes mitochondria, endoplasmic reticulum and ribosomes; activity of mitochrondrial respiratory enzymes; glycogen in hepatocytes; serum cortisol	1, 10 mT 1 h d^{-1}, 10 d	Structural changes in hepatocytes mitochondria, endoplasmic reticulum and ribosomes; increased activity of NADH dehydro-genase, succinic dehydro-genase, cytochrome oxidase; increase in glycogen in hepatocytes; high serum cortisol.	The reported changes may be due to temporary alterations in liver cell organelles.

(Parafiniuk et al., 1992)	Guinea pig	Structural changes in hepatocytes mitochondria	5, 300 mT 1 h d^{-1}, 3-7 wk	Structural changes in hepatocytes mitochondria.	

7.2.2.8 Conclusions

Few studies have been carried out on the effects of static electric fields. The evidence indicates that the surface electric charge can be perceived, and there is weak evidence to suggest that if the static field is sufficiently intense (> 40 kV m^{-1} in rats), then this may induce aversive behaviour.

There is good evidence that the movement of laboratory rodents in static magnetic fields equal to or greater than 4 T may be unpleasant, inducing aversive responses and conditioned avoidance. Such effects are thought to be consistent with magnetohydrodynamic effects on the endolymph of the vestibular apparatus. Otherwise, the data on behaviour are variable.

There is some evidence that several vertebrate and invertebrate species are able to use static magnetic fields, at levels as low as geomagnetic field strengths, for orientation. However, these responses are not thought to be relevant to human health.

There is some evidence of a stimulating effect on bone formation of static magnetic fields in the millitesla range. Stronger proof is present for such effects of tesla-strength static magnetic fields in a model system, but this treatment needs to be confirmed *in vivo*.

There is good evidence that exposure to fields greater than about 1 T (0.1 T in larger animals) will induce flow potentials around the heart and major blood vessels, but the physiological consequences of this remain unclear. Several hours of exposure to very high flux densities of up to 8 T in the heart region did not result in any cardiovascular effects in pigs. In rabbits, short and long exposure to fields ranging from geomagnetic levels to the millitesla range were reported to affect the cardiovascular system, although the evidence is not strong.

The results from one group suggested that the static magnetic fields of millitesla intensities may suppress early blood pressure elevation via hormonal regulatory system. The same group has reported that low-intensity SMF of up to 0.2 T may induce local effects on blood flow that may lead to improvement of microcirculation. In addition, another group reported that high static magnetic field flux densities of up to 10 T may lead to reduced skin blood flow and temperature. In all these cases, however, the end points are rather labile, a situation that may have been complicated by pharmacological manipulation, including anaesthesia in some cases, and immobilisation. In general, it is difficult to reach any firm conclusion without some independent replication.

There are several studies describing possible effects of magnetic field exposure on blood cells and the haemopoietic system. However, the results are equivocal, limiting the conclusions that can be drawn. The available evidence regarding effects of static magnetic field exposure on enzymatic and ionic constituents in serum comes primarily from one laboratory. These findings need to be confirmed by independent laboratories before conclusions can be drawn.

With regard to effects on the endocrine system, several studies from one laboratory suggest that static magnetic field exposure can affect pineal synthesis and melatonin content. However, some studies performed at other laboratories have been unable to demonstrate an effect. It is possible that differences in the study designs, e.g. exposure circumstances, species, outcome measures, or timing of exposure, can explain the conflicting results. The finding of a suppressive effect of static magnetic field exposure on melatonin production needs to be confirmed in further research before firm conclusions can be drawn. On the whole, few studies have investigated static magnetic field effects on endocrine systems other than the pineal and no consistent effects have emerged.

Reproduction and development is a very important issue in MRI exposure, for both patients and clinical staff. On this subject, only a few good studies of static magnetic field effects are available at field values above 1 T. MRI studies *per se* are uninformative in this respect, because it is difficult to distinguish the effects of the static fields from those of the other MRI fields. Further examination of the possible effects of static field exposure is urgently needed for the assessment of health risk.

With regard to genotoxicity and cancer, so few animal studies have been carried out that it is not possible to draw any firm conclusions.

8   HUMAN RESPONSES

8.1   Laboratory studies

Experimental studies using volunteers, including those exposed to EMFs, are restricted for ethical reasons to the investigation of transient physiological phenomena that can be determined to be harmless in the controlled conditions of a laboratory. The advantage of volunteer experiments is that they indicate the likely response of people exposed under similar conditions. Disadvantages of volunteer studies include the innocuous nature of the effects that can be investigated, the often short duration of exposure and investigation, the small number of subjects usually examined, and thus limited statistical power to detect an effect. In addition, it is difficult to create an identical physical environment for unexposed sessions for MRI studies, and the fields inside the magnet might interfere with measurements of the biological endpoints. Experiments on human subjects are naturally subject to stringent ethical constraints. The subjects are usually screened for medical fitness and, therefore, may not reflect the responses of potentially more susceptible members of society. Within this limited context, however, volunteer studies can give valuable insight into the physiological effects of exposure to an agent.

The majority of laboratory studies have examined static magnetic field effects, recently often in connection with MRI exposures. However, a few studies on the perceptual effects of surface charge generated by static electric fields have been carried out.

8.1.1   Static electric fields

Blondin et al. (1996) investigated human perception of electric fields and ion currents during conditions simulating those present in the vicinity of a high-voltage DC transmission line, with the purpose to establish the sensory thresholds for detection. Healthy volunteers were recruited through advertisements in local newspapers (23 men, 25 women). The electric fields and ion current generating system was located in the ceiling of the exposure chamber which could expose subjects to uniform DC fields of up to 50 kV m^{-1} and uniform ion current densities of up to 300 nA m^{-2}. Fields were presented either alone or in combination with some specified level of ions. Subjects presented with continuous series of successive trials, each trial lasting about 25 seconds. Half of the trials were non-signal, 'blank' trials. The median detection thresholds were 45.1 kV m^{-1} in the non-ion condition, and 36.9 kV m^{-1} with a high ion-concentration condition. There was a large variation in individual thresholds; 33% had thresholds under 40 kV m^{-1} and 66% under 50 kV m^{-1}. Two subjects had thresholds under 20 kV m^{-1}. With a simultaneous high ion current density (120 nA m^{-2}), 33% of subjects detected fields < 20 kV m^{-1}, and 10% could detect a 10 kV m^{-1} field.

A study by Clairmont et al. (1989) investigated the effect of interactions between AC and DC fields when placing AC and DC high-voltage lines in the same power line corridor. A small part of the study was an experiment where human subjects described sensation levels at different exposure conditions. Observations were made under a hybrid (both AC and DC) test line. Each person rated various sensations at measurement locations along the lateral profile of the test line, while the DC field, AC field, and ion current density were simultaneously monitored at each of the locations. The authors concluded that the combination of AC and DC fields caused relatively large increases in sensation of the fields, compared to each field condition alone. However, there was no adequate description of how the experiments were conducted; i.e. the number of subjects, selection of subjects, and characteristics of subjects are all unknown, exposure conditions are poorly described, and subjects were not blinded to the exposure condition.

Table 36. Static electric fields

Authors	Endpoint	Exposure	Results	Comments
(Blondin et al., 1996)	Human perception of electric fields and ion currents	Electric field: 0 - 50 kV m^{-1} Ion current density: 0, 60 or 120 nA m^{-2}	Median detection threshold 45.1 kV m^{-1} in non-ion condition, 36.9 kV m^{-1} in high ion-concentration condition. 33% had thresholds < 40 kV m^{-1}, 66% < 50 kV m^{-1}. Two subjects had thresholds < 20 kV m^{-1}. With a ion current density of 120 nA m^{-2}, 33% detected fields < 20 kV m^{-1}, 10% detected a 10 kV m^{-1} field.	
(Clairmont et al., 1989)	Effects on human sensation by combination of DC and AC electric fields	DC field: 0 - 40 kV m^{-1} AC field: 0, 2, 5, 10, or 15 kV m^{-1}	Increased sensation in combined fields.	Experiment poorly described, not systematic, unknown number of subjects, not blinded.

8.1.2   Static magnetic fields

8.1.2.1 Neurobehavioural studies

Possible effects on the nervous system can be studied at several different levels, from a simple level to the more complex. Effects on properties of the peripheral nervous system, such as conduction velocity, are readily investigated and may be relevant to effects seen at higher levels of organization. Measurement of evoked potentials recorded from the brain, usually in response to an auditory, visual or somatic signal, takes this process further and include measuring potential effects on signal transduction and central nervous system processing. Measurement of the electrical activity of the brain (EEG) reflects spontaneous activity, possibly in different mental states, but the results are notoriously difficult to interpret. Tests of cognition, mood and other behaviours assess the integrated output of the brain, and so are directly relevant to well being.

8.1.2.1.1 Human peripheral nerve function

Hong (1987) studied peripheral motor nerve conduction velocity and nerve excitability in 10 volunteers after short exposure (5, 10, 15 sec) to 1 T. No changes were found in nerve conduction velocity, whereas a transient increase in the nerve excitability index (measured as the ratio of the compound muscle action potential seen during or after exposure compared to that measured before exposure) was observed. This change was observed 5 sec or more after exposure, and disappeared within the following 3 min. The authors concluded that motor nerve excitability is increased during such exposure.

Vogl et al. (1991) studied nerve conduction velocity in 10 subjects before, during and after exposure to static magnetic fields of 1 T, and to combined MRI and RF fields. They found no effects of either static field exposure alone or from MRI imaging.

Table 37. Peripheral nerve conduction velocity

Authors	Endpoint	Exposure	Results	Comments
Static magnetic field studies				
(Hong, 1987)	Nerve function	1 T 5, 10, 15 sec	No effect on nerve conduction velocity; temporary increase of excitability index: effect not present 3 min after exposure.	

MRI or combined exposure studies				
(Vogl et al., 1991)	Peripheral nerve conduction velocities	1 T 1 h	Evoked potentials, as measured here, are not affected by MRI exposure.	

8.1.2.1.2 Evoked and spontaneous brain activity

Electrical responses (potentials) evoked in the brain by exposure of a subject to a sensory stimulus such as an auditory noise or visual signal can be used as a diagnostic tool to indicate conduction problems in a nerve pathway, including nerves and synapses within the central nervous system. Hong and Shellock (1990) measured latencies of somatosensory evoked potentials in 11 normal subjects exposed to a static field of 1.5 T without detecting any differences in the latency or amplitude of evoked waveform when comparing measurements before and during exposure.

Dobson, Fuller and collaborators studied spontaneously occurring activity as measured in epileptic patients by EEG after exposure to fields in the mT range. Using the technique of comparing to individual baselines, they reported increased epileptiform activity in six out of nine presurgical epileptic patients. No effect was seen in one other patient and the results in the last two could not be interpreted. One non-epileptic volunteer was also included in the study (Fuller et al., 1995). In a study of 10 mesial temporal lobe epilepsy patients, Dobson et al. (2000a), making the critical assumption that epileptiform activity is a time-invariant Poisson process, found an alteration in epileptiform activity in five out of 10 patients, although the stimulation protocol resulting in these alterations differing between patients. A very complex field protocol makes the evaluation of the exposure difficult. Dobson et al. (2000b) also studied three patients with mesial temporal lobe epilepsy. Significant alterations in epileptiform activity were observed in 2 of the three subjects, while magnetic stimulation resulted in cessation of interictal spike/wave trains in the third.

Müller and Hotz (1990) measured possible delays in brainstem auditory evoked potentials after exposure to up to 2 T MRI imaging without finding any significant difference in a sample of 11 patients when comparing to measurements made before the exposure. In addition, one healthy volunteer was exposed during three hours of increasing exposure from 0 to 2 T MRI (Hotz et al., 1992). No effect was found on brainstem response in this person.

Vogl et al. (1991) recorded auditory (N=6), visual (N=20) and somatosensory evoked potentials (N=20) before, during and after exposure to static magnetic fields of 1 T and to combined MRI and RF fields without seeing any effect on latency and waveform for any of the exposure conditions.

Metabolic activity is another way of assessing neural activity in the brain. Volkow et al. (2000) measured brain metabolic activity in 12 healthy volunteers during MRI exposure, simulated MRI exposure (using a PET scanner modified to look like an MRI unit), and during a regular PET scan. The real and simulated MRI exposures were associated with lower metabolic activity compared to the regular PET scan. The authors suggest that this was due to differences in the visual field of the MRI and PET scanner, and that it also indicated that the subjects had habituated to the pulsed gradient field noise of the MRI scan.

Table 38. Evoked and spontaneous brain activity

Authors	Endpoint	Exposure	Results	Comments
Static magnetic field studies				
(Hong & Shellock, 1990)	Somato-sensory evoked potentials (SEP). Difference in latency of N20 and P25.	1.5 T duration not specified	No effects on short-latency of SEP.	Applied t-statistic does not look sound.
(Fuller et al., 1995)	EEG of epileptic patients	0.1, 0.9, 1.3, 1.8 mT 20 sec	Generation of epileptiform activity in the range of 0.9 - 1.8 mT in 6 of 7 exposed patients.	Dosimetry at the target (hippocampus) is questionable. Protocol is based on the assumption that there is no time trend in the epileptiform activity.
(Dobson et al., 2000a)	EEG of epileptic patients. Interictal spike counts	1 - 4 mT repeatedly for 5, 20 sec	No overall effect attributable to SMF exposure. Claim that 50% of subjects had significant alteration in at least one protocol (5/30 significant protocols).	Experimental protocol complex and difficult to interpret. Baseline before sub-protocols not consistent. Overall evaluation questionable. No sham exposures. Possible time trends.

| (Dobson et al., 2000b) | EEG of epileptic patients. Interictal spike counts | 0.9, 1.3, 1.8 mT repeatedly for 2, 5,10, 20 sec | Generation of epileptiform activity at 1.8 mT in two of three patients. | Experimental protocol complex and difficult to interpret. Insufficient data to draw conclusions. Very inhomogeneous results, even within the three subjects. |

MRI or combined exposure studies

(Müller & Hotz, 1990; Hotz et al., 1992)	Brainstem auditory evoked potentials (BAEP)	1.5 T 14 - 67 min	No change in relative BAEP inter-peak latency after exposure to MRI.	
(Hotz et al., 1992)	Brainstem auditory evoked potentials (BAEP)	0, 0.5, 1, 1.5, 2 T 3 h	No change.	N=1.
(Vogl et al., 1991)	Somato-sensory, visual, and auditory evoked potentials and peripheral nerve conduction velocities	1 T 1 h	Evoked potentials, as measured here, are not affected by MRI exposure.	
(Volkow et al., 2000)	Brain glucose metabolism	4 T 35 min	Metabolism lowered in real and simulated MRI environment: no effect of SMF (but effect of visual stimulation).	Possibility that sound stimulus is responsible for differences between MRI and PET. Small gradient fields present with SMF.

Studies considered to be uninformative

(von Klitzing, 1989)
(von Klitzing & Tessmann, 1989)
(von Klitzing, 1987)

8.1.2.1.3 Sensory perception

Schenck et al. (1992) reported 'dose-dependent' sensations of vertigo, nausea and a metallic taste in the mouth in 11 volunteers exposed to static magnetic fields of 1.5 and 4 T, and another group of 24 subjects with 1.5 T exposure, in an MRI system. Similar sensations have been anecdotally noted by other groups during volunteer and patient exposures (Kangarlu et al., 1999; Chakeres et al., 2003b; Crozier & Liu, 2005). These sensations occurred during movement of the head through a gradient field. In addition, magnetic phosphenes could sometimes be seen during eye movement in a field of at least 2 T. These effects may well be attributable to the weak electric fields induced by movement within the gradient field. The vertigo however, may be specifically attributable to magnetohydrodynamic forces acting on the endolymph of the semi-circular canals (Schenck, 2000).

In a study of auditory function, Winther (1999) found no effect on hearing and balance in 11 healthy male subjects following their exposure to a static magnetic field of 2 - 7 mT for 9 h. The subjects slept near the magnet during one night. Hearing and balance were measured in the evening before, and in the morning after the exposure.

Table 39. Sensory perception

Authors	Endpoint	Exposure	Results	Comments
Static magnetic field studies				
(Schenck et al., 1992)	Sensory experiences during motion in the field	1.5, 4 T total exposure, 1 - 35 h over one year	At 4 T more vertigo, nausea, metallic taste, magneto-phosphenes.	Results consistent with induced electric fields and/or with direct effect on vestibular organ.
(Winther et al., 1999)	Inner ear function	2 - 7 mT 9 h	No effect on any parameter.	

8.1.2.1.4 Cognitive studies

With regard to cognitive studies, two studies using a battery of cognitive test have been recently carried out during exposure to fields of 1.5 and 8 T (see Chakeres & de Vocht, 2005 for a review). Chakeres et al. (2003a) studied the effect of an 8 T static field exposure on the cognitive function of 25 healthy volunteers aged between 20 and 51 years. Cognitive function was assessed using seven standard neuropsychological tests of short-term memory, working memory, attention, and auditory reaction time. The tests were conducted inside and outside of the magnet, and the order of exposure condition was randomized. No effects were found, except for a small decline in the performance of a short-term memory task.

De Vocht et al. (2003) examined the effect of exposure to a 1.5 T static magnetic field on 6 standard measures of sensory function, cognitive function and motor co-ordination in 17 healthy volunteers. The head of the exposed subjects was in a field of 700 mT. The subjects did all tests at a session before the start of the experiment, to minimize the learning effect. Four different exposure conditions were used; 1st week unexposed with no movements, 2nd week unexposed with movements, 3rd week exposed with movements, and 4th week exposed with no movements. The authors found significant declines in the performance of a hand-eye coordination task (4%) and a near visual contrast sensitivity task (16%) when subjects were exposed to static and gradient fields.

Preece et al. (1998) also examined static field effects on cognitive function in 16 subjects during exposure to a static magnetic field of 0.5 mT (or to a 50 Hz, 0.5 mT magnetic field) in a randomized three-way cross over study. No effects were found during static field exposure, although exposure to the 50 Hz field resulted in a decline in numeric working memory sensitivity and word recognition sensitivity.

Other studies have generally reported a lack of effect on cognitive function following static magnetic fields or MRI exposure. In a study of 10 subjects, Kangarlu et al. (1999) found no effects on executive, cognitive, language and motor functions tested immediately after a one hour exposure to an 8 T pure static field when compared to tests performed shortly before the exposure session. The study design did not take possible learning effects into account.

Brockway and Bream (1992) included a total of 421 patients and volunteers in four experiments on the effect of MRI exposure on memory. In the first two experiments, 100 subjects were tested before and after MRI exposure. The last two experiments included exposed subjects and an unexposed control group. In experiment one, a reduced face and name identification ability was found, which the authors attributed to the order in which the tests were performed. A similar effect was found in experiment four, but this was seen in both the exposed and unexposed groups.

Besson et al. (1984) compared scores from 7 subjects on 7 psychometric tests performed before exposure to a NMR brain imaging procedure and respective test scores 1-5 days after the exposure. Exposure duration was 10 minutes, and the corresponding static field was 0.04 T; RF fields were also present. An improvement in two tests was found. However, this may be due to a learning effect.

Sweetland et al. (1987) assigned 150 volunteers either to an MRI imaging procedure (0.15 T static field and RF), a sham condition without any field, or a control condition outside the MRI unit. Exposure duration was 47 minutes. A battery of psychometric tests was performed before exposure, immediately after exposure, and three months later. Analyses of differences in the test scores did not indicate an exposure effect. Given the large number of tests that were analysed, a few statistically significant results were probably due to chance.

These data did not show effects of exposure on neurophysiological responses and cognitive functions in stationary volunteers during exposure to static magnetic fields of up to 8 T, nor can they rule out such effects. However, a dose dependent induction of vertigo and nausea was found in workers and volunteers during movement in static fields greater than 2 - 3 T. The possibility that eye-hand coordination and near visual contrast sensitivity are reduced in fields adjacent to a 1.5 T MRI unit should be further investigated. The presence of a magnetic field gradient was more commonly associated with these types of neurophysiological responses. All available studies are based on small numbers with limited power to detect modest effects, and have methodological limitations.

Table 40. Cognitive functions

Authors	Endpoint	Exposure	Results	Comments
Static magnetic field studies				
(Chakeres et al., 2003a)	11 different standardised neuro-cognitive tests, and an auditory motor reaction time test	0.05, 8 T ~ 1 h	No effect, except for small negative effect on short-term memory.	
(de Vocht et al., 2003)	Evaluation of cognitive-motor, cognitive and sensory function	0, 1.5 T 1 h	No effect, except for 4% reduction in performance of eye-hand coordination tests and 16% reduction in near visual contrast.	
(Preece et al., 1998)	Cognitive function	0.6 mT ~ 1 h	No effect.	Exposure duration not given. Presumed to be throughout the behavioural test.
(Kangarlu et al., 1999)	Cognitive, language and motor function	8 T 1 h	No effects. Some reports of vertigo and metallic taste in the mouth during movement.	The study design did not take into account possible learning effects.

MRI or combined exposure studies				
(Brockway & Bream, Jr., 1992)	Memory loss: specifically recall tests for faces, common objects, lexical items and digit span	0, 1.5 T duration unspecified	Some decline in memory performance in patients compared to controls, but not attributed to exposure, since effects were independent of body location (e.g. head or foot) being imaged.	RF (and presumably switched gradient fields) also present. Effect cannot be ascribed to SMF alone.
(Sweetland et al., 1987)	Six standardised tests of cognitive function	0.15 T ~ 1 h	No apparent effect on human cognition. However, anxiety scores increased and digit span scores decreased following MRI exposure. Interpretation of effects difficult: no difference between exposed and control groups.	Switched gradient and RF fields also present.
(Besson et al., 1984)	Four standardised tests of cognitive function	0.04 T 10 min	Increase in verbal and full scale IQ following exposure.	Switched gradient fields and RF fields also present

8.1.2.2 Circulatory system

It is known that flow potentials, which can be easily recorded on ECGs (see chapter 5), are induced around the major blood vessels and hearts of exposed patients during MRI. In addition, calculations suggest that magnetohydrodynamic forces will impede the flow of blood in major vessels at very high flux densities (~ 5% at 10 T; see section 5.1.3). The possible consequences of these effects have been explored in studies of high-intensity static magnetic field with intensities between 1 and 8 T associated with MRI-investigations. Other studies focused on the physiotherapeutic devices already in clinical use with intensities < 100 mT. Exposure durations have varied from 10 min up to 1 h.

8.1.2.2.1 Cardiac function, blood flow and blood pressure in volunteers

A number of volunteer studies have recently been carried out to test these calculations. Kangarlu et al. (1999) found that 10 volunteers exposed to an 8 T field for 1 hour showed no change in heart rate, or diastolic or systolic blood pressure, measured after exposure, compared to measurements taken before the exposure. The ECG recorded during exposure was regarded as uninterpretable due to the superposition of the potential generated by aortic blood flow and smaller potentials generated by blood flow in other vessels, but no change was observed when comparing ECG measurements taken before and after the exposure. More detailed studies by the same group have recently been published. One of these involved a study of 25 subjects and reported a lack of clinically significant effects of exposure to fields of up to 8 T on heart rate, respiratory rate, systolic and diastolic blood pressure, finger pulse oxygenation levels and core body temperature (Chakeres et al., 2003b). There was a statistically significant trend for systolic pressure to increase with flux density. At 8 T this was about 4 mm Hg, which is consistent with a haemodynamic compensation for a magnetohydrodynamic reduction in blood flow (Chakeres & de Vocht, 2005), but was also approximately one half of the difference seen when the subjects moved from a supine to a sitting body position. Blood pressure returned to normal after cessation of exposure. It is not clear whether the change in blood pressure was caused by the static field exposure or to other circumstances during the experiment, as no sham exposed group was included. No ectopic beats or cardiac arrhythmias were reported in either study.

Hinman (2002) reported the effects of exposure on heart rate and blood pressure associated with short-term exposure to 100 mT static magnetic fields. The exposure was local; the subjects laid down on 42 small permanent magnets. Seventy-five healthy adults were assigned to one of three treatment groups (positive versus negative polarity and control) in a double blind, randomized controlled trial. Heart rate and blood pressure were monitored prior to exposure, at 1 min, 5 min, 10 min and 15 min intervals during exposure, and again 5 min after exposure. Slight, non-significant decreases in heart rate and blood pressure were observed. An earlier study (Jehenson et al., 1988), conducted at a flux density of 2 T, investigated cardiac rhythm changes in 12 healthy volunteers for 1 hour before exposure, 1 hour during exposure, and 22 hours after exposure. In addition, four subjects were exposed to 1 T, and nine control subjects were exposed to 0 T. A significant 17% increase in cardiac cycle length was observed after 10 minutes of exposure at 2 T and during the reminder of the exposure period. The cardiac cycle was back to pre-exposure values 10 minutes after exposure. No significant effects were observed at 1 or 0 T.

No effects on blood flow were seen in a number of other studies (Stick et al., 1991; Mayrovitz et al., 2001; Martel et al., 2002). All of these studies used small, locally placed, permanent magnets, e.g. on the forearm or on the hand.

186

Shellock and Crues (1987) included 50 patients for clinical MRI imaging that were evaluated for heart rate and blood pressure. The study was done with a 1.5 T system, and the RF component gave whole body average SAR of 0.4 - 1.2 W/kg. There was no change in average heart rate or blood pressure immediately before and after MRI exposure. The authors concluded that whole body MRI exposure at 1.5 T is not associated with significant changes in heart rate or blood pressure.

Table 41. Cardiac function, blood flow and blood pressure

Authors	Endpoint	Exposure	Results	Comments
Static magnetic field studies				
(Kangarlu et al., 1999)	Body temperature, heart rate, respiratory rate, blood pressure, cognitive changes and ECG	8 T 1 h	No effect; although ECG changes were noted within normal range.	ECG's obtained during exposure could not be interpreted.
(Chakeres et al., 2003b)	ECG, heart rate, respiratory rate, systolic and diastolic blood pressures, finger pulse oxygenation levels, core body temperature	1.5 - 8 T 5 min	No clinically significant changes in vital signs. Systolic blood pressure increased with 8 T exposure. ECG rhythm strip analysis showed no significant post-exposure changes.	
(Hinman, 2002)	Heart rate and blood pressure	< 100 mT 15 min	No effect.	
(Jehenson et al., 1988)	Cardiac rhythm	1 - 2 T 1 h	Temporary increase in cardiac cycle length: 17% at 2 T, 10% at 1 T, and 0% at 0 T.	Harmless for healthy subjects, possible safety problem in dysrhythmic patients.
(Stick et al., 1991)	Blood flow in single thumb or forearm	0.4 - 0.5, 0.9 - 1 T 10 min	No blood flow change in the skin of the thumb and at the forearm.	No statistics.

(Mayrovitz et al., 2001)	Laser Doppler flowmetry (LDF) or laser Doppler imaging (LDI) perfusion in single hand	0.1 T 36 min	No detectable effect on skin blood perfusion in healthy subjects.	
(Martel et al., 2002)	Resting forearm blood flow and vascular resistance	30 min	No effect.	
(Weikl et al., 1989)	ECG	0.5 - 4 T 10 or 30 min	No arrhythmias, no changes in heart rate. Small reversible changes in ECG due to Hall effect.	
MRI or combined exposure studies				
(Shellock & Crues, 1987)	Heart rate and blood pressure	1.5 T 15 min	Whole body average SAR > 0.4 W/kg. Heart rate and average mean blood pressure not altered.	MRI exposure conditions.
Studies considered to be uninformative				
(Barker & Cain, 1985)				
(Sud & Sekhon, 1989)				
(Sakhnini & Khuzaie, 2001)				

8.1.2.2.2 Serum proteins and hormone levels

Male volunteers (N=35), 25 to 49 years old, were exposed to a static magnetic field of 9.6 mT during 40 minutes (Schmidt et al., 1999). A set of Helmholtz coils was used to produce the static field, which also created a ripple of time-varying magnetic fields 0.2 - 0.6% of the static field (19 - 57 µT). The subjects also spent a 40 min control period inside the coils without exposure, with one week between the two sessions. Urine and blood samples were taken before and after exposure and control sessions. An increase in serum and urinary creatinine was found after exposure. No change in calcium levels was observed. However, it is not possible to separate effects of the static magnetic field from the time varying field.

Healthy male volunteers (N=11), 23 - 43 years old, were exposed during the night to a static magnetic field from a 0.5 T interventional MRI unit (Haugsdal et al., 2001). Three beds were set up in the vicinity of the super-conducting coil, and exposure ranged from 1.2 - 13.7 mT at different locations in the beds. Total daily urine production was collected in four time intervals during the exposure day, the day after exposure and the control day 7 days after the exposure day. No effect on the excretion of 6-sulfatoxymelatonin was found. However, the number of subjects was too small to detect modest effects on melatonin production. The exposure situation did not resemble ordinary working conditions around an MRI system in terms of movements in varying static magnetic fields.

Table 42. Serum hormones and proteins

Authors	Endpoint	Exposure	Results	Comments
Static magnetic field studies				
(Schmidt et al., 1999)	Creatinine, calcium	9.6 mT 40 min	Increase in serum and urinary creatinine. No change in calcium levels.	Paper in Norwegian. Exposure to SMF + time varying field.
(Haugsdal et al., 2001)	Melatonin	1.2 - 13.7 mT 9 h	No effect on the excretion of 6-sulfatoxymelatonin.	Number of subjects too small to detect modest effects on melatonin levels. Nocturnal situation is not equal to normal work environments (e.g. movement while working, time varying fields).

8.1.2.3 Body and skin temperature

The effect of exposure to 1.5 T pure static magnetic fields for 20 min or 60 min on human body and skin temperature was investigated in three experiments performed by Shellock et al. (1986; 1989). The group size varied from 6 to 11 healthy volunteers for different experiments. Skin temperature was measured on the following sites: abdomen, forehead, upper arm, forearm, chest, thigh, calf and sublingual area. Body temperature was measured via an oesophageal tube. No significant temperature changes were found.

Chakeres et al. (2003b) studied 25 healthy volunteers, aged 24 - 53 years, exposed to static magnetic field strengths of 1.5, 3, 4.5, 6, and 8 T. Core body temperature was measured before, during, and after exposure. No change in core body temperature was found.

Shellock and Crues (1987) included 50 patients for clinical MRI imaging that were evaluated for core and skin temperatures. The study was done with a 1.5 T system, and the RF component gave a whole body average SAR of 0.4 - 1.2 W kg^{-1}. There was an average increase of core body temperature of 0.2 °C, but there was no correlation between change in body temperature and SAR.

The influence on deep body core and superficial body temperature of humans as the result of exposure to 0.35 T and 1.5 T pure static and RF fields was investigated in a total of 20 subjects in several experiments (Vogl et al., 1988). Outcomes were measured before, during and after exposure. No influence on the central body temperature (oesophagus and rectum), or on the superficial temperature (venous intravascular), was seen.

Table 43. Body and skin temperature

Authors	Endpoint	Exposure	Results	Comments
Static magnetic field studies				
(Shellock et al., 1986)	Body temperature	1.5 T 20, 60 min	No changes in core body temperature.	
(Shellock et al., 1989)	Body and skin temperatures	1.5 T 20 min	No significant changes of surface temperature at abdomen, forehead, upper arm, forearm, chest, thigh, calf and sublingual.	
(Chakeres et al., 2003b)	Core body temperature	1.5 - 8 T 5 min	No effect on core temperature.	
MRI or combined exposure studies				
(Shellock & Crues, 1987)	Temperature	1.5 T 15 min	Whole body average SAR > 0.4 W/kg. Core body temperature increased on average 0.2 °C.	MRI exposure conditions.
(Vogl et al., 1986) (Vogl et al., 1988)	Deep and superficial body temperatures	0.35 or 1.5 T exposure to SMF followed by imaging sequences	No temperature change due to MRI procedure, no change of core temperature (oesophagus, rectum) nor of the superficial temperature (venous intravascular).	No conclusion for skin and subcutaneous temperatures.

8.1.2.4 Dental exposure

Orthodontic magnets and implants are tools sometimes used nowadays in dental and oral medicine. Questions have been asked about the potential adverse health effects of static fields from these implants.

Bondemark et al. (1995; 1998) examined the effects of orthodontic magnets on the oral mucosa, the dental pulp and the gingival in a total of 15 patients (two studies, $N_1=7$, $N_2=8$ patients). The endpoints of those examinations were morphological and histological alterations of the surrounding tissue. The magnet and the demagnetised control magnet were bonded on molars on either side of the mouth. The static magnetic fields from the implants varied between 10 and 140 mT. The maximum observation period was 9 months. Some inflammations were detected in tissue close to both the magnet and demagnetised magnet, but not in other sites. Those were attributed to contact irritation rather than to the static magnetic field.

Table 44. Dental exposure

Authors	Endpoint	Exposure	Conclusions	Comments
Static magnetic field studies				
(Bondemark et al., 1995)	Tissue changes	10 - 90 mT 8 wk	No histologically detectable changes in human dental pulp or gingival tissues.	
(Bondemark et al., 1998)	Morphological, histological and immunohisto-chemical changes	80 - 140 mT 9 months	No difference found between control and test tissues. Observed minor tissue reactions were attributed to contact irritation with the magnet body.	

8.1.2.5 Therapeutic treatment

The impact of magnetism on human tissues and human health and its use in the therapeutic treatment is an ancient and contentious subject (Schenck, 2005) that remains so to the present (Whitaker & Adderly, 1998; Park, 2000). The studies are listed in Table 45.

Many of the studies on therapeutic effects share a number of methodological limitations, the most important being potential placebo effects due to lack of blinding and the fact that the field strengths were not adequately characterized.

Table 45. Therapeutic treatment
Authors
Studies considered to be uninformative
(Hong et al., 1982)
(Lin et al., 1985)
(Ivanov et al., 1990)
(Lud & Demeckiy, 1990)
(Caselli et al., 1997)
(Dexter, Jr., 1997)
(Vallbona et al., 1997)
(Bernhold & Bondemark, 1998)
(Man et al., 1999)
(Collacott et al., 2000)
(Holcomb et al., 2000)
(Alfano et al., 2001)
(Segal et al., 2001)
(Thomas et al., 2001)
(Suomi & Koceja, 2001)
(Carter et al., 2002)
(Hinman et al., 2002)
(Weintraub et al., 2003)

8.1.2.6 Conclusions

There are only very limited data available from human experimental studies on the potential effects of exposure to static electric fields. The results of the one small study that has investigated detection thresholds for static electric fields indicated that the perception threshold in people depends on various factors and ranges between 10 and 45 kV m^{-1}. Thresholds for annoyance from such sensations are probably equally variable, but have not been systematically studied. The study of combined electric fields from DC and AC high voltage power lines indicated the possibility of increased sensations of the combined exposure, but limitations of the experimental design, and lack of confirmative data, prevent any conclusions.

The available data do not indicate that there are effects of static magnetic field exposure on neurophysiological responses and cognitive functions in stationary volunteers, nor can they rule out such effects (since most of the performed studies are small and have several methodological limitations). A dose-dependent induction of vertigo and nausea was found in workers, patients and volunteers during movement in static fields greater than about 2 T. One study suggested that eye-hand coordination and near visual contrast sensitivity are reduced in fields adjacent to a 1.5 T MRI unit. The occurrence of all of these effects is likely to be dependent on the gradient of the field and the movement of the subject.

Flow potentials are induced in the major blood vessels and in the heart by the flow of blood with a static magnetic field. These electrical potentials are largest in the aorta, and occur during the T-wave of the cardiac cycle. In addition, the flow of blood in a vessel will experience a force opposing its motion. It has been estimated that the flow potentials will generate currents at the sino-atrial node of about 110 - 120 mA m^{-2} at 5 T, and about 200 mA m^{-2} at 10 T. It was predicted that the magnetohydrodynamic effect could lead to a reduction in blood flow in the aorta estimated to about 1% and 5%, respectively. A small change in blood pressure and heart rate was observed in some studies, but these were in the range of normal physiological variability.

There is no evidence of effects of static magnetic fields on other aspects of cardiovascular physiology, or on serum proteins and hormones. Exposure to static magnetic fields of up to 8 T does not appear to induce temperature changes in humans. However, most of the studies were very small, based on convenience samples, and often included non-comparable groups. Thus, it is not possible to draw any conclusions regarding the wide variety of end-points examined in this report.

Because of methodological limitations in available studies, it is not possible to draw any conclusions regarding the wide variety of reported therapeutic end-points.

8.2   Epidemiological studies

Epidemiological studies can provide direct information on the health of people exposed to static fields, and are therefore given the greatest weight in health risk assessment by WHO and IARC (Repacholi & Cardis, 1997). However, their observational nature makes it difficult to infer causal relationships, except when the evidence is strong or when findings are supported by experimental data. This is because they may be subject to bias (such as when the quality of information on EMF exposures obtained directly from diseased people differs from that obtained from people without the disease) and confounding factors. The latter may occur, for example, when workers exposed to EMFs are also exposed to other agents in the workplace that are strongly correlated to static fields and could affect disease risk.

Studies have been carried out almost exclusively on workers exposed to static magnetic fields generated by equipment using large DC currents (see chapter 3). Most workers were exposed to moderate static magnetic fields of up to several 10's mT either as welders, aluminium smelters, or workers in various industrial plants using large electrolytic cells in chemical separation processes. However, such work is also likely to have involved exposure to a variety of potentially hazardous fumes and aerosols, confounding interpretation. Health endpoints studied in these workers have included cancer incidence, haematological changes and related outcomes, chromosome aberration frequency, reproductive outcomes and musculoskeletal disorders. In addition, one study examined fertility and pregnancy outcome in female MRI operators, where the potential to have been exposed to relatively large static fields of up to ~ 1 T may have existed.

8.2.1 Cancer

8.2.1.1 Welders

A large number of studies have investigated cancer risks among welders. Unfortunately, none of the studies contained adequate exposure assessment for static fields and they thus do not allow for a meaningful analysis. Welders are also exposed to a varying degree to other potentially harmful agents, e.g. welding fumes, ELF and RF magnetic fields. Furthermore, most of the studies did not provide enough information to determine the type of welding used, further limiting the usefulness of this data in the review of potential health effects of static magnetic field exposure. Thus, the studies of welders are not reviewed in any detail. However, these studies are important, given a relatively high exposure to static fields in some of the welding processes. Two meta-analyses provide the most information. A meta-analysis of brain tumors in 38 studies of occupational EMF exposure (Kheifets et al., 1995) reported a small but significantly elevated risk for welders (relative risk [RR] = 1.25; 95% confidence interval [CI]: 1.06 - 1.47). Another meta-analysis of 29 occupational studies of leukaemia found no risk increase in welders (Kheifets et al., 1997).

8.2.1.2 Aluminium Workers

Various studies investigated the cancer risk in aluminium plant workers. In 1982 Andersen et al. reported overall mortality and cancer incidence in 7,410 male employees from 4 Norwegian aluminium plants (Andersen et al., 1982). The mortality in the cohort was compared to the general population, and the cancer incidence was compared to the incidence in the population living in the counties where the aluminium plants were located. Only lung cancer incidence was increased, but the risk was essentially confined to two production subgroups: workers with a short duration of employment and workers with a very long duration of employment in older plants. The interpretation of the results is restricted due to the healthy worker effects and the incomplete smoking histories.

Rockette and Arena (1983) studied a cohort of 27,829 male aluminium workers employed for ≥ 5 years between 1946 and 1977 in 14 reduction plants in the USA, comparing the mortality among aluminium workers to that of the general US male population. They reported a slightly higher than expected, but not statistically significant mortality from pancreatic, genito-urinary and lymphohaematopoietic cancers. Deaths from lymphohaematopoietic cancer were not confined to one subcategory of disease, or to one industrial process. As would be expected from a healthy worker effect, they found a reduced mortality from all cases of death, and also for several major causes of death such as all malignant neoplasms combined, cardiovascular disease, and diabetes mellitus. The healthy worker effect makes the modestly increased risks for some cancer sites interesting, despite the lack of statistical significance. Static magnetic fields were not measured, and other exposures (e.g. polycyclic aromatic hydrocarbons, PAH) were present in the same jobs. As a result, these could not be separated from exposure to static magnetic fields.

In a cohort study of aluminium reduction workers in France, Mur et al. (1987) analysed the mortality between 1950 and 1976 of 6,455 workers in order to assess occupational risks. The study focused on lung cancer risks from air pollutants. Cancer mortality (standardised mortality ratio [SMR] = 1.09; 95%-CI: 0.97 - 1.22) and mortality from all causes (SMR = 0.85; 95%-CI: 0.80 - 0.91) was not significantly increased compared to the general population. Although not statistically significant, an SMR of about 2 was observed for malignant tumours in the liver, brain, bone, skin and bladder. Analysis of workers involved in electrolysis, maintenance or smelting yielded statistically nonsignificant SMRs of 1.09, 1.03, and 0.80, respectively. The cancer risk of electrolysis workers decreased with length of employment. No exposure levels to static magnetic fields were reported. In addition to exposure to static magnetic fields, the workers were exposed to numerous chemicals such as coal tar pitch and PAH, substances that are known to increase the risk of some of these cancers. Only limited information about other confounding factors, e.g. smoking, was available. Information about cause of death could only be obtained for 71% of the cohort.

A cohort study was carried out in British Columbia, Canada, involving 4,213 male workers with ≥ 5 years of work experience at an aluminium reduction plant between 1954 and 1985 (Spinelli et al., 1991). The static magnetic fields usually generated in the plant ranged between 1 - 10 mT. The potential exposure to magnetic fields and to coal-tar pitch volatiles was determined for each job by industrial hygienists using a job-exposure matrix. Mortality and incidence rates were compared to the general male population. Potential confounding from smoking was controlled for in the analyses. The SMR in the total cohort was 0.77 (90% CI: 0.70 - 0.84) for all causes of death, and 2.2 (90% CI: 1.2 - 3.7) for tumours of the brain and central nervous system (International Code of Disease (ICD)-9 191, 192) and 1.8 (90% CI: 0.8 - 3.3) for leukaemia (ICD-9 204 - 208). For cancer incidence ascertained from 1970 onwards, the standardized incidence ratio (SIR) was 1.9 (90% CI: 0.97 - 3.5) for brain cancer (ICD-9 191), and 0.76 (90% CI: 0.21 - 2.0) for leukaemia. However, no individual cause of cancer death or incident cancer was related to cumulative exposure to magnetic fields, as estimated from the job-exposure matrix. The incidence of bladder cancer was strongly related to cumulative exposure to coal-tar pitch volatiles.

In 1995 Rønneberg and Andersen determined cancer morbidity in a cohort of 1,137 men working in a prebake smelter for at least 6 months during the period 1922 - 1975 (Rønneberg, 1995; Rønneberg & Andersen, 1995). The cohort was followed in the Norwegian Cancer registry during the period 1953 - 1991. In the prebake process, the anodes made from coke and coal tar paste are fabricated in a separate facility and then introduced into the electrolysis vessel. This is likely to result in reduced concentrations of air-borne polycyclic aromatic hydrocarbons and coal tar particulate volatiles as compared to the newer Söderberg process, where the electrodes are introduced as a liquid paste and hardened in the electrolysis vessel itself. The intensity of exposure to coal tar pitch volatiles, asbestos, pot emissions, heat stress, and magnetic fields had been previously assessed for all jobs at the smelter (Rønneberg, 1995). The cancer incidence in the cohort was compared to the incidence in the general male population. No association was found between static magnetic field exposure and cancers of the nervous system or haematopoietic system, but the number of observed cases was very small. There is probably some overlap between this study and the study by Andersen et al. (1982).

Rønneberg et al. (1999) studied cancer incidence in a population composed of 2,647 male short-term workers and two cohorts of men employed for at least four years in a Norwegian aluminium smelter (2,888 production workers and 373 maintenance workers). Of the 5,962 men who initially satisfied the inclusion criteria, six had died before the observation period started in 1953 and 48 were lost to follow-up. The remaining 5,908 men were linked to the files of the Norwegian Cancer Registry and followed up from 1953 (or date of first employment) until date of death or emigration, or the end of 1993. There was an association between exposure to coal tar pitch volatiles and bladder cancer. There was no association between static magnetic fields and cancers of the brain or lymphatic and haematopoietic tissues. Cancer incidence was not elevated in any of the cohorts when compared with the expected incidence calculated on the basis of the age- and calendar year-specific cancer incidence of all men in Norway applied to the person-years at risk among cohort members. In contrast, there was a significant positive association between employment as a maintenance electrician working mainly with 220-V alternating current and lymphatic and haematopoietic cancer, and a statistically nonsignificant association between PAH and lung cancer. The healthy worker effect may have caused an underestimation of potential effects. There was only limited control of confounding variables.

Milham (1982) calculated proportionate mortality ratios (PMR) for leukaemia and non-Hodgkin's lymphoma with respect to the occupation. In extended analyses of a larger material additional cancer sites were analysed (Milham, 1985). Elevated PMRs were found among aluminium workers for several cancer sites; pancreatic, lung, and haematological malignancies. The highest PMR was seen for acute leukaemia (PMR = 233) and for other lymphomas (PMR = 260). This study has numerous limitations, including cross-sectional design, unknown contribution of different exposure sources, and confounding from other exposures.

8.2.1.3 Chloralkali Plants

Barregård et al. (1985) studied cancer mortality and cancer incidence in a group of 157 male workers at a Swedish chloralkali plant compared to the general Swedish male population. The employees had all worked regularly or permanently for at least one year during the period 1951 - 1983 in the cell room where the electrolysis process took place and where they had been exposed to static magnetic fields (average: 14 mT). The investigators reported no excess incidence of, or mortality from, cancer. The results might be due to the healthy worker effect. Only unspecific outcomes were studied (all causes of death, all types of cancers combined). The study had poor statistical power.

The study was later expanded to include workers at eight chloralkali plants, a total of 1,190 men (Barregård et al., 1990). This study was focused on exposure to inorganic mercury, and no magnetic field measurements were made. An increased risk of lung cancer was observed. Workers at some of the plants were also exposed to asbestos, which could explain some of the observed risk increase. A slightly higher mortality from circulatory diseases was also noted. The healthy worker effect may have also affected the results in the expanded study. Information about smoking habits was not available. The statistical power was poor for specific cancer types.

Ellingsen et al. (1993) studied cancer incidence and mortality in 674 workers employed for the first time before 1980 at two Norwegian chloralkali plants. Cancer incidence and mortality were compared to expected rates in the general Norwegian male population, based on five year age groups and calendar years from 1953 - 1989. The main hypothesis concerned mercury vapour, and no magnetic field measurements were taken. A modest increase in lung cancer incidence was found. No risk increases were found for cancers of the nervous system or lymphatic and haematopoietic tissues. The overall mortality was close to that expected and there were no increased risk for any specific cause of death. The healthy worker effect is likely to have affected the results. There was no control for confounding factors, other than age and calendar. The study had poor statistical power.

8.2.2 Haematology, Immune Status and Blood Pressure

After the identification of a cluster of B-cell lymphoma in an aluminium reduction plant, Davis and Milham (1990) used a pilot study to investigate the immune status of 23 workers, as immuno-deficiency is a known risk factor for B-cell lymphoma. Out of the 350 employees, 44 volunteered for the study but only 23 could be included. Twenty of these workers worked in the potroom, where there was potential for high exposure to static magnetic fields as well as coal tar pitch. Three workers were considered as unexposed because they had never worked in the potroom. Potroom workers had significantly higher T8 levels (mean = 1,227 cells/µl) than non-potroom workers (mean = 558 cells/µl) or in comparison to normal for the general population values (median = 450 cells/µl). T4 levels were higher for potroom workers (mean = 1,017 cells/µl) than for non potroom workers (mean = 597 cells/µl) ($p < 0.1$) or normal values (median = 756 cells/µl). The subject selection procedure was not well described. In addition, there were only 3 unexposed subjects. Population values are reported as medians, which are likely to be lower than mean values. Smoking may be a confounding variable, but even the non-smoking potroom workers had higher T8 counts than the general population.

Tuschl et al. (2000) studied immune parameters in hospital personnel exposed to different sources of EMF. The immune parameters of 10 MRI workers (generally exposed to static magnetic fields of 0.5 mT in the operator room and occasionally to higher field strengths) did not differ from those of the control group (23 persons). Other immune parameters examined that showed no difference between exposed and unexposed workers included relative and absolute numbers of lymphocytic subsets, the proliferative activity of T and B cells, the production of interleukin 2, interferon gamma and tumour necrosis factor alpha, serum immunoglobulins, non-specific immunity of monocytes and granulocytes. The subject selection procedure was not well described. The MRI workers were an average of 10 years younger than the other groups, and smoking was half as prevalent. The actual individual exposure for the working group could not be measured and could only be roughly estimated.

Marsh et al. (1982) studied 320 exposed and 186 unexposed workers in various industrial plants using large electrolytic cells in chemical separation processes. The averaged static field level in the exposed work environment was 7.6 mT and the maximum field was 14.6 mT. Based on theoretical considerations, the authors separately examined vertical and horizontal components of magnetic fields. Horizontal fields were considered as most relevant with respect to induced currents. Vertical fields may be relevant for processes with a certain latency period, as only vertical fields remain constant over time in a moving upright body. The authors did not find major health problems in this population. While the mean values of both the exposed and unexposed groups were within the normal range, white cell counts were decreasing with increasing horizontal magnetic fields. The percentage of lymphocyte and percentage of monocyte increased with increasing horizontal magnetic field. An increase in the systolic and diastolic blood pressure with increasing exposure to the vertical component of the magnetic field was observed in black subjects. The opposite trend was observed in the whole study population, with a tendency for a decreasing systolic and diastolic pressure with increasing vertical magnetic field strength (p = 0.08). Results for whites and Hispanics were not reported. It was noted that the description of the results in the text did not always correspond to the numbers reported in the specified models. The subject selection procedure was not well described. The 320 exposed workers were likely to have been exposed to mercury and chlorine as well, whereas the unexposed group was not. Only large long-term health effects could have been detected in this small study population.

8.2.3 Chromosome Aberrations

Skyberg et al. (1993) compared chromosome aberration in the lymphocytes of 13 high voltage laboratory cable splicers with 20 referents not exposed to electric and magnetic fields. The cable splicers were generally exposed to static and alternating magnetic field strength of 5 - 15 μT. They could also occasionally be exposed to magnetic fields strengths up to 10 mT by touching the cable. Generally, no differences between exposed and unexposed workers were found. However, exposed smokers had more chromosome breaks than smokers, in comparison to the control group (based on 7 exposed smokers). It is not known what property of the EMF exposure, if any, was responsible for the observed effect. In addition, there were only a small number of subjects.

8.2.4 Reproduction

Several indicators of reproductive health were studied in aluminium and metal workers, as well as MRI operators.

Mur et al. (1998) compared the birth-rate of 692 potroom male workers exposed to static magnetic fields ranging from 4 - 30 mT to that from 588 unexposed male workers from the same aluminium plants (all blue-collar workers). The birth rate was calculated for each couple by dividing the number of children by the number of years since marriage. To control for cultural differences, only French men were included in the study. The authors found a statistically significant increase in the birth rate (relative birth-rate ratio of 1.1; $p < 0.001$). This result was interpreted as an indicator that the fertility of the male workers was not decreased due to exposure to static magnetic fields or heat. However, the age of the husband/wife was not controlled for in the analysis.

Irgens et al. (1997) studied the male proportion in offspring of workers in metal smelters, welders and workers involved in production of electric wires during the period 1970 - 1993. The male proportion among offspring to fathers and mothers not working in any of the investigated occupations were used as a reference. In total, 1.2 million births were included. Aluminium workers were exposed to static magnetic fields of up to 10 mT and to alternating fields of up to 0.1 mT. Workers in plants producing magnesium, nickel or iron were assumed to be exposed to 50 Hz magnetic fields up to 2 mT. The production of electric wire is associated with 50 Hz magnetic fields up to 0.015 mT, and occasional exposure of the hand to static and alternating magnetic fields of up to 10 mT. Common static and alternating field strengths to which the welders were reported to be exposed were 0.001 - 0.05 mT. The offspring of male aluminium workers or welders had a proportion of males similar to that of the unexposed population (RR = 0.98; 95% CI: 0.94 - 1.03, and RR = 1.01; 95% CI: 0.99 - 1.03, respectively). The offspring of women working in the smelter industry had a significantly reduced male proportion, which was particularly reduced for women working in the aluminium plants (RR = 0.72; 95% CI: 0.59 - 0.90, based on 81 exposed births). Exposure misclassification was very likely in this study because the job title was reported only every 10 years by an imprecise three digit coding system. There was no o control of any confounding factors, not even the age of the parents.

Evans et al. (1993) investigated infertility and pregnancy outcome in a cross-sectional study among MRI workers in the USA: 1,915 female

MRI operators reported 1,421 pregnancies, of which 287 pregnancies occurred during work as an MRI operator, the remaining during work in another job or while being a homemaker. The risk of miscarriage for pregnancies during MRI work was slightly (but not statistically significantly) increased compared to work in other jobs, and was considerably higher than the risk of homemakers. Minor differences were found for early delivery and low birth weight when compared to homemakers, but not when compared to other workers. The gender ratio of offspring in the same study was not changed (Kanal et al., 1993). There was no control for age: for example, women with pregnancies during work as MRI operators were markedly older than other groups. Homemakers below 30 years of age at pregnancy had a very low miscarriage rate, which may have influenced the risk estimate. Selection bias and reporting bias cannot be ruled out in this study, as it cannot be determined what proportion of the total female MRI workers participated in the study.

Baker et al. (1994) carried out limited follow-up of 20 children with a variety of abnormalities imaged *in utero* with 0.5 T echo planar MRI. Only case reports are presented, with no comparison group.

Myers et al. (1998) investigated effects on intrauterine growth following *in utero* exposure to MRI. A total of 74 pregnant volunteer women were recruited through advertisements, and underwent up to five MRI scans during pregnancy. A control group consisted of 148 unexposed pregnant women matched on maternal age, parity, ethnic origin, smoking history, and postcode. No effect was found on gestational age-adjusted birth weight, although unadjusted birth weights and gestational age were significantly lower in the MRI group. The study is small, and the results are difficult to interpret.

Clements et al. (2000) followed 20 children exposed to MRI for four times between 20 weeks to term and 35 unexposed children, from birth until 9 month of age. A small decrease in length was found in exposed children, and an increase in gross motor function. No other effects were found. It is unclear how the subjects were selected to be participants in the study, and no participation rates were reported. It seems likely that this was not a random sample, and that selection bias may therefore have affected the results. The statistical analyses were questionable. Furthermore, the number of children is very small, and thus only very large effects could have been detected.

8.2.5 *Musculoskeletal Symptoms*

A retrospective cohort study in an aluminium plant compared the occurrence of musculoskeletal symptoms during 1986 to 1991 among an exposed (N = 342) and an unexposed group (N = 277) of workers (Moen et al., 1995). Employees were exposed in potrooms to static magnetic fields between 3 and 20 mT, and to ripple components (alternating currents) as well. The unexposed group consisted of workers from the cast house, the rolling mill and transport workers. The exposed and unexposed groups had similar exposures to other risk factors for musculoskeletal disorders, e.g. chemical substances, vibration, work load, etc. The analysis was based on the symptoms reported to the occupational health care unit in 1986 and 1991. No difference was found between the exposed and unexposed groups. Further analyses focusing on sick leave due to musculoskeletal disorders also failed to detect an association to the exposure with static magnetic field (Moen et al., 1996). Selection bias may have been present if health is a consideration in the selection of workers to work in the potroom. Minor health problems may not have been included in this study, because they probably did not get reported to the health care unit.

8.2.6 Conclusions

The few epidemiological studies published to date leave a number of unresolved issues concerning the possibility of increased cancer risk from exposure to static magnetic fields. Assessment of exposure has been poor, and the number of participants in some of the studies has been very small, and thus these studies are able to detect only very large risks for such rare diseases. Most of the studies were conducted in aluminium plants or other smelter plants. The inability of these studies to provide useful information is supported by the lack of clear evidence for other, more established carcinogenic factors present in some of the work environments studies. Other non-cancerous health effects have been considered even more sporadically. Most of these studies are based on very small numbers and have numerous methodological limitations. Other environments with a potential for high fields have not been adequately evaluated, e.g. MRI operators. In short, there is insufficient material for a health evaluation.

Table 46. Epidemiology

Authors	Population	Endpoint	Type	Exposure	Results	Comments
Cancer						
Aluminium workers						
(Andersen et al., 1982)	7,410 male employees from 4 Norwegian aluminium plants	Mortality and cancer incidence	Cohort	SMF: no levels stated	Increased lung cancer incidence; essentially only in workers with short duration of employment and workers with very long duration of employment in older plants.	Interpretation of results restricted due to healthy worker effects and incomplete smoking histories.
(Rockette & Arena, 1983)	21,829 workers in the aluminium industry	Mortality	Cohort	SMF: 4 - 50 mT	Cancer of pancreas (p<0.01); leukaemia (n.s.).	Healthy worker effect makes modestly increased risks for some cancer sites interesting despite lack of statistical significance. SMF not measured. Other exposures, e.g. PAH, could not be separated from SMF exposure.

(Mur et al., 1987)	6,455 workers in French aluminium plants between 1950 and 1976	Mortality	Cohort	SMF: no levels stated	No increased cancer mortality and mortality from all causes.	No SMF exposure levels reported. Also exposure to numerous chemicals such as coal tar pitch and PAH, that are known to increase risk of some cancers. Limited information on other confounding factors, e.g. smoking. Information on cause of death only obtained for 71% of the cohort.
(Spinelli et al., 1991)	4,213 workers of an aluminium plant in BC, Canada	Mortality and cancer incidence	Cohort	SMF: no levels stated	All causes of mortality: SMR=0.77; all cancer: SMR=0.92; brain cancer: SMR=2.2 (1.2 - 3.1); bladder cancer: SMR=1.7 (1.1 - 2.6).	
(Rønneberg & Andersen, 1995) (Rønneberg et al., 1999)	5,908 workers in Norwegian aluminium smelters	Mortality and cancer morbidity	Cohort	SMF: 2 - 10 mT ELF: 0.3 - 10 µT	No increased risk for brain cancer and lymphatic and haemopoietic tissue cancer. Increased leukaemia risk for employment as an electrician.	Possible underestimation of potential effects due to healthy worker effect. Limited confounding control. Probably some overlap with Andersen et al., (1982).

(Milham, 1985)	12,714 death records of 'electrical' workers	Mortality	Cross-sectional	SMF: possible exposure	Acute leukaemia: PMR=162; other lymphomas: PMR=164.	Numerous limitations, e.g. cross-sectional design, unknown contribution of different exposure sources.

Chloralkali Plants

(Barregård et al., 1985)	157 exposed men in a chloralkali plant engaged in the electrolytic production of chlorine	Cancer mortality and incidence	Cohort	SMF: 4 - 29 mT	Mortality: SMR= 0.8 (0.4 - 1.3); cancer: SIR=0.8 (0.3 - 1.9).	Results might be due to healthy worker effect. Unspecific outcomes (all causes of death, all types of cancers combined). Poor statistical power.
(Barregård et al., 1990)	1,190 exposed men in eight chloralkali plants	Mortality and cancer incidence	Cohort	SMF: no levels stated	Slightly increased cardio-vascular mortality, increased lung cancer incidence.	Healthy worker effect possible, comparison to general population. Poor statistical power for specific cancer types. Limited confounding control.
(Ellingsen et al., 1993)	674 exposed men in two chloralkali plants	Mortality and cancer incidence	Cohort	SMF: no levels stated	Slightly increased lung cancer risk. Incidence of all cancers combined and total mortality close to unity.	Healthy worker effect possible, comparison to general population. Poor statistical power. Limited confounding control.

Haematology, immune status and blood pressure

(Davis & Milham, 1990)	20 exposed potroom workers and 3 unexposed worker from the same plant	Immune status	Cross-sectional	SMF: no levels stated	More T8 cells ($p<0.05$) and T4 cells ($p<0.1$).	Selection procedure not well described. Only 3 unexposed subjects. Population values reported as medians (likely to be lower than means). Smoking may be a confounding factor, but even non-smoking potroom workers had higher T8 counts than general population value.
(Tuschl et al., 2000)	Hospital personnel: 10 MRI worker 10 workers at induction heaters 23 controls	Immune para-meters	Cross-sectional	MRI: SMF: 0.5 T (operator room) Induction heater: ELF/IF (50 Hz - 21.3 kHz): 2 mT	No effects on number of natural killer cells and oxidative burst in monocytes in MRI workers.	Selection procedure not well described. Exposed and unexposed groups not comparable in terms of age and smoking habits.

(Marsh et al., 1982)	320 workers exposed to SMF from electrolytic cells and 186 unexposed workers	General health indicators	Cross-sectional	SMF: mean = 7.6 mT, max = 14.6 mT	Decrease in white cell counts. Increase in lymphocyte and monocyte percentages. No effects on red cell count haemoglobin and haematocrit reading. Only in people of colour: increase in systolic and diastolic pressure.	Selection procedure not well described. SMF-exposed workers likely to be also exposed to mercury and chlorine, whereas unexposed group was not. Exposure to magnesium dust likely for exposed and unexposed workers.
Chromosome aberrations						
(Skyberg et al., 1993)	13 high voltage laboratory employees and 20 referents	Chromosome aberrations	Cross-sectional	Static or 50 Hz B-field: 5 - 15 µT, sometimes up to 10 mT Static or alternating E-field 5 - 10 kV/m	More chromosome aberrations in exposed smokers than in non-exposed smokers.	Small numbers of subjects. Not known what property of EMF exposure, if any, is responsible for observed effect.
Reproduction						
(Mur et al., 1998)	692 potroom workers in aluminium plants and 588 controls from the same plants	Birth rate	Cross-sectional	SMF: 4 - 30 mT	Birth rate ratio exposed/ control: 1.1 (p<0.001).	Not controlled for the age of husband/wife.

(Irgens et al., 1997)	Norwegian workers in metal reduction plants and electric wire production	Offspring sex ratio	Register	SMF: up to 10 mT ELF: up to 1 mT	Male: smelter works: RR=0.97 (0.92 - 1.02) wire production: RR=0.92 (0.80 - 1.05) welders: RR=1.01 (0.99 - 1.03) Female: aluminium works: RR=0.72 (0.59 - 0.90) all smelter works: RR=0.88 (0.79 - 0.99)	Exposure misclassificati on very likely, because job title reported only every 10 years by an imprecise three digit coding system. No control of confounding factors, not even age of parents.
(Evans et al., 1993) (Kanal et al., 1993)	1,915 female MRI technol- ogists and nurses from USA	Infertility and pregnancy outcome	Cross- sectional	SMF: 6% of working hours: 0.5 - 2 T 6% of working hours: 10 mT remaining time: < 10mT	MRI vs other workers: miscarriage: relative risk ratio (RRR)=1.3 (0.9 - 1.8) early delivery: RRR=1.2 (0.8 - 1.9) low birthweight: RRR=1.0 (0.5 - 2.0) MRI vs home- makers: miscarriage: RRR=3.2 (1.7 - 6.0) early delivery: RRR=1.7 (0.9 - 3.4) low birthweight: RRR=1.5 (0.5 - 4.41)	Women with pregnancies during work as an MRI operator markedly older than other groups. Pregnant homemakers below age 30 had a very low miscarriage rate - may have influenced risk estimate. Possible selection and reporting bias. Unknown participation rate of female MRI workers.

(Baker et al., 1994)	20 exposed children, no un-exposed comparison group	Hearing deficit	Appear to be case reports	0.5 T echo planar MRI	No effect found at 8 months hearing test.	No quantitative data. Varying follow-up time. Sound levels not reported.
(Myers et al., 1998)	74 children exposed to MRI *in utero*	Intra-uterine growth	Cohort	Up to five MRI scans *in utero*	No effect on gestational age-adjusted birth weight. Lower unadjusted birth weight and lower gestational age in exposed children.	Exposed participants recruited through advertisement
(Clements et al., 2000)	20 children exposed to MRI *in utero*, and 35 unexposed children	Develop-ment at 9 month of age	Cohort	Four MRI scans *in utero*	Small decrease in length, increase in gross motor function.	Subject selection procedure not described. Statistical analyses are questionable.
Musculoskeletal system						
(Moen et al., 1995) (Moen et al., 1996)	342 exposed potroom workers in an aluminium plant and 277 unexposed workers from the same plants	Symptoms of musculo-skeletal system	Cohort	SMF: 3 - 20 mT and ELF ripple components	Musculo-skeletal symptoms from neck, shoulders, arms: OR=0.9 (0.3 - 4.0). Musculo-skeletal symptoms from back, hips, legs: OR=1.1 (0.3 - 3.2).	Possible exposure to coal tar pitch. Selection bias may be present if health is a consideration in the selection of workers to work in the potroom. Minor health problems may not be included in study (probably not reported to health care unit).

9 HEALTH RISK ASSESSMENT

In this chapter, the possible impact on human health from exposure to static electric or static magnetic fields is assessed from the reviews of the epidemiological and biological data, along with the information on exposure indicated in the preceding chapters.

9.1 Static electric field effects

Static electric fields occur naturally in the atmosphere. Values of up to 3 kV m-1 can occur under thunderclouds, but in fair weather they generally are of order of 100 V m^{-1}. The most common cause of human exposure is charge separation as a result of friction. For example, , charge potentials of several kilovolts can be accumulated when walking on non-conducting carpets, generating local fields of up to 500 kV m^{-1}. Direct current (DC) power transmission can produce static electric field strengths of up to 20 kV m^{-1}, rail systems using DC can generate fields of up to 300 V m^{-1} inside the train, and VDUs create electric fields of around 10 - 20 kV m^{-1} at a distance of 30 cm.

Static electric fields do not penetrate electrically conductive objects such as the human body. The field induces a surface electric charge and is always perpendicular to the body surface. A sufficiently large surface charge density may be perceived through its interaction with body hair and by other effects such as spark discharges (microshocks). The perception threshold in people depends on various factors and can range between 10 - 45 kV m^{-1}. Thresholds for annoyance from such sensations are probably equally variable, but have not been systematically studied. Painful microshocks can be expected when a person who is well insulated from the ground touches a grounded object, or when a grounded person touches a conductive object that is well insulated from ground. However, the threshold static electric field values will vary depending on the degree of insulation and other factors.

Few animal studies of static electric field effects have been carried out. The overall results do not suggest that exposure is associated with adverse health effects.

There are no studies on exposure to static electric fields from which to make any conclusion on chronic or delayed effects. IARC (2002) noted that there was insufficient evidence to determine the carcinogenicity of static electric fields.

9.2 Static magnetic field effects

The geomagnetic field varies over the Earth's surface between about 35 - 70 µT and is implicated in the orientation and migratory behaviour of certain animal species. Man-made static magnetic fields are generated wherever DC currents are used, such as in some transportation systems powered by electricity, industrial processes such as aluminium production, and in arc welding. Magnetic flux densities of up to 2 mT have been reported inside electric trains and in modern magnetic levitation (MagLev) systems. Workers are exposed to larger fields in arc welding, where fields of around 5 mT are present close to the welding cables, and in the electrolytic reduction of alumina where fields of up to around 60 mT are encountered.

The advent of superconductors in the 1970's and 80's facilitated the use of much larger magnetic fields in medical diagnosis through the development of magnetic resonance imaging (MRI) and spectroscopy (MRS). It is estimated that some 200 million MRI scans have been performed worldwide. Most scanners operate at 1 to 3 T, and MRI exposures include pulsed magnetic and radiofrequency fields. Typically, static magnetic flux density is only 0.5 mT at the operator's console, but it may be higher. However, occupational exposure > 1 T can occur during the construction, testing and maintenance of these devices, as well as during certain medical procedures carried out in MRI. Machines of 7 - 8 T are being installed at a few sites and the first 9.4 T MRI system was installed in 2003. Both are associated with higher exposures. Various research and high energy technologies also employ superconductors where workers can be repeatedly exposed to fields as high as 2 T for periods of up to a few hours per day.

A major difficulty in the assessment of the effects of exposure to static magnetic fields is the paucity of relevant data. There have been few studies of possible long-term health effects in exposed people, particularly in fields of ~ 1 T and above. The likelihood of there being such effects can be assessed, in the first instance, from a consideration of physical interaction mechanisms. Three broad categories of effects can be recognized; namely, a) electrodynamic interactions with ionic conduction currents; b) magnetomechanical effects, including the orientation of magnetically anisotropic structures in a uniform field and the translation of paramagnetic and ferromagnetic materials in magnetic field gradients; and c) effects on the electron spin states of radical pair intermediates in certain types of metabolic reactions. The second effect represents generally weak interactions because the magnetic susceptibility of most biological material is very small and therefore significant mostly at flux densities greater than 1 T.

Ionic currents interact with static magnetic fields as a result of the Lorentz forces exerted on moving charge carriers, giving rise to an induced electric field and exerting a force opposing the motion. Examples of such processes are the ionic currents associated with the flow of blood, and the movement of ions through channels in cell membranes. Thresholds for significant interactions with the movement of ions in ion channels are thought to be around 24 T. However, measurable flow potentials are generated in major blood vessels around the heart in fields above ~ 0.1 T and their possible physiological consequences are discussed below. The magnetohydrodynamic forces opposing the blood flow could become increasingly physiologically significant at much higher flux densities.

Movement of the whole or part of the body, e.g. eyes and head, in a static magnetic field gradient will also induce an electric field and current during the period of movement. Dosimetric calculation suggests that such induced electric fields will be substantial during normal movement around or within fields > 2 - 3 T, and may account for the numerous anecdotal reports of vertigo and occasional magnetic phosphenes experienced by patients, volunteers and workers during movement in the field. These effects are discussed in greater detail below.

Magnetomechanical interactions in a magnetic field exert a torque on macromolecules and structurally ordered molecular assemblies that exhibit magnetic anisotropy, causing them to tend to rotate. Such effects can be seen *in vitro* at fields > 1 T and may play a role in orientation of magnetotactic bacteria and other organisms sensitive to the geomagnetic field. The significance of this, if any, to human health is unclear. A second major type of magnetomechanical interaction is the translation of paramagnetic and ferromagnetic substances in static magnetic field spatial gradients. However, most biological materials are only weakly diamagnetic. A few, for example de-oxygenated red blood cells, are weakly paramagnetic, but the force exerted on them even at 4 T is very small compared to gravity. The forces exerted on ferromagnetic objects such as metal tools pose dangers due to their acceleration in strong magnetic field gradients. Of particular concern in MRI, are electromagnetic interference (EMI) with the normal functioning of pacemakers and other implantable medical devices, and the physical forces on these and other implanted metal objects (such as aneurysm clips).

Several classes of organic chemical reactions can be influenced by static magnetic fields in the range from 10 to 100 mT as a result of effects on the electron spin states of the reaction intermediates. Studies carried out *in vitro* have shown that some metabolic reactions of this type can be affected. It is considered that it is unlikely that there will be major effects of physiological consequence, or even long-term mutagenic effects, arising from magnetic field induced changes in free radical concentration or fluxes.

9.2.1 Physiological responses

Mechanistic considerations and volunteer studies of acute effects from short-term exposure to static fields in the tesla range and field gradients point to the following effects: the induction of electrical potentials (flow potentials) around the major blood vessels close to and within the heart, and an increase in the resistance to blood flow in these vessels; and the induction of electrical potentials and eddy currents in the body caused by physical movement within an high static field gradient, resulting for example in vertigo and nausea during head movement. These latter effects have also been attributed to magnetohydrodynamic effects on the vestibular organs of the inner ear.

9.2.1.1 Flow potentials and reduced blood flow

Flow potentials result from Lorentz forces acting on moving charges and are generally associated with ventricular contraction and the ejection of blood into the aorta in animals and humans. The Lorentz interaction also results in a 'magnetohydrodynamic' force opposing the flow of blood. The reduction in aortic blood flow predicted at 5, 10 and 15 T is about 1%, 5% and 10%, respectively.

Theoretical considerations indicate that flow potentials generated by blood flow in coronary arteries may be of greater physiological significance than those generated in the aorta. The consequences of flow potentials for health are less clear. Three possibilities have been considered: changing the rate of excitation of the heart by acting on the sinoatrial pacemaker tissues, inducing the ectopic initiation of activity at sites that are not normally endogenously active, and altering the pattern of action potential propagation through the ventricular myocardium, which could be potentially arrhythmogenic. Calculations on healthy hearts suggest that the first two effects have thresholds in excess of 8 T. It is more difficult to assess the threshold for initiating potentially lethal re-entrant arrhythmias by disturbing the pattern of action potential propagation. It is important to note that these calculations have not been validated by experimental investigation, although the paper of Chakares (2005) contains some information on this.

Changes in blood pressure and heart rate were observed in some studies of healthy volunteers, but not in others. The observed changes were within the range of normal physiology. The methodological limitations of the available studies are such, however, that it is not generally possible to draw conclusions about the effects of static magnetic fields on these endpoints.

Mammalian studies do not provide strong evidence for or against effects on the cardiovascular system when exposed to static magnetic fields up to 8 T.

9.2.1.2 Movement-induced electric potentials and related effects

Physical movement within a static field gradient, such as that occurring at the entrance to an MRI scanner and head movement within the scanner, has been reported to induce transient sensations of vertigo and nausea, and sometimes phosphenes and a metallic taste in the mouth. Occurrence of these effects is likely to be dependent on the gradient of the field and the movement of the subject. Such effects have been reported in volunteers, workers and patients exposed to static fields in excess of about 2-4 T. Such effects are also consistent with the results of animal studies in which aversive behaviour and conditioned avoidance was induced in laboratory rodents following exposure to static fields of 4 T and above.

It is conceivable that such effects, although only transient, may adversely affect people within such magnetic fields and field gradients. The available studies do not indicate that there are effects of static magnetic field exposure on neurophysiological responses and cognitive functions in stationary volunteers, nor can they rule out such effects. One study suggested that eye-hand coordination and near visual contrast sensitivity are reduced in fields adjacent to a 1.5 T MRI unit. The potential of such effects affecting the optimal performance of workers carrying out delicate procedures (e.g. surgeons) must be highlighted. Steps taken to mitigate these effects include moving slowly in and around magnets. However, the electric fields and currents induced in people working in such fields have not been clearly defined.

9.2.1.3 Other physiological responses

With regard to effects on the circulatory system, a number of researchers have reported that exposure of laboratory animals to fields up to several tesla (but sometimes as weak as the geomagnetic field of 35 - 70 µT) variously affect skin blood flow, arterial blood pressure and other cardiovascular parameters. However, these endpoints are rather labile, a situation which may have been complicated by pharmacological manipulation (including anaesthesia in some cases) and immobilisation.

A few studies in rats indicated a possible temporary or weak dysfunction of the blood brain barrier following a short clinical MRI procedure. At present, there is inadequate data to evaluate risks to human health.

Some laboratories have looked for effects of static magnetic fields on hormones, mostly the production and release of melatonin from the pineal gland. Several studies from one laboratory suggested that the inversion of the horizontal component of the geomagnetic field can affect pineal melatonin synthesis and content.

It is difficult to reach any firm conclusion without independent replication of these studies.

9.2.2 Reproduction and development

The available evidence from epidemiological studies is not sufficient to draw any conclusions about potential reproductive and developmental effects of exposure to static magnetic fields encountered in occupational environments, including MRI. The few studies that were available had severe methodological limitations.

Studies of possible reproductive and developmental effects on mammalian species are most relevant to humans. No adverse effects have been demonstrated in such studies, but few have been carried out, especially in excess of 1 T. The MRI studies, taken as a whole, were inconclusive. The animal numbers were small, the data variable and the effect, if any, impossible to disentangle from the effects of pulsed gradient magnetic or RF fields, or other potential stressors.

9.2.3 Cancer and genotoxicity

The few epidemiological studies published to date concerning the possibility of increased cancer risk from exposure to static magnetic fields leave a number of unresolved issues. Assessment of exposure has been poor, and the numbers of participants in these studies have been very small. Most of the studies were conducted in aluminium and other smelter plants. Inability of these studies to provide useful information is supported by lack of clear evidence for other, more established, carcinogenic factors present in some of the work environments. The evidence from animal studies concerning carcinogenesis is inconclusive, since too few studies have been carried out.

From the limited number of animal studies that have been published, there is no evidence that static fields of less than 1 T are genotoxic. However, while one study reported an increased frequency of micronuclei following exposure at fields of 3 or 4.7 T, there has been no replication of this work.

No genotoxic effects have been seen in *in vitro* studies following static magnetic field exposures of up to 7 T. Investigations of the combined action of static magnetic field exposure and known mutagens have shown variable results. Conclusions about synergistic effects on genotoxicity cannot be made without confirmation in mammalian studies.

9.3 Conclusions

9.3.1 Chronic and delayed effects

Electric fields

There are no studies of exposure to static electric fields from which to make any conclusion on chronic or delayed effects. IARC (2002) noted that there was insufficient evidence to determine the carcinogenicity of static electric fields.

Magnetic fields

With regard to static magnetic fields, the available evidence from epidemiological and laboratory studies is not sufficient to draw any conclusions about chronic and delayed effects. IARC (2002) concluded that there was inadequate evidence in humans for the carcinogenicity of static magnetic fields, and no relevant data available from experimental animals. They are therefore not at present classifiable as to their carcinogenicity to humans.

9.3.2 Acute effects

Electric fields

Few studies of static electric field effects have been carried out. On the whole, the results suggest that the only adverse acute health effect is associated with direct perception of fields and discomfort from microshocks.

Magnetic fields

Short-term exposure to static magnetic fields in the tesla range and associated field gradients revealed a number of acute effects.

Cardiovascular responses, such as changes in blood pressure and heart rate, have been occasionally observed in human volunteer and animal studies. However, these were within the range of normal physiology for exposure to static magnetic fields up to 8 T.

Although not experimentally verified, it is important to note that calculations suggest three possible effects of induced flow potentials: minor changes in the rate of heart beat (which may be considered to have no health consequences), the induction of ectopic heart beats (which may be more physiologically significant), and an increase in the likelihood of re-entrant arrhythmia (possibly leading to ventricular fibrillation). The first two effects are thought to have thresholds in excess of 8 T, while threshold values for the third are difficult to assess at present because of modelling complexity. Some 5 - 10 per 10,000 people are particularly susceptible to re-entrant arrhythmia, and the risk to such people may be increased by exposure to static magnetic fields and gradient fields.

The limitations of the available data are such, however, that it is not possible to draw firm conclusions about the effects of static magnetic fields on the endpoints considered above.

Physical movement within a static field gradient is reported to induce sensations of vertigo and nausea, and sometimes phosphenes and a metallic taste in the mouth, for static fields in excess of about 2 - 4 T. Although only transient, such effects may adversely affect people. Together with possible effects on eye-hand coordination, the optimal performance of workers executing delicate procedures (e.g. surgeons) could be reduced, along with a concomitant reduction in safety.

Effects on other physiological responses have been reported, but it is difficult to reach any firm conclusion without independent replication.

This risk assessment for static fields has been conducted with all the scientific information available. This has involved identifying whatever health risks can be determined and quantified. Nonetheless, the severe lack of information has meant that it has not been possible to properly characterise the risks from static field exposure. There are indications, from modelling studies and/or some observations in people, of field levels that could elicit acute effects. However, the information on long-term and delayed effects is insufficient to characterize risk, only general statements can be made, and these rely on very few well-conducted studies. Having identified large gaps in knowledge, research recommendations have been made in Chapter 1.

10   RECOMMENDATIONS FOR NATIONAL AUTHORITIES

It is recommended that national authorities implement programs that protect both the public and workers from any untoward effects of static fields. However, given that the main effect of static electric fields is discomfort from electric discharge to tissues of the body, the protective program could merely be the provision of information about situations that could lead to exposure to large electric fields and how to avoid them.

A program is needed to protect against established acute effects of static magnetic fields. Because insufficient information is currently available on possible long-term or delayed effects of exposure, cost-effective precautionary measures may be needed to limit exposures of workers and the public. Basic protective measures needed to avoid direct and ancillary effects of exposure, and information on exposure standards, form the main protective measures for people exposed to strong static magnetic fields.

National authority recommendations are reported below:

10.1   Exposure guidelines and standards

National authorities should adopt standards based on sound science that limit the exposure of people to static magnetic fields. Implementation of health-based standards provides the primary protective measure for workers and the public.

International standards exist for static magnetic fields (ICNIRP, 1994) and are described in Appendix 1. However, WHO recommends that these be reviewed in light of more recent evidence from the scientific literature.

10.2   Device standards

WHO urges technical standards bodies to continue the development of appropriate technical standards related to the design and manufacture of devices that use static magnetic fields, especially MRI units.

To ensure patient safety, standards should continue to be updated on MRI compatibility of medical implanted devices (see: http://www.astm.org/).

10.3   Protective measures and ancillary hazards

National authorities should establish or complement existing programs that provide protection against possible effects from exposure to static magnetic fields. As described below, protective measures for the

218

industrial and scientific use of magnetic fields can be categorized as engineering design controls, the use of separation distance, and administrative controls. Another general category of hazard control measures, namely personal protective equipment (e.g., special garments and face masks), is not effective for magnetic fields.

Protective measures against the ancillary hazards from magnetic interference with surgical and dental implants or with emergency or medical electronic equipment are a special area of concern. In addition, the mechanical forces imparted to ferromagnetic implants and loose ferromagnetic objects in high-field facilities also require that precautions be taken.

The techniques to prevent needless exposure to high intensity magnetic fields generally fall into three categories, namely,

(a)   **Distance and time**

This entails limiting human access to and/or length of occupancy in locations where field strengths may pose a significant risk. Since the external magnetic flux density decreases with distance from the source, separation distance is a fundamental protective measure. For example, at large distances from a static magnetic field dipole source (i.e. distance >> diameter of source), the field decreases approximately as the reciprocal of the cube of the separation distance.

(b)   **Magnetic shielding**

The use of ferromagnetic core materials restricts the spatial extent of external flux lines of a magnetic device. External enclosures of ferromagnetic materials can also 'capture' flux lines and reduce external flux densities. However, shielding is normally an expensive control measure and of limited use for scientific instruments. Furthermore, it has not generally been shown to be cost-effective when compared with the use of separation distance for large installations (Hassenzahl et al., 2004).

(c)   **Administrative measures**

There are a number of administrative measures that can lead to significant reductions in exposure to magnetic fields:

•   pre-employment or pre-placement medical examinations are needed to ensure that any prospective staff member has no medical condition that would preclude working around strong magnetic fields, or has no implanted medical devices or metallic implants that could be affected by the magnetic field and lead to some adverse health outcome;

- educational programs for staff who need to work around static magnetic fields are needed so that they can have the information necessary to minimize their exposure and be able to work safely around strong magnetic fields;

- warning signs should be posted and special access areas identified to limit exposure of personnel near strong magnet facilities;

- loose ferromagnetic and paramagnetic objects can be converted into dangerous missiles when subjected to magnetic field gradients. Avoidance of this hazard can only be achieved by removing loose metallic objects from the area of the magnet and from personnel;

- in some circumstances, for example in MRI facilities, a combination of shielding, restricted access, and the use of metal detectors may be appropriate to avoid detrimental effects from exposure to magnetic fields.

10.4 Ancillary hazards: implantable medical devices

Electromagnetic interference (EMI) with the normal functioning of pacemakers and other implantable medical devices, and the physical forces on these and other implanted metal objects such as aneurysm clips, etc. are of particular concern in MRI. Certain types of cardiac pacemakers exhibit malfunctions in response to EMI.

Pacemaker malfunctions can also be caused by MRI static magnetic fields, which produce closure of a reed relay switch used to test the pacemaker's performance while operating in a fixed rate pacing mode.

This indicates a requirement for effective controls to prevent patients bearing medical implants from being adversely affected by the fields present in MRI devices.

In addition, possible effects of fields on medical implants should be addressed by competent technical bodies.

10.5 Optimal performance of workers in static magnetic fields

Movement-induced electric potentials and related effects during physical movement within static magnetic field gradients could lead to induced sensations of vertigo and nausea, phosphenes and metallic taste in the mouth, as well as possible effect on eye-hand coordination and near visual contrast sensitivity.

These effects can occur during body or head movement within the magnetic field, thereby having a possible negative influence on the performance of workers during critical procedures at that time. This also poses a potential safety risk.

Steps that can be taken to mitigate these effects should focus on general recommendations to move slowly and to limit sudden head movements, and on awareness notification and training.

10.6 Precautionary measures

Since there is still considerable uncertainty in the available information about possible health effects from exposure to static magnetic fields, national authorities might want to consider implementing precautionary measures that ensure that peoples' exposures are well below the standards. However, such precautionary measures should not undermine the scientific base of the limits by arbitrary reductions in the limits values. Rather, various engineering, administrative and work practice measures should be considered.

WHO is developing a precautionary framework for the reasonable and cost-effective development of precautionary options. Readers should refer to: www.who.int/emf for the latest version of this framework.

10.7 Patient exposure to MRI

WHO recognizes the benefit received by patients undergoing magnetic resonance procedures. However, the static magnetic and other fields to which the patient is exposed are greatly in excess of those normally encountered by the general public or by workers. WHO therefore recommends that patients (and volunteers) undergoing such procedures should be informed of the nature of the associated benefits and risks. The risks are those associated with the direct effects of the fields on the body, as reviewed and assessed in this document, and those associated with indirect effects such as the electromagnetic interference on implanted medical devices and the movement of metal objects in the body.

10.8 Protection program

The American College of Radiology has published a comprehensive set of safety and protective measures for working in MRI units and for patient management (Kanal et al., 2002). These should be implemented as part of a basic protective program for MRI units.

10.9 Licensing

National authorities should consider licensing MRI units in order to ensure that protective measures are implemented. This would also allow additional requirements to be complied with for MRI units with strengths in excess of local national standards or 2 T. Such requirements relate to provision of information on patients and workers, and any incidents or injuries resulting from the strong magnetic fields.

10.10 Research

Given the large gaps in knowledge that pertain to the safety of people exposed to static magnetic fields, national authorities should fund research to fill these gaps. Recommendations for further research form part of this document and are posted on the WHO web site: www.who.int/emf. Researchers should be funded to conduct studies recommended in this WHO research agenda.

Since higher and higher magnetic field strengths are being introduced, and little scientific information is available regarding their safety, it is recommended that national authorities fund MRI units to:

- collect information on worker exposure to static magnetic fields and make it available for epidemiological studies;

- collect information on patients subjected to MRI procedures. This information should be in a form useful for future epidemiological studies;

- require that facilities operating MRI units collect and provide, to a central agency, any information on incidents and injuries that result from use of MRI units with strengths in excess of 3 T.

National authorities should fund databases collecting information on exposures to workers where high long-term exposures occur, such as those involved in the manufacture of MRI or similarly high strength magnets, and new technologies such as MagLev trains.

11. REFERENCES

ABLE K.P. & ABLE M.A. (1993) Daytime calibration of magnetic orientation in a migratory bird requires a view of skylight polarization. Nature, **364** 523-525.

ACGIH - AMERICAN CONFERENCE OF GOVERNMENTAL INDUSTRIAL HYGIENISTS (2001) Documentation of the Threshold Limit Values and Biological Exposure Indices, 7th ed. Cincinnati, OH: American Conference of Governmental Industrial Hygienists.

ADAIR R.K. (1991) Constraints on biological effects of weak extremely-low-frequency electromagnetic fields. Phys Rev A, **43**(2): 1039-1048.

ADAIR R.K. (2000) Static and low-frequency magnetic field effects: health risks and therapies. Rep Prog Phys, **63** 415-454.

AGNIR - ADVISORY GROUP ON NON-IONISING RADIATION (1994) Health Effects related to the use of Visual Display Units. Report of and Advisory Group on Non-Ionising Radiation. Doc NRPB, **5**(2).

AGNIR - ADVISORY GROUP ON NON-IONISING RADIATION (2001) ELF electromagnetic fields and the risk of cancer. Doc NRPB, **12**(1).

ALDINUCCI C., GARCIA J.B., PALMI M., SGARAGLI G., BENOCCI A., MEINI A., PESSINA F., ROSSI C., BONECHI C. & PESSINA G.P. (2003a) The effect of exposure to high flux density static and pulsed magnetic fields on lymphocyte function. Bioelectromagnetics, **24**(6): 373-379.

ALDINUCCI C., GARCIA J.B., PALMI M., SGARAGLI G., BENOCCI A., MEINI A., PESSINA F., ROSSI C., BONECHI C. & PESSINA G.P. (2003b) The effect of strong static magnetic field on lymphocytes. Bioelectromagnetics, **24**(2): 109-117.

ALFANO A.P., TAYLOR A.G., FORESMAN P.A., DUNKL P.R., MCCONNELL G.G., CONAWAY M.R. & GILLIES G.T. (2001) Static magnetic fields for treatment of fibromyalgia: a randomized controlled trial. J Altern Complement Med, **7**(1): 53-64.

ALPEN E.L. (1979) Magnetic field exposure guidelines. In: Magnetic field effects on biological systems (ed. Tenforde, T. S.), pp. 25-32. New York, London: Plenum Press.

ANDERSEN A., DAHLBERG B.E., MAGNUS K. & WANNAG A. (1982) Risk of cancer in the Norwegian aluminium industry. Int J Cancer, **29**(3): 295-298.

AOKI H., YAMAZAKI H., YOSHINO T. & AKAGI T. (1990) Effects of static magnetic fields on membrane permeability of a cultured cell line. Res Commun Chem Pathol Pharmacol, **69**(1): 103-106.

ASASHIMA M., SHIMADA K. & PFEIFFER C.J. (1991) Magnetic shielding induces early developmental abnormalities in the newt, Cynops pyrrhogaster. Bioelectromagnetics, **12**(4): 215-224.

ASTM - AMERICAN SOCIETY FOR TESTING AND MATERIALS (2003a) Standard test method for measurement of magnetically induced displacement force on medical devices in the magnetic resonance environment. West Conshohocken, PA: ASTM International (F2052-02).

ASTM - AMERICAN SOCIETY FOR TESTING AND MATERIALS (2003b) Standard test method for measurement of magnetically induced torque on passive implants in the magnetic resonance environment. West Conshohocken, PA: ASTM International (F2213-04).

ATEF M.M., ABD EL-BASET M.S., EL KAREEM A., AIDA S. & FADEL M.A. (1995) Effects of a static magnetic field on haemoglobin structure and function. Int J Biol Macromol, **17**(2): 105-111.

AYRAPETYAN S.N., GRIGORIAN K.V., AVANESIAN A.S. & STAMBOLTSIAN K.V. (1994) Magnetic fields alter electrical properties of solutions and their physiological effects. Bioelectromagnetics, **15**(2): 133-142.

AZANZA M.J. (1989) Steady magnetic fields mimic the effect of caffeine on neurons. Brain Res, **489**(1): 195-198.

AZANZA M.J. & DEL MORAL A. (1994) Cell membrane biochemistry and neurobiological approach to biomagnetism. Prog Neurobiol, **44**(6): 517-601.

BAILEY W.H. & CHARRY J.M. (1986) Behavioral monitoring of rats during exposure to air ions and DC electric fields. Bioelectromagnetics, **7**(3): 329-339.

BAKER P.N., JOHNSON I.R., HARVEY P.R., GOWLAND P.A. & MANSFIELD P. (1994) A three-year follow-up of children imaged in utero with echo-planar magnetic resonance. Am J Obstet Gynecol, **170**(1 Pt 1): 32-33.

BALABAN P.M., BRAVARENKO N.I. & KUZNETZOV A.N. (1990) Influence of a stationary magnetic field on bioelectric properties of snail neurons. Bioelectromagnetics, **11**(1): 13-25.

BARKER A.T. & CAIN M.W. (1985) The claimed vasodilatory effect of a commercial permanent magnet foil: results of a double-blind trial. Clin Phys Physiol Meas, **6**(3): 261-263.

BARNOTHY M.F. & BARNOTHY J.M. (1970) Magnetic fields and the number of blood platelets. Nature, **225**(238): 1146-1147.

BARNOTHY M.F. & SUMEGI I. (1969) Abnormalities in organs of mice induced by a magnetic field. Nature, **221**(177): 270-271.

BARREGÅRD L., JARVHOLM B. & UNGETHUM E. (1985) Cancer among workers exposed to strong static magnetic fields. Lancet, **2**(8460): 892.

BARREGÅRD L., SALLSTEN G. & JARVHOLM B. (1990) Mortality and cancer incidence in chloralkali workers exposed to inorganic mercury. Br J Ind Med, **47**(2): 99-104.

BATTOCLETTI J.H., SALLES-CUNHA S., HALBACH R.E., NELSON J., SANCES A., JR. & ANTONICH F.J. (1981) Exposure of rhesus monkeys to 20 000 G steady magnetic field: effect on blood parameters. Med Phys, **8**(1): 115-118.

BAUM J.W. & NAUMAN C.H. (1984) Influence of strong magnetic fields on genetic endpoints in Tradescantia tetrads and stamen hairs. Environ Mutagen, **6**(1): 49-58.

BEASON R. & SEMM P. (1996) Does the avian ophthalmic nerve carry magnetic navigational information? J Exp Biol, **199**(Pt 5): 1241-1244.

BEASON R.C., WILTSCHKO R. & WILTSCHKO W. (1997) Pigeon homing: effects of magnetic pulses on initial orientation. Auk, **114** 405-415.

BEAUGNON E. & TOURNIER R. (1991) Levitation of water and organic substances in high static magnetic fields. J Phys III, **1** 1423-1428.

BEERS G.J., PHILLIPS J.L., PRATO F.S. & NAIR I. (1998) Biologic effects of low-level electromagnetic fields: current issues and controversies. Magn Reson Imaging Clin N Am, **6**(4): 749-774.

BEHARI J. & MATHUR R. (1997) Exposure effects of static magnetic field on some physiological parameters of developing rats. Indian J Exp Biol, **35**(8): 894-897.

BEHR K.P., TIFFE H.W., HINZ K.H., LUDERS H., FRIEDERICHS M., RYLL M. & HUNDESHAGEN H. (1991) [The effect of magnetic resonance treatment on chicken embryos]. Dtsch Tierarztl Wochenschr, **98**(4): 149-152.

BEISCHER D.E. (1969) Vectorcardiogram and aortic blood flow of squirrel monkeys (Sciamiri sciureus) in a strong superconducting electromagnet. In: Biological effects of magnetic fields. Volume 2 (ed. Barnothy, M. F.), pp. 241. New York: Plenum Press.

BEISCHER D.E. & KNEPTON J.C., JR. (1964) Influence of strong magnetic fields on the electrocardiogram of squirrel monkeys (Saimiri sciureus). Aerosp Med, **35** 939-944.

BELLOSSI A. (1983) No-effect of a static uniform magnetic field on mouse trypanosomiasis. Radiat Environ Biophys, **22**(4): 311-313.

BELLOSSI A. (1984) The effect of a static uniform magnetic field on mice: a study of methylcholanthren carcinogenesis. Radiat Environ Biophys, **23**(2): 107-109.

BELLOSSI A. (1986a) Effect of static magnetic fields on survival of leukaemia-prone AKR mice. Radiat Environ Biophys, **25**(1): 75-80.

BELLOSSI A. (1986b) Lack of an effect of static magnetic field on calcium efflux from isolated chick brains. Bioelectromagnetics, **7**(4): 381-386.

BELLOSSI A. (1986c) The effect of a static non-uniform magnetic field on mice. A study of Lewis tumour graft. Radiat Environ Biophys, **25**(3): 231-234.

BELLOSSI A., BELLOSSI G. & DE CERTAINES J. (1981) The effect of a constant and uniform magnetic field on mouse brain: a study by magnetic nuclear resonance. Aviat Space Environ Med, **52**(9): 537-539.

BELLOSSI A., SUTTER-DUB M.T. & SUTTER B.C. (1984) Effects of constant magnetic fields on rats and mice: a study of weight. Aviat Space Environ Med, **55**(8): 725-730.

BELLOSSI A. & TOUJAS L. (1982) The effect of a static uniform magnetic field on mice. A study of a Lewis tumour graft. Radiat Environ Biophys, **20**(2): 153-157.

BELOUSOVA L.E. (1965) Possible braking or arrest of blood by a magnetic field. Biophysics, **10** 404-405.

BELYAEV I.Y., ALIPOV Y.D. & HARMS-RINGDAHL M. (1997) Effects of zero magnetic field on the conformation of chromatin in human cells. Biochim Biophys Acta, **1336**(3): 465-473.

BENSON D.E., GRISSOM C.B., BURNS G.L. & MOHAMMAD S.F. (1994) Magnetic field enhancement of antibiotic activity in biofilm forming Pseudomonas aeruginosa. ASAIO J, **40**(3): M371-M376.

BERNHOLD M. & BONDEMARK L. (1998) A magnetic appliance for treatment of snoring patients with and without obstructive sleep apnea. Am J Orthod Dentofacial Orthop, **113**(2): 144-155.

BESSON J.A., FOREMAN E.I., EASTWOOD L.M., SMITH F.W. & ASHCROFT G.W. (1984) Cognitive evaluation following NMR imaging of the brain. J Neurol Neurosurg Psychiatry, **47**(3): 314-316.

BHATIA A.L. (1999) Static magnetic field as biological modifier: a study on temperature dependent influence. Indian J Biochem Biophys, **36**(5): 361-364.

BINHI V.N. (2002) Magnetobiology: underlying physical problems. Academic Press.

BINHI V.N., ALIPOV Y.D. & BELYAEV I.Y. (2001) Effect of static magnetic field on E. coli cells and individual rotations of ion-protein complexes. Bioelectromagnetics, **22**(2): 79-86.

BINHI V.N. & SAVIN A.V. (2003) Effects of weak magnetic fields on biological systems: physical aspects. Physics Uspekhi, **46**(3): 259-291.

BLAKEMORE R. (1975) Magnetotactic bacteria. Science, **190**(4212): 377-379.

BLANK M. & SOO L. (1992) Threshold for inhibition of Na, K-ATPase by ELF alternating currents. Bioelectromagnetics, **13**(4): 329-333.

BLANK M. & SOO L. (1996) The threshold for Na,K-ATPase stimulation by electromagnetic fields. Bioeletrochem Bioenerg, **40** 63-65.

BLONDIN J.P., NGUYEN D.H., SBEGHEN J., GOULET D., CARDINAL C., MARUVADA P.S., PLANTE M. & BAILEY W.H. (1996) Human perception of electric fields and ion currents associated with high-voltage DC transmission lines. Bioelectromagnetics, **17**(3): 230-241.

BONDEMARK L., KUROL J. & LARSSON A. (1998) Long-term effects of orthodontic magnets on human buccal mucosa--a clinical, histological and immunohistochemical study. Eur J Orthod, **20**(3): 211-218.

BONDEMARK L., KUROL J. & WISTEN A. (1995) Extent and flux density of static magnetic fields generated by orthodontic samarium-cobalt magnets. Am J Orthod Dentofacial Orthop, **107**(5): 488-496.

BOURLAND J.D., NYENHUIS J.A. & SCHAEFER D.J. (1999) Physiologic effects of intense MR imaging gradient fields. Neuroimaging Clin N Am, **9**(2): 363-377.

BOWMAN J.D. & METHNER M.M. (2000) Hazard surveillance for industrial magnetic fields: II. Field characteristics from waveform measurements. Ann Occup Hyg, **44**(8): 615-633.

BRACKEN T.D. (1979) The HVDC transmission line environment. In: Proceedings of the Workshop on Electrical and Biological Effects Related to HVDC Transmission PNL-3121. Springfield, VA: National Technical Information Service.

BRAGANZA L.F., BLOTT B.H., COE T.J. & MELVILLE D. (1984) The superdiamagnetic effect of magnetic fields on one and two component multilamellar liposomes. Biochim Biophys Acta, **801**(1): 66-75.

BRANDT T. (2003) Vertigo: its multisensory syndromes. London, New York: Springer.

BRAS W., DIAKUN G.P., DIAZ J.F., MARET G., KRAMER H., BORDAS J. & MEDRANO F.J. (1998) The susceptibility of pure tubulin to high magnetic fields: a magnetic birefringence and x-ray fiber diffraction study. Biophys J, **74**(3): 1509-1521.

BRASSART J., KIRSCHVINK J.L., PHILLIPS J.B. & BORLAND S.C. (1999) Ferromagnetic material in the eastern red-spotted newt notophthalmus viridescens. J Exp Biol, **202** Pt 22 3155-3160.

BREWER H.B. (1979) Some preliminary studies of the effects of a static magnetic field on the life cycle of the Lebistes reticulatus (guppy). Biophys J, **28**(2): 305-314.

BROCKLEHURST B. & MCLAUCHLAN K.A. (1996) Free radical mechanism for the effects of environmental electromagnetic fields on biological systems. Int J Radiat Biol, **69**(1): 3-24.

BROCKWAY J.P. & BREAM P.R., JR. (1992) Does memory loss occur after MR imaging? J Magn Reson Imaging, **2**(6): 721-728.

BRODY A.S., SORETTE M.P., GOODING C.A., LISTERUD J., CLARK M.R., MENTZER W.C., BRASCH R.C. & JAMES T.L. (1985) AUR memorial Award. Induced alignment of flowing sickle erythrocytes in a magnetic field. A preliminary report. Invest Radiol, **20**(6): 560-566.

BRUCE G.K., HOWLETT C.R. & HUCKSTEP R.L. (1987) Effect of a static magnetic field on fracture healing in a rabbit radius. Preliminary results. Clin Orthop,(222): 300-306.

BUEMI M., MARINO D., DI PASQUALE G., FLOCCARI F., SENATORE M., ALOISI C., GRASSO F., MONDIO G., PERILLO P., FRISINA N. & CORICA F. (2001) Cell proliferation/cell death balance in renal cell cultures after exposure to a static magnetic field. Nephron, **87**(3): 269-273.

BULL A.W., CHERNG S. & JENROW K.A. (1993) Weak magnetostatic field alter calmodulin-dependent cyclic nucleotide phosphodiesterase activity. In: Electricity and Magnetism in Biology and Medicine (ed. Blank, M.), pp. 319-322. San Francisco: San Francisco Press.

BULLARD E.C. (1948) On the secular change of the earth's magnetic field. Mont Not R A S geophys Suppl, **5** 248.

CAMILLERI S. & MCDONALD F. (1993) Static magnetic field effects on the sagittal suture in Rattus norvegicus. Am J Orthod Dentofacial Orthop, **103**(3): 240-246.

CARNES K.I. & MAGIN R.L. (1996) Effects of in utero exposure to 4.7 T MR imaging conditions on fetal growth and testicular development in the mouse. Magn Reson Imaging, **14**(3): 263-274.

CARSON J.J., PRATO F.S., DROST D.J., DIESBOURG L.D. & DIXON S.J. (1990) Time-varying magnetic fields increase cytosolic free Ca2+ in HL-60 cells. Am J Physiol, **259**(4 Pt 1): C687-C692.

CARTER R., ASPY C.B. & MOLD J. (2002) The effectiveness of magnet therapy for treatment of wrist pain attributed to carpal tunnel syndrome. J Fam Pract, **51**(1): 38-40.

CASELLI M.A., CLARK N., LAZARUS S., VELEZ Z. & VENEGAS L. (1997) Evaluation of magnetic foil and PPT Insoles in the treatment of heel pain. J Am Podiatr Med Assoc, **87**(1): 11-16.

CAVOPOL A.V., WAMIL A.W., HOLCOMB R.R. & MCLEAN M.J. (1995) Measurement and analysis of static magnetic fields that block action potentials in cultured neurons. Bioelectromagnetics, **16**(3): 197-206.

CHADWICK P. & LOWES F. (1998) Magnetic fields on British trains. Ann Occup Hyg, **42**(5): 331-335.

CHAKERES D.W., BORNSTEIN R. & KANGARLU A. (2003a) Randomized comparison of cognitive function in humans at 0 and 8 Tesla. J Magn Reson Imaging, **18**(3): 342-345.

CHAKERES D.W. & DE VOCHT F. (2005) Static magnetic field effects on human subjects related to magnetic resonance imaging systems. Prog Biophys Mol Biol, **87**(2-3): 255-265.

CHAKERES D.W., KANGARLU A., BOUDOULAS H. & YOUNG D.C. (2003b) Effect of static magnetic field exposure of up to 8 Tesla on sequential human vital sign measurements. J Magn Reson Imaging, **18**(3): 346-352.

CHEN I.I.H. & SAHA S. (1985) Analysis of an intensive magnetic field on blood flow: part 2. J Bioelectr, **4**(1): 55-61.

CHEW S., AHMADI A., GOH P.S. & FOONG L.C. (2001) The effects of 1.5 T magnetic resonance imaging on early murine in-vitro embryo development. J Magn Reson Imaging, **13**(3): 417-420.

CHIGNELL C.F. & SIK R.H. (1995a) Magnetic field effects on the photohaemolysis of human erythrocytes by ketoprofen and protoporphyrin IX. Photochem Photobiol, **62**(1): 205-207.

CHIGNELL C.F. & SIK R.H. (1995b) Magnetic field effects on the photohemolysisphotohaemolysis of human erythrocytes by ketoprofen and protoporphyrin IX. Photochem Photobiol, **62**(1): 205-207.

CHIGNELL C.F. & SIK R.H. (1995c) Magnetic field effects on the photohemolysisphotohaemolysis of human erythrocytes by ketoprofen and protoporphyrin IX. Photochem Photobiol, **62**(1): 205-207.

CHIGNELL C.F. & SIK R.H. (1995d) Magnetic field effects on the photohemolysisphotohaemolysis of human erythrocytes by ketoprofen and protoporphyrin IX. Photochem Photobiol, **62**(1): 205-207.

CHIGNELL C.F. & SIK R.H. (1998a) The effect of static magnetic fields on the photohaemolysis of human erythrocytes by ketoprofen. Photochem Photobiol, **67**(5): 591-595.

CHIGNELL C.F. & SIK R.H. (1998b) The effect of static magnetic fields on the photohemolysisphotohaemolysis of human erythrocytes by ketoprofen. Photochem Photobiol, **67**(5): 591-595.

CHIGNELL C.F. & SIK R.H. (1998c) The effect of static magnetic fields on the photohemolysisphotohaemolysis of human erythrocytes by ketoprofen. Photochem Photobiol, **67**(5): 591-595.

CHILES C., HAWROT E., GORE J. & BYCK R. (1989) Magnetic field modulation of receptor binding. Magn Reson Med, **10**(2): 241-245.

CHOLERIS E., DEL SEPPIA C., THOMAS A.W., LUSCHI P., GHIONE G., MORAN G.R. & PRATO F.S. (2002) Shielding, but not zeroing of the ambient magnetic field reduces stress- induced analgesia in mice. Proc R Soc Lond B Biol Sci, **269**(1487): 193-201.

CLAIRMONT B.A., JOHNSON G.B., ZAFFANELLA L.E. & ZELINGHER S. (1989) The effects of HVAC-HVDC line separation in a hybrid corridor. IEEE Trans Power Deliv, **4** 1338-1.

CLEMENTS H., DUNCAN K.R., FIELDING K., GOWLAND P.A., JOHNSON I.R. & BAKER P.N. (2000) Infants exposed to MRI in utero have a normal paediatric assessment at 9 months of age. Br J Radiol, **73**(866): 190-194.

COHLY H.H., ABRAHAM G.E., III, NDEBELE K., JENKINS J.J., THOMPSON J. & ANGEL M.F. (2003) Effects of static electromagnetic fields on characteristics of MG-63 osteoblasts grown in culture. Biomed Sci Instrum, **39** 454-459.

COLLACOTT E.A., ZIMMERMAN J.T., WHITE D.W. & RINDONE J.P. (2000) Bipolar permanent magnets for the treatment of chronic low back pain: a pilot study. JAMA, **283**(10): 1322-1325.

COOKE P. & MORRIS P.G. (1981) The effects of NMR exposure on living organisms. II. A genetic study of human lymphocytes. Br J Radiol, **54**(643): 622-625.

CORDEIRO P.G., SECKEL B.R., MILLER C.D., GROSS P.T. & WISE R.E. (1989) Effect of a high-intensity static magnetic field on sciatic nerve regeneration in the rat. Plast Reconstr Surg, **83**(2): 301-308.

COULTON L.A., BARKER A.T., VAN LIEROP J.E. & WALSH M.P. (2000) The effect of static magnetic fields on the rate of calcium/calmodulin- dependent phosphorylation of myosin light chain. Bioelectromagnetics, **21**(3): 189-196.

COZENS F.L. & SCAIANO J.C. (1993) A comparative study of magnetic field effects on the dynamics of germinate and random radical pair processes in micelles. J Am Chem Soc, **115**(5204): 5211.

CREIM J.A., LOVELY R.H., WEIGEL R.J., FORSYTHE W.C. & ANDERSON L.E. (1993) Rats avoid exposure to HVdc electric fields: a dose response study. Bioelectromagnetics, **14**(4): 341-352.

CREIM J.A., LOVELY R.H., WEIGEL R.J., FORSYTHE W.C. & ANDERSON L.E. (1995) Failure to produce taste-aversion learning in rats exposed to static electric fields and air ions. Bioelectromagnetics, **16**(5): 301-306.

CROZIER S. & DODDRELL D.M. (1997) Compact MRI magnet design by stochastic optimization. J Magn Reson, **127**(2): 233-237.

CROZIER S. & LIU F. (2005) Numerical evaluation of the fields induced by body motion in or near high-field MRI scanners. Prog Biophys Mol Biol, **87**(2-3): 267-278.

DANIELYAN A.A. & AYRAPETYAN S.N. (1999) Changes of hydration of rats' tissues after in vivo exposure to 0.2 Tesla steady magnetic field. Bioelectromagnetics, **20**(2): 123-128.

DANIELYAN A.A., MIRAKYAN M.M., GRIGORYAN G.Y. & AYRAPETYAN S.N. (1999) The static magnetic field effects on ouabain H3 binding by cancer tissue. Physiol Chem Phys Med NMR, **31**(2): 139-144.

DARENDELILER M.A., DARENDELILER A. & SINCLAIR P.M. (1997) Effects of static magnetic and pulsed electromagnetic fields on bone healing. Int J Adult Orthodon Orthognath Surg, **12**(1): 43-53.

DARENDELILER M.A., SINCLAIR P.M. & KUSY R.P. (1995) The effects of samarium-cobalt magnets and pulsed electromagnetic fields on tooth movement. Am J Orthod Dentofacial Orthop, **107**(6): 578-588.

DAVIS H.P., MIZUMORI S.J., ALLEN H., ROSENZWEIG M.R., BENNETT E.L. & TENFORDE T.S. (1984) Behavioral studies with mice exposed to DC and 60-Hz magnetic fields. Bioelectromagnetics, **5**(2): 147-164.

DAVIS R.L. & MILHAM S. (1990) Altered immune status in aluminum reduction plant workers. Am J Ind Med, **18**(1): 79-85.

DAWSON T.W. & STUCHLY M.A. (1998) High resolution organ dosimetry for human exposure to low frequency magnetic fields. IEEE Trans Magnet, **34** 1-11.

DE LATOUR C. (1973) Magnetic separation in water pollution control. IEEE Trans Magnet, **9**(3): 314-316.

DE VOCHT F., WENDEL DE JOODE B., ENGELS H. & KROMHOUT H. (2003) Neurobehavioral effects among subjects exposed to high static and gradient magnetic fields from a 1.5 Tesla magnetic resonance imaging system--a case-crossover pilot study. Magn Reson Med, **50**(4): 670-674.

DEL MORAL A. & AZANZA M.J. (1992) Model for the effects of static magnetic fields on isolated neurons. J Magnetism Magn Mat, **114**(3): 240-242.

DEL SEPPIA C., LUSCHI P., GHIONE S., CROSIO E., CHOLERIS E. & PAPI F. (2000) Exposure to a hypogeomagnetic field or to oscillating magnetic fields similarly reduce stress-induced analgesia in C57 male mice. Life Sci, **66**(14): 1299-1306.

DENEGRE J.M., VALLES J.M., JR., LIN K., JORDAN W.B. & MOWRY K.L. (1998) Cleavage planes in frog eggs are altered by strong magnetic fields. Proc Natl Acad Sci U S A, **95**(25): 14729-14732.

DEUTSCHLANDER M.E., BORLAND S.C. & PHILLIPS J.B. (1999a) Extraocular magnetic compass in newts. Nature, **400**(6742): 324-325.

DEUTSCHLANDER M.E., PHILLIPS J.B. & BORLAND S.C. (1999b) The case for light-dependent magnetic orientation in animals. J Exp Biol, **202** (Pt 8) 891-908.

DEXTER D., JR. (1997) Magnetic therapy is ineffective for the treatment of snoring and obstructive sleep apnea syndrome. Wis Med J, **96**(3): 35-37.

DIETRICH, F. M. and JACOBS, W. L. (1999) Survey and assessment of electric and magnetic field public exposure in the transportation environment. US Department of Transportation, Federal Railroad Adminstration (Report nr PB99-130908).

DOBSON J., ST PIERRE T., WIESER H.G. & FULLER M. (2000a) Changes in paroxysmal brainwave patterns of epileptics by weak-field magnetic stimulation. Bioelectromagnetics, **21**(2): 94-99.

DOBSON J., ST PIERRE T.G., SCHULTHEISS-GRASSI P.P., WIESER H.G. & KUSTER N. (2000b) Analysis of EEG data from weak-field magnetic stimulation of mesial temporal lobe epilepsy patients. Brain Res, **868**(2): 386-391.

DOLEZALEK H. (1979) Atmospheric electricity. In: Handbook of chemistry and physics. Cleveland, OH: Chemical Rubber Publishing Co.

DUDA D., GRZESIK J. & PAWLICKI K. (1991) Changes in liver and kidney concentration of copper, manganese, cobalt and iron in rats exposed to static and low-frequency (50 Hz) magnetic fields. J Trace Elem Electrolytes Health Dis, **5**(3): 181-186.

EC - EUROPEAN COMMISSION (1996) Non-ionizing radiation - Sources, exposure and health effects. Luxemburg: Office for Official Publications of the European Communities.

EDMONDS D.T. (1996) A sensitive optically detected magnetic compass for animals. Proc R Soc Lond B Biol Sci, **263**(1368): 295-298.

EDWARDS M.J., SAUNDERS R.D. & SHIOTA K. (2003) Effects of heat on embryos and foetuses. Int J Hyperthermia, **19**(3): 295-324.

EGUCHI Y., OGIUE-IKEDA M. & UENO S. (2003) Control of orientation of rat Schwann cells using an 8-T static magnetic field. Neurosci Lett, **351**(2): 130-132.

EICHWALD C. & WALLECZEK J. (1996) Activation-dependent and biphasic electromagnetic field effects: model based on cooperative enzyme kinetics in cellular signaling. Bioelectromagnetics, **17**(6): 427-435.

EICHWALD C. & WALLECZEK J. (1998) Magnetic field perturbations as a tool for controlling enzyme-regulated and oscillatory biochemical reactions. Biophysical Chemistry, **74** 209-224.

ELLINGSEN D.G., ANDERSEN A., NORDHAGEN H.P., EFSKIND J. & KJUUS H. (1993) Incidence of cancer and mortality among workers exposed to mercury vapour in the Norwegian chloralkali industry. Br J Ind Med, **50**(10): 875-880.

EMURA R., ASHIDA N., HIGASHI T. & TAKEUCHI T. (2001) Orientation of bull sperms in static magnetic fields. Bioelectromagnetics, **22**(1): 60-65.

ENGSTRÖM S. (1997) What is the time scale of magnetic field interaction in biological systems? Bioelectromagnetics, **18**(3): 244-249.

ENGSTRÖM S. & FITZSIMMONS R. (1999) Five hypotheses to examine the nature of magnetic field transduction in biological systems. Bioelectromagnetics, **20**(7): 423-430.

ENGSTRÖM S., MARKOV M.S., MCLEAN M.J., HOLCOMB R.R. & MARKOV J.M. (2002) Effects of non-uniform static magnetic fields on the rate of myosin phosphorylation. Bioelectromagnetics, **23**(6): 475-479.

ESFORMES I., KUMMER F.J. & LIVELLI T.J. (1981) Biological effects of magnetic fields generated with CoSm magnets. Bull Hosp Jt Dis Orthop Inst, **41** 81-87.

ESPINAR A., PIERA V., CARMONA A. & GUERRERO J.M. (1997) Histological changes during development of the cerebellum in the chick embryo exposed to a static magnetic field. Bioelectromagnetics, **18**(1): 36-46.

EVANS J.A., SAVITZ D.A., KANAL E. & GILLEN J. (1993) Infertility and pregnancy outcome among magnetic resonance imaging workers. J Occup Med, 35(12): 1191-1195.

EVESON R.W., TIMMEL C.R., BROCKLEHURST B., HORE P.J. & MCLAUCHLAN K.A. (2000) The effects of weak magnetic fields on radical recombination reactions in micelles. Int J Radiat Biol, 76(11): 1509-1522.

FAM W.Z. (1981) Prolonged exposure of mice to 350 kV/m electrostatic field. IEEE Trans Biomed Eng, 28(6): 453-459.

FANELLI C., COPPOLA S., BARONE R., COLUSSI C., GUALANDI G., VOLPE P. & GHIBELLI L. (1999) Magnetic fields increase cell survival by inhibiting apoptosis via modulation of Ca2+ influx. FASEB J, 13(1): 95-102.

FEINENDEGEN L.E. & MUHLENSIEPEN H. (1987) In vivo enzyme control through a strong stationary magnetic field--the case of thymidine kinase in mouse bone marrow cells. Int J Radiat Biol Relat Stud Phys Chem Med, 52(3): 469-479.

FISCHER J.H., FREAKE M.J., BORLAND S.C. & PHILLIPS J.B. (2001) Evidence for the use of magnetic map information by an amphibian. Anim Behav, 62 1-10.

FLIPO D., FOURNIER M., BENQUET C., ROUX P., LE BOULAIRE C., PINSKY C., LABELLA F.S. & KRZYSTYNIAK K. (1998) Increased apoptosis, changes in intracellular Ca2+, and functional alterations in lymphocytes and macrophages after in vitro exposure to static magnetic field. J Toxicol Environ Health A, 54(1): 63-76.

FORBES L.K., CROZIER S. & DODDRELL D.M. (1997) Rapid computation of static fields produced by thick circular solenoids. IEEE Trans Magnet, 33 4405-4410.

FRANKEL R.B. & LIBURDY R.P. (1996) Biological effects of static magnetic fields. In: Handbook of Biological Effects of Electromagnetic Fields (eds. Polk, C. & Postow, E.), pp. 149-183. Boca Raton, FL: CRC Press.

FUJITA N. & TENFORDE T.S. (1982) Portable magnetic field dosimeter with data acquisition capabilities. Rev Sci Inst, 53 326-331.

FULLER M., DOBSON J., WIESER H.G. & MOSER S. (1995) On the sensitivity of the human brain to magnetic fields: evocation of epileptiform activity. Brain Res Bull, 36(2): 155-159.

GAFFEY, C. T. and TENFORDE, T. S. (1979) Changes in the electrocardiograms of rats and dogs exposed to DC magnetic fields. Berkeley, CA: University of California, Lawrence Berkeley Laboratory (report nr LBL-9085).

GAFFEY C.T. & TENFORDE T.S. (1981) Alterations in the rat electrocardiogram induced by stationary magnetic fields. Bioelectromagnetics, 2(4): 357-370.

GAFFEY C.T. & TENFORDE T.S. (1983) Bioelectric properties of frog sciatic nerves during exposure to stationary magnetic fields. Radiat Environ Biophys, 22(1): 61-73.

GAFFEY C.T., TENFORDE T.S. & DEAN E.E. (1980) Alterations in the electrocardiograms of baboons exposed to DC magnetic fields. Bioelectromagnetics, 1 209.

GAFFNEY B.J. & MCCONNEL H.M. (1974) Effect of a magnetic field on phospholipid membranes. Chem Phys Lett, 24 310-313.

GAUSS C.F. (1839) Allegemeine Theorie des Erdmagnetismus. Leipzig.

GEARD C.R., OSMAK R.S., HALL E.J., SIMON H.E., MAUDSLEY A.A. & HILAL S.K. (1984) Magnetic resonance and ionizing radiation: a comparative evaluation in vitro of oncogenic and genotoxic potential. Radiology, 152(1): 199-202.

GMITROV J. & OHKUBO C. (2002a) Artificial static and geomagnetic field interrelated impact on cardiovascular regulation. Bioelectromagnetics, 23(5): 329-338.

GMITROV J. & OHKUBO C. (2002b) Verapamil protective effect on natural and artificial magnetic field cardiovascular impact. Bioelectromagnetics, 23(7): 531-541.

GMITROV J., OHKUBO C. & OKANO H. (2002) Effect of 0.25 T static magnetic field on microcirculation in rabbits. Bioelectromagnetics, 23(3): 224-229.

GOODMAN E.M., GREENEBAUM B. & MARRON M.T. (1995) Effects of electromagnetic fields on molecules and cells. Int Rev Cytol, **158** 279-338.

GORCZYNSKA E. (1986) The effect of static magnetic field on fibrinogen degradation products level in rabbits with thrombosis. J Hyg Epidemiol Microbiol Immunol, **30**(3): 269-273.

GORCZYNSKA E. (1987a) Liver and spleen morphology, ceruloplasmin activity and iron content in serum of guinea pigs exposed to the magnetic field. J Hyg Epidemiol Microbiol Immunol, **31**(4): 357-363.

GORCZYNSKA E. (1987b) The process of myelopoiesis in guinea pigs under conditions of a static magnetic field. Acta Physiol Pol, **38**(5): 425-432.

GORCZYNSKA E. (1988) Fibrinolytical processes in rabbits activated by the magnetic field. J Hyg Epidemiol Microbiol Immunol, **32**(4): 391-396.

GORCZYNSKA E., GALKA G., WEGRZYNOWICZ R. & MIKOSZA H. (1986) Effect of magnetic field on the process of cell respiration in mitochondria of rats. Physiol Chem Phys Med NMR, **18**(1): 61-69.

GORCZYNSKA E. & WEGRZYNOWICZ R. (1983) The effect of magnetic fields on platelets, blood coagulation and fibrinolysis in guinea pigs. Physiol Chem Phys Med NMR, **15**(6): 459-468.

GORCZYNSKA E. & WEGRZYNOWICZ R. (1984) The effect of static magnetic field on protein concentration in serum of guinea-pigs. J Hyg Epidemiol Microbiol Immunol, **28**(3): 257-260.

GORCZYNSKA E. & WEGRZYNOWICZ R. (1985) Activity of acid and alkali phosphatase in guinea pigs exposed to the static magnetic fields. J Hyg Epidemiol Microbiol Immunol, **29**(2): 135-139.

GORCZYNSKA E. & WEGRZYNOWICZ R. (1986a) Effect of chronic exposure to static magnetic field upon the K+, Na+ and chlorides concentrations in the serum of guinea pigs. J Hyg Epidemiol Microbiol Immunol, **30**(2): 121-126.

GORCZYNSKA E. & WEGRZYNOWICZ R. (1986b) Effect of chronic exposure to static magnetic field upon the serum glutamic pyruvic transaminase activity GPT and morphology of the cardiac muscle, skeletal muscles, kidneys, cerebellum and lung tissue in guinea pigs. J Hyg Epidemiol Microbiol Immunol, **30**(3): 275-281.

GORCZYNSKA E. & WEGRZYNOWICZ R. (1989) Effect of static magnetic field on some enzymes activities in rats. J Hyg Epidemiol Microbiol Immunol, **33**(2): 149-155.

GORCZYNSKA E. & WEGRZYNOWICZ R. (1991a) Glucose homeostasis in rats exposed to magnetic fields. Invest Radiol, **26**(12): 1095-1100.

GORCZYNSKA E. & WEGRZYNOWICZ R. (1991b) Structural and functional changes in organelles of liver cells in rats exposed to magnetic fields. Environ Res, **55**(2): 188-198.

GOWLAND P.A. (2005) Present and future magnetic resonance sources of exposure to static fields. Prog Biophys Mol Biol, **87**(2-3): 175-183.

GRANDOLFO M. (1989) Magnetic field strengths in the high speed train ETR450. In: Proceedings of the 26th National Congress of the Italian Radiation Protection Association (AIRP).

GRAY J.R., FRITH C.H. & PARKER J.D. (2000) In vivo enhancement of chemotherapy with static electric or magnetic fields. Bioelectromagnetics, **21**(8): 575-583.

GRISSOM C.B. (1995) Magnetic field effects in biology: survey of possible mechanisms with emphasis on radical-pair recombination. Chem Rev, **95** 3-24.

GRZESIK J., BORTEL M., DUDA D., KUSKA R., LUDYGA K., MICHNIK J., SMOLKA B., SOWA B., TRZECIAK H. & ZIELINSKI G. (1988) Influence of a static magnetic field on the reproductive function, certain biochemical indices and behaviour of rats. Pol J Occup Med, **1**(4): 329-339.

GUISASOLA C., DESCO M., MILLAN O., VILLANUEVA F.J. & GARCIA-BARRENO P. (2002a) Biological dosimetry of magnetic resonance imaging. J Magn Reson Imaging, **15**(5): 584-590.

GUISASOLA C., DESCO M., MILLAN O., VILLANUEVA F.J. & GARCIA-BARRENO P. (2002b) Biological dosimetry of magnetic resonance imagingThis work has not been presented at any ISMRM meeting nor has it been accepted for presentation at a future meeting. J Magn Reson Imaging, **15**(5): 584-590.

HANZLIK M., HEUNEMANN C., HOLTKAMP-ROTZLER E., WINKLHOFER M., PETERSEN N. & FLEISSNER G. (2000) Superparamagnetic magnetite in the upper beak tissue of homing pigeons. Biometals, **13** 325-331.

HARKINS T.T. & GRISSOM C.B. (1994) Magnetic field effects on B12 ethanolamine ammonia lyase: evidence for a radical mechanism. Science, **263**(5149): 958-960.

HARKINS T.T. & GRISSOM C.B. (1995) The magnetic field dependent step in B12 ethanolamine ammonia-lyase is radical pair recombination. J Am Chem Soc, **117**(1): 566-567.

HASSENZAHL, W., MAHAFFY, M., and WEINROFEN, J. (1978) Evaluation of environmental control technologies for magnetic fields. Springfield, Virginia: US Department of Energy, National Technical Information Service (NTIS report DOE/EV-0029).

HASSENZAHL, W., MAHAFFY, M., and WEINROFEN, J. (2004) Evaluation of environmental control technologies for magnetic fields. Springfield, VA: National Technical Information Service (NTIS report DOE/EV-0029).

HAUGSDAL B., TYNES T., ROTNES J.S. & GRIFFITHS D. (2001) A single nocturnal exposure to 2-7 millitesla static magnetic fields does not inhibit the excretion of 6-sulfatoxymelatonin in healthy young men. Bioelectromagnetics, **22**(1): 1-6.

HEINE J., SCHEINICHEN D., JAEGER K., HERZOG T., SUMPELMANN R. & LEUWER M. (1999) Effect of magnetic resonance imaging on human respiratory burst of neutrophils. FEBS Lett, **446**(1): 15-17.

HEINRICHS W.L., FONG P., FLANNERY M., HEINRICHS S.C., CROOKS L.E., SPINDLE A. & PEDERSEN R.A. (1988) Midgestational exposure of pregnant BALB/c mice to magnetic resonance imaging conditions. Magn Reson Imaging, **6**(3): 305-313.

HELFRICH W. (1973) Lipid bilayer spheres - deformation and birefringence in magnetic fields. Phys Lett A, **43**(5): 409-410.

HIGASHI T., SAGAWA S., ASHIDA N. & TAKEUCHI T. (1996) Orientation of glutaraldehyde-fixed erythrocytes in strong static magnetic fields. Bioelectromagnetics, **17**(4): 335-338.

HIGASHI T., YAMAGISHI A., TAKEUCHI T. & DATE M. (1995) Effects of static magnetic fields on erythrocyte rheology. Bioelectrochem Bioenerg, **36** 101-108.

HIGASHI T., YAMAGISHI A., TAKEUCHI T., KAWAGUCHI N., SAGAWA S., ONISHI S. & DATE M. (1993) Orientation of erythrocytes in a strong static magnetic field. Blood, **82**(4): 1328-1334.

HIGH W.B., SIKORA J., UGURBIL K. & GARWOOD M. (2000) Subchronic in vivo effects of a high static magnetic field (9.4 T) in rats. J Magn Reson Imaging, **12**(1): 122-139.

HINMAN M.R. (2002) Comparative effect of positive and negative static magnetic fields on heart rate and blood pressure in healthy adults. Clin Rehabil, **16**(6): 669-674.

HINMAN M.R., FORD J. & HEYL H. (2002) Effects of static magnets on chronic knee pain and physical function: a double-blind study. Altern Ther Health Med, **8**(4): 50-55.

HIRAI T., NAKAMICHI N. & YONEDA Y. (2002) Activator protein-1 complex expressed by magnetism in cultured rat hippocampal neurons. Biochem Biophys Res Commun, **292**(1): 200-207.

HIRAOKA M., MIYAKOSHI J., LI Y.P., SHUNG B., TAKEBE H. & ABE M. (1992) Induction of c-fos gene expression by exposure to a static magnetic field in HeLaS3 cells. Cancer Res, **52**(23): 6522-6524.

HIROSE H., NAKAHARA T. & MIYAKOSHI J. (2003a) Orientation of human glioblastoma cells embedded in type I collagen, caused by exposure to a 10 T static magnetic field. Neurosci Lett, **338**(1): 88-90.

HIROSE H., NAKAHARA T., ZHANG Q.M., YONEI S. & MIYAKOSHI J. (2003b) Static magnetic field with a strong magnetic field gradient (41.7 T/m) induces c-Jun expression in HL-60 cells. In Vitro Cell Dev Biol Anim, **39**(8-9): 348-352.

HO M.W., STONE T.A., JERMAN I., BOLTON J., BOLTON H., GOODWIN B.C., SAUNDERS P.T. & ROBERTSON F. (1992) Brief exposures to weak static magnetic field during early embryogenesis cause cuticular pattern abnormalities in Drosophila larvae. Phys Med Biol, **37**(5): 1171-1179.

241

HÖJEVIK P., SANDBLOM J., GALT S. & HAMNERIUS Y. (1995) Ca2+ ion transport through patch-clamped cells exposed to magnetic fields. Bioelectromagnetics, 16(1): 33-40.

HOLCOMB R.R., WORTHINGTON W.B., MCCULLOUGH B.A. & MCLEAN M.J. (2000) Static magnetic field therapy for pain in the abdomen and genitals. Pediatr Neurol, 23(3): 261-264.

HOLDEN A.V. (2005) The sensitivity of the heart to static magnetic fields. Prog Biophys Mol Biol, 87(2-3): 289-320.

HONG C.Z. (1987) Static magnetic field influence on human nerve function. Arch Phys Med Rehabil, 68(3): 162-164.

HONG C.Z., HARMON D. & YU J. (1986) Static magnetic field influence on rat tail nerve function. Arch Phys Med Rehabil, 67(10): 746-749.

HONG C.Z., HUESTIS P., THOMPSON R. & YU J. (1988) Learning ability of young rats is unaffected by repeated exposure to a static electromagnetic field in early life. Bioelectromagnetics, 9(3): 269-273.

HONG C.Z., LIN J.C., BENDER L.F., SCHAEFFER J.N., MELTZER R.J. & CAUSIN P. (1982) Magnetic necklace: its therapeutic effectiveness on neck and shoulder pain. Arch Phys Med Rehabil, 63(10): 462-466.

HONG C.Z. & SHELLOCK F.G. (1990) Short-term exposure to a 1.5 tesla static magnetic field does not affect somato-sensory-evoked potentials in man. Magn Reson Imaging, 8(1): 65-69.

HONG F.T., MAUZERALL D. & MAURO A. (1971) Magnetic anisotropy and the orientation of retinal rods in a homogeneous magnetic field. Proc Natl Acad Sci USA, 68(6): 1283-1285.

HORE P.J. (2005) Rapporteur's report: sources and interaction mechanisms. Prog Biophys Mol Biol, 87(2-3): 205-212.

HORIUCHI S., ISHIZAKI Y., OKUNO K., ANO T. & SHODA M. (2001) Drastic high magnetic field effect on suppression of Escherichia coli death. Bioelectrochemistry, 53(2): 149-153.

HORIUCHI S., ISHIZAKI Y., OKUNO K., ANO T. & SHODA M. (2002) Change in broth culture is associated with significant suppression of Escherichia coli death under high magnetic field. Bioelectrochemistry, 57(2): 139.

HOTZ M.A., MULLER S., ALLUM J.H. & PFALTZ C.R. (1992) Human auditory-evoked potentials before and after magnetic resonance imaging. Eur Arch Otorhinolaryngol, **249**(2): 85-86.

HOUPT T.A., PITTMAN D.W., BARRANCO J.M., BROOKS E.H. & SMITH J.C. (2003) Behavioral effects of high-strength static magnetic fields on rats. J Neurosci, **23**(4): 1498-1505.

IARC WORKING GROUP ON THE EVALUATION OF CARCINOGENIC RISKS TO HUMANS (2002) Non-ionizing radiation, Part 1: static and extremely low-frequency (ELF) electric and magnetic fields. IARC Monogr Eval Carcinog Risks Hum, **80** 1-395.

ICHIOKA S., IWASAKA M., SHIBATA M., HARII K., KAMIYA A. & UENO S. (1998) Biological effects of static magnetic fields on the microcirculatory blood flow in vivo: a preliminary report. Med Biol Eng Comput, **36**(1): 91-95.

ICHIOKA S., MINEGISHI M., IWASAKA M., SHIBATA M., NAKATSUKA T., ANDO J. & UENO S. (2003) Skin temperature changes induced by strong static magnetic field exposure. Bioelectromagnetics, **24**(6): 380-386.

ICHIOKA S., MINEGISHI M., IWASAKA M., SHIBATA M., NAKATSUKA T., HARII K., KAMIYA A. & UENO S. (2000) High-intensity static magnetic fields modulate skin microcirculation and temperature in vivo. Bioelectromagnetics, **21**(3): 183-188.

ICNIRP - INTERNATIONAL COMMISSION ON NON-IONIZING RADIATION PROTECTION (1994) Guidelines on limits of exposure to static magnetic fields. Health Phys, **66** 100-106.

ICNIRP - INTERNATIONAL COMMISSION ON NON-IONIZING RADIATION PROTECTION (1996) Non-ionizing radiation. Proceedings of the Third International Non-ionizing Radiation Workshop, Baden, Austria. Oberschleissheim: International Commission on Non-ionizing Radiation Protection.

ICNIRP - INTERNATIONAL COMMISSION ON NON-IONIZING RADIATION PROTECTION (1998) Guidelines on limits of exposure to time-varying electric, magnetic and electromagnetic fields (1 Hz - 300 GHz). Health Phys, **74**(4): 494-522.

ICNIRP - INTERNATIONAL COMMISSION ON NON-IONIZING RADIATION PROTECTION (2003) Exposure to static and low frequency electromagnetic fields, biological effects and health consequences (0 - 100 kHz). Oberschleissheim: International Commission on Non-ionizing Radiation Protection (publication ICNIRP 13/2003).

IEEJ - INSTITUTE OF ELECTRICAL ENGINEERS OF JAPAN (1998) The evaluation of health effects by exposure to electric and magnetic fields and determined future studies. (in Japanese). Tokyo: Denki Gakkai (The Institute of Electrical Engineers of Japan).

IINO M. (1997) Effects of a homogeneous magnetic field on erythrocyte sedimentation and aggregation. Bioelectromagnetics, 18(3): 215-222.

IINO M. & OKUDA Y. (2001) Osmolality dependence of erythrocyte sedimentation and aggregation in a strong magnetic field. Bioelectromagnetics, 22(1): 46-52.

IKEHATA M., KOANA T., SUZUKI Y., SHIMIZU H. & NAKAGAWA M. (1999) Mutagenicity and co-mutagenicity of static magnetic fields detected by bacterial mutation assay. Mutat Res, 427(2): 147-156.

IMAJO Y., HIRATSUKA J., MATSUMIYA A., YAMAMOTO M. & NISHISHITA S. (1989) [The effect of a static magnetic field on hamsters bearing melanoma-- cell cycle analysis by flow cytometry]. Nippon Gan Chiryo Gakkai Shi, 24(6): 1261-1265.

INNIS N.K., OSSENKOPP K.P., PRATO F.S. & SESTINI E. (1986) Behavioral effects of exposure to nuclear magnetic resonance imaging: II. Spatial memory tests. Magn Reson Imaging, 4(4): 281-284.

IRGENS A., KRUGER K., SKORVE A.H. & IRGENS L.M. (1997) Male proportion in offspring of parents exposed to strong static and extremely low-frequency electromagnetic fields in Norway. Am J Ind Med, 32(5): 557-561.

ISHIZAKI Y., HORIUCHI S., OKUNO K., ANO T. & SHODA M. (2001) Twelve hours exposure to inhomogeneous high magnetic field after logarithmic growth phase is sufficient for drastic suppression of Escherichia coli death. Bioelectrochemistry, 54(2): 101-105.

ITEGIN M., GUNAY I., LOGOGLU G. & ISBIR T. (1995) Effects of static magnetic field on specific adenosine-5'- triphosphatase activities and bioelectrical and biomechanical properties in the rat diaphragm muscle. Bioelectromagnetics, 16(3): 147-151.

IVANOV S.G., SMIRNOV V.V., SOLOV'EVA F.V., LIASHEVSKAIA S.P. & SELEZNEVA L.I. (1990) [The magnetotherapy of hypertension patients]. Ter Arkh, 62(9): 71-74.

IWASAKA M., MIYAKOSHI J. & UENO S. (2003) Magnetic field effects on assembly pattern of smooth muscle cells. In Vitro Cell Dev Biol Anim, 39(3-4): 120-123.

IWASAKA M. & UENO S. (2003) Detection of intracellular macromolecule behavior under strong magnetic fields by linearly polarized light. Bioelectromagnetics, 24(8): 564-570.

IWASAKA M., UENO S. & TSUDA H. (1994) Enzymatic activity of plasmin in strong magnetic fields. IEEE Trans Magnet, 30(6): 4701-4703.

JACKSON J.D. (1999) Classical Electrodynamics, 3rd ed. New York: Wiley.

JAJTE J., GRZEGORCZYK J., ZMYSLONY M. & RAJKOWSKA E. (2002) Effect of 7 mT static magnetic field and iron ions on rat lymphocytes: apoptosis, necrosis and free radical processes. Bioelectrochemistry, 57(2): 107-111.

JAJTE J., ZMYSLONY M. & RAJKOWSKA E. (2003) [Protective effect of melatonin and vitamin E against prooxidative action of iron ions and static magnetic field]. Med Pr, 54(1): 23-28.

JANKOVIC B.D., JOVANOVA-NESIC K., NIKOLIC V. & NIKOLIC P. (1993) Brain-applied magnetic fields and immune response: role of the pineal gland. Int J Neurosci, 70(1-2): 127-134.

JANKOVIC B.D., MARIC D., RANIN J. & VELJIC J. (1991) Magnetic fields, brain and immunity: effect on humoral and cell- mediated immune responses. Int J Neurosci, 59(1-3): 25-43.

JANKOVIC B.D., NIKOLIC P., CUPIC V. & HLADNI K. (1994) Potentiation of immune responsiveness in aging by static magnetic fields applied to the brain. Role of the pineal gland. Ann N Y Acad Sci, 719 410-418.

JEHENSON P., DUBOC D., LAVERGNE T., GUIZE L., GUERIN F., DEGEORGES M. & SYROTA A. (1988) Change in human cardiac rhythm induced by a 2-T static magnetic field. Radiology, 166(1 Pt 1): 227-230.

JOVÉ M., TORRENTE M., GILABERT R., ESPINAR A., COBOS P. & PIERA V. (1999) Effects of static electromagnetic fields on chick embryo pineal gland development. Cells Tissues Organs, 165(2): 74-80.

KALE P.G. & BAUM J.W. (1979) Genetic effects of strong magnetic fields in Drosophila melanogaster: I. Homogeneous fields ranging from 13,000 to 37,000 Gauss. Environ Mutagen, 1(4): 371-374.

KALE P.G. & BAUM J.W. (1980) Genetic effects of strong magnetic fields in Drosophila melanogaster: II. lack of interaction between homogeneous fields and fission neutron- plus-gamma radiation. Environ Mutagen, 2(2): 179-186.

KANAL E., BORGSTEDE J.P., BARKOVICH A.J., BELL C., BRADLEY W.G., FELMLEE J.P., FROELICH J.W., KAMINSKI E.M., KEELER E.K., LESTER J.W., SCOUMIS E.A., ZAREMBA L.A. & ZINNINGER M.D. (2002) American College of Radiology White Paper on MR Safety. Am J Roentgenol, 178(6): 1335-1347.

KANAL E., GILLEN J., EVANS J.A., SAVITZ D.A. & SHELLOCK F.G. (1993) Survey of reproductive health among female MR workers. Radiology, 187(2): 395-399.

KANGARLU A., BURGESS R.E., ZHU H., NAKAYAMA T., HAMLIN R.L., ABDULJALIL A.M. & ROBITAILLE P.M. (1999) Cognitive, cardiac, and physiological safety studies in ultra high field magnetic resonance imaging. Magn Reson Imaging, 17(10): 1407-1416.

KANGARLU A. & ROBITAILLE P.M.L. (2000) Biological effects and health implications in magnetic resonance imaging. Concepts Magn Reson, 12 321-359.

KAY H.H., HERFKENS R.J. & KAY B.K. (1988) Effect of magnetic resonance imaging on Xenopus laevis embryogenesis. Magn Reson Imaging, 6(5): 501-506.

KELTNER J.R., ROOS M.S., BRAKEMAN P.R. & BUDINGER T.F. (1990) Magnetohydrodynamics of blood flow. Magn Reson Med, 16(1): 139-149.

KHAR'KOVA N.A., KAZANIN V.I., VOLKOVA Z.S. & RED'KO A.F. (1976) [Effect of a steady magnetic field on several properties of a pathogenetic staphylococcus]. Zh Mikrobiol Epidemiol Immunobiol,(1): 145-146.

KHEIFETS L.I., AFIFI A.A., BUFFLER P.A. & ZHANG Z.W. (1995) Occupational electric and magnetic field exposure and brain cancer: a meta-analysis. J Occup Environ Med, 37(12): 1327-1341.

KHEIFETS L.I., AFIFI A.A., BUFFLER P.A., ZHANG Z.W. & MATKIN C.C. (1997) Occupational electric and magnetic field exposure and leukemia. A meta-analysis. J Occup Environ Med, 39 1074-1091.

KHOORY R. (1987) Compensation of the natural magnetic field does not alter N-acetyltransferase activity and melatonin content of rat pineal gland. Neurosci Lett, 76(2): 215-220.

KIMCHI T. & TERKEL J. (2001) Magnetic compass orientation in the blind mole rat Spalax ehrenbergi. J Exp Biol, 204(Pt 4): 751-758.

KINOUCHI Y., YAMAGUCHI H. & TENFORDE T.S. (1996) Theoretical analysis of magnetic field interactions with aortic blood flow. Bioelectromagnetics, 17(1): 21-32.

KIRSCHVINK J.L., KOBAYASHI-KIRSCHVINK A., DIAZ-RICCI J.C. & KIRSCHVINK S.J. (1992) Magnetite in human tissues: a mechanism for the biological effects of weak ELF magnetic fields. Bioelectromagnetics, Suppl 1 101-113.

KIRSCHVINK J.L., WALKER M.M. & DIEBEL C.E. (2001) Magnetite-based magnetoreception. Curr Opin Neurobiol, 11(4): 462-467.

KLIMOVSKAIA L.D. & SMIRNOVA N.P. (1975) [Autonomic reactions in rabbits exposed to a constant magnetic field]. Kosm Biol Aviakosm Med, 9(3): 18-22.

KLIMOVSKAIA L.D. & SMIRNOVA N.P. (1976) [Change in the evoked potentials of the brain exposed to a constant magnetic field]. Biull Eksp Biol Med, 82(8): 907-910.

KLOIBER O., OKADA Y. & HOSSMANN K.A. (1990) [A 4.7 T static magnetic field has no effect on the electric activity of the brain in cats]. EEG EMG Z Elektroenzephalogr Elektromyogr Verwandte Geb, 21(4): 229-232.

KOANA T., IKEHATA M. & NAKAGAWA M. (1995) Estimation of genetic effects of a static magnetic field by a somatic cell test using mutagen-sensitive mutants of Drosophila melanogaster. Bioelectrochem Bioenerg, 36 95-100.

KOANA T., OKADA M.O., IKEHATA M. & NAKAGAWA M. (1997) Increase in the mitotic recombination frequency in Drosophila melanogaster by magnetic field exposure and its suppression by vitamin E supplement. Mutat Res, **373**(1): 55-60.

KOLIN A. (1945) An alternating field induction flow meter of high sensitivity. Rev Sci Inst, **16** 109-116.

KOLIN A. (1952) Improved apparatus and technique for electromagnetic determination of blood flow. Rev Sci Inst, **23** 235-242.

KONERMANN G. & MONIG H. (1986) [Effect of static magnetic fields on the prenatal development of the mouse]. Radiologe, **26**(10): 490-497.

KÖNIG H.L., KRUEGER A.P., LANG S. & SÖNNIG W. (1981) Biological effects of environmental magnetism. New York, NY: Springer Verlag New York, Inc.

KOTANI H., IWASAKA M., UENO S. & CURTIS A. (2000) Magnetic orientation of collagen and bone mixture. J Appl Phys, **87**(9): 6191-6193.

KOTANI H., KAWAGUCHI H., SHIMOAKA T., IWASAKA M., UENO S., OZAWA H., NAKAMURA K. & HOSHI K. (2002) Strong static magnetic field stimulates bone formation to a definite orientation in vitro and in vivo. J Bone Miner Res, **17**(10): 1814-1821.

KOWALCZUK C.I., SIENKIEWICZ Z.J. & SAUNDERS R.D. (1991) Biological effects of exposure to non-ionising electromagnetic fields and radiation. Chilton, Didcot: National Radiological Protection Board (publication nr NRPB-R238).

KROEKER G., PARKINSON D., VRIEND J. & PEELING J. (1996) Neurochemical effects of static magnetic field exposure. Surg Neurol, **45**(1): 62-66.

KUMAR V. (1978) Exact analysis for calculating hemodynamic parameters in unsteady blood flow in arteries in the presence of a static magnetic field. Stud Biophys, **72** 43-50.

KURINOBU S. & UCHIYAMA S. (1982) Recovery of plankton from red tide by HGMS. IEEE Trans Magnet, **18** 1526-1528.

KWONG-HING A., SANDHU H.S., PRATO F.S., FRAPPIER J.R. & KAVALIERS M. (1989) Effects of magnetic resonance imaging (MRI) on the formation of mouse dentin and bone. J Exp Zool, **252**(1): 53-59.

LEASK M.J.M. (1977) Physicochemical mechanism for magnetic field detection by migratory birds and homing pigeons. Nature, **267** 144-145.

LERCHL A., NONAKA K.O. & REITER R.J. (1991) Pineal gland "magnetosensitivity" to static magnetic fields is a consequence of induced electric currents (eddy currents). J Pineal Res, **10**(3): 109-116.

LERCHL A., NONAKA K.O., STOKKAN K.A. & REITER R.J. (1990) Marked rapid alterations in nocturnal pineal serotonin metabolism in mice and rats exposed to weak intermittent magnetic fields. Biochem Biophys Res Commun, **169**(1): 102-108.

LEVIN M. & ERNST S.G. (1997) Applied DC magnetic fields cause alterations in the time of cell divisions and developmental abnormalities in early sea urchin embryos. Bioelectromagnetics, **18**(3): 255-263.

LEVINE R.L. & BLUNI T.D. (1994) Magnetic field effects on spatial discrimination learning in mice. Physiol Behav, **55**(3): 465-467.

LEVINE R.L., DOOLEY J.K. & BLUNI T.D. (1995) Magnetic field effects on spatial discrimination and melatonin levels in mice. Physiol Behav, **58**(3): 535-537.

LIBOFF A.R., CHERNG S., JENROW K.A. & BULL A. (2003) Calmodulin-dependent cyclic nucleotide phosphodiesterase activity is altered by 20 microT magnetostatic fields. Bioelectromagnetics, **24**(1): 32-38.

LIBURDY R.P., TENFORDE T.S. & MAGIN R.L. (1986) Magnetic field-induced drug permeability in liposome vesicles. Radiat Res, **108**(1): 102-111.

LIN J.C., SINGLETON G.W., SCHAEFFER J.N., HONG C.Z. & MELTZER R.J. (1985) Geophysical variables and behavior: XXVII. Magnetic necklace: its therapeutic effectiveness on neck and shoulder pain: 2. Psychological assessment. Psychol Rep, **56**(2): 639-649.

LINDER-ARONSON A., FORSBERG C.M., RYGH P. & LINDSKOG S. (1996) Tissue response to space closure in monkeys: a comparison of orthodontic magnets and superelastic coil springs. Eur J Orthod, **18**(6): 581-588.

LINDER-ARONSON A. & LINDSKOG S. (1995) Effects of static magnetic fields on human periodontal fibroblasts in vitro. Swed Dent J, **19**(4): 131-137.

LINDER-ARONSON A., LINDSKOG S. & RYGH P. (1992) Orthodontic magnets: effects on gingival epithelium and alveolar bone in monkeys. Eur J Orthod, **14**(4): 255-263.

LINDER-ARONSON A., RYGH P. & LINDSKOG S. (1995) Effects of orthodontic magnets on cutaneous epithelial thickness and tibial bone growth in rats. Acta Odontol Scand, **53**(4): 259-263.

LINDER-ARONSON S. & LINDSKOG S. (1991) A morphometric study of bone surfaces and skin reactions after stimulation with static magnetic fields in rats. Am J Orthod Dentofacial Orthop, **99**(1): 44-48.

LIU F. & CROZIER S. (2004) Electromagnetic fields inside a lossy, multilayered spherical head phantom excited by MRI coils: models and methods. Phys Med Biol, **49**(10): 1835-1851.

LIU F., EDGE R., HENBEST K., TIMMEL C.R., HORE P.J. & GAST P. (2005) Magnetic field effect on singlet oxygen production in a biochemical system. Chem Commun, **2** 174-176.

LIU F., ZHAO H. & CROZIER S. (2003a) Calculation of electric fields induced by body and head motion in high-field MRI. J Magn Reson, **161**(1): 99-107.

LIU F., ZHAO H. & CROZIER S. (2003b) On the induced electric field gradients in the human body for magnetic stimulation by gradient coils in MRI. IEEE Trans Biomed Eng, **50**(7): 804-815.

LOCKWOOD D.R., KWON B., SMITH J.C. & HOUPT T.A. (2003) Behavioral effects of static high magnetic fields on unrestrained and restrained mice. Physiol Behav, **78**(4-5): 635-640.

LOHMANN K.J., CAIN S.D., DODGE S.A. & LOHMANN C.M. (2001) Regional magnetic fields as navigational markers for sea turtles. Science, **294**(5541): 364-366.

LOHMANN K.J. & JOHNSEN S. (2000) The neurobiology of magnetoreception in vertebrate animals. Trends Neurosci, **23**(4): 153-159.

LOHMANN K.J., WILLOWS A.O. & PINTER R.B. (1991) An identifiable molluscan neuron responds to changes in earth-strength magnetic fields. J Exp Biol, **161** 1-24.

LUD G.V. & DEMECKIY A.M. (1990) Use of permanent magnetic field in reconstructive surgery of the main arteries (experimental study). Acta Chir Plast, **32**(1): 28-34.

MAGIN R.L., LEE J.K., KLINTSOVA A., CARNES K.I. & DUNN F. (2000) Biological effects of long-duration, high-field (4 T) MRI on growth and development in the mouse. J Magn Reson Imaging, 12(1): 140-149.

MAHDI A., GOWLAND P.A., MANSFIELD P., COUPLAND R.E. & LLOYD R.G. (1994) The effects of static 3.0 T and 0.5 T magnetic fields and the echo- planar imaging experiment at 0.5 T on E. coli. Br J Radiol, 67(802): 983-987.

MALININ G.I., GREGORY W.D., MORELLI L., SHARMA V.K. & HOUCK J.C. (1976) Evidence of morphological and physiological transformation of mammalian cells by strong magnetic fields. Science, 194(4267): 844-846.

MALKO J.A., CONSTANTINIDIS I., DILLEHAY D. & FAJMAN W.A. (1994) Search for influence of 1.5 Tesla magnetic field on growth of yeast cells. Bioelectromagnetics, 15(6): 495-501.

MAN D., MAN B. & PLOSKER H. (1999) The influence of permanent magnetic field therapy on wound healing in suction lipectomy patients: a double-blind study. Plast Reconstr Surg, 104(7): 2261-2266.

MARET G. & DRANSFELD K. (1977) Macromolecules and membranes in high magnetic fields. Physica B, 86-88: 1077-1083.

MARET G., SCHICKFUS M.V., MAYER A. & DRANSFELD K. (1975) Orientation of nucleic acids in high magnetic fields. Phys Rev Lett, 35 397-400.

MARIANI F., CAPPELLI G., EREMENKO T. & VOLPE P. (2001) Influence of static magnetic fields on cell viability, necrosis and apoptosis. Boll Soc Ital Biol Sper, 77(4-6): 71-84.

MARKOV M.S., RYABY J.T. & WANG S. (1992) Extremely weak AC and DC magnetic fields significantly affect myosin phosphorylation. In: Charge and Field Effects in Biosystems, Vol. 3 (eds. Allen, M. J. & Cleary, S. F.), pp. 225-230. Boston, MA: Birkhauser Press.

MARKOV M.S., WANG S. & PILLA A.A. (1993) Effects of weak low frequency sinusoidal and DC magnetic fields on myosin phosphorylation in a cell-free preparation. Bioelectrochem Bioenerg, 30 119-125.

MARSH J.L., ARMSTRONG T.J., JACOBSON A.P. & SMITH R.G. (1982) Health effect of occupational exposure to steady magnetic fields. Am Ind Hyg Assoc J, **43**(6): 387-394.

MARTEL G.F., ANDREWS S.C. & ROSEBOOM C.G. (2002) Comparison of static and placebo magnets on resting forearm blood flow in young, healthy men. J Orthop Sports Phys Ther, **32**(10): 518-524.

MATRONCHIK A.I., ALIPOV E.D. & BELIAEV I.I. (1996) [A model of phase modulation of high frequency nucleoid oscillations in reactions of E. coli cells to weak static and low-frequency magnetic fields]. Biofizika, **41**(3): 642-649.

MAYROVITZ H.N., GROSECLOSE E.E., MARKOV M. & PILLA A.A. (2001) Effects of permanent magnets on resting skin blood perfusion in healthy persons assessed by laser Doppler flowmetry and imaging. Bioelectromagnetics, **22**(7): 494-502.

MCDONALD F. (1993) Effect of static magnetic fields on osteoblasts and fibroblasts in vitro. Bioelectromagnetics, **14**(3): 187-196.

MCLAUCHLAN K.A. (1989) Magnetokinetics, mechanistics and synthesis. Chem Br, **25**: 895-898.

MCLAUCHLAN K.A. & STEINER U.E. (1991) The spin-correlated radical pair as a reaction intermediate. Molecular Physics, **73** 241-263.

MCLEAN M.J., HOLCOMB R.R., WAMIL A.W., PICKETT J.D. & CAVOPOL A.V. (1995) Blockade of sensory neuron action potentials by a static magnetic field in the 10 mT range. Bioelectromagnetics, **16**(1): 20-32.

MELVILLE D. (1975) Direct magnetic separation of red cells from whole blood. Nature, **255**(5511): 706.

MESSMER J.M., PORTER J.H., FATOUROS P., PRASAD U. & WEISBERG M. (1987) Exposure to magnetic resonance imaging does not produce taste aversion in rats. Physiol Behav, **40**(2): 259-261.

MESZAROS K. (1991) Magnetic field elicits hypotension mediated by platelet activating factor in rats injected with iron beads. Biochem Biophys Res Commun, **180**(1): 315-322.

MEVISSEN M., BUNTENKOTTER S. & LOSCHER W. (1994) Effects of static and time-varying (50-Hz) magnetic fields on reproduction and fetal development in rats. Teratology, **50**(3): 229-237.

MEVISSEN M., STAMM A., BUNTENKOTTER S., ZWINGELBERG R., WAHNSCHAFFE U. & LOSCHER W. (1993) Effects of magnetic fields on mammary tumor development induced by 7,12-dimethylbenz(a)anthracene in rats. Bioelectromagnetics, **14**(2): 131-143.

MILD K.H., SANDSTRÖM M. & LOVTRUP S. (1981) Development of Xenopus laevis embryos in a static magnetic field. Bioelectromagnetics, **2**(2): 199-201.

MILHAM S. (1982) Mortality from leukemia in workers exposed to electrical and magnetic fields. N Engl J Med, **307**(4): 249.

MILHAM S. (1985) Mortality in workers exposed to electromagnetic fields. Environ Health Perspect, **62** 297-300.

MILHAM S., HATFIELD J.B. & TELL R. (1999) Magnetic fields from steel-belted radial tires: implications for epidemiologic studies. Bioelectromagnetics, **20**(7): 440-445.

MILLER G. (1987) Exposure guidelines for magnetic fields. Am Ind Hyg Assoc J, **48**(12): 957-968.

MIYAMOTO H., YAMAGUCHI H., IKEHARA T. & KINOUCHI Y. (1996) Effects of electromagnetic fields on K+ (Rb+) uptake by HeLa cells. In: Biological Effects of Magnetic and Electromagnetic Fields (ed. Ueno, S.), pp. 101-119. New York: Plenum Press.

MNAIMNEH S., BIZRI M. & VEYRET B. (1996) No effect of exposure to static and sinusoidal magnetic fields on nitric oxide production by macrophages. Bioelectromagnetics, **17**(6): 519-521.

MOEN B.E., DRABLOS P.A., PEDERSEN S., SJOEN M. & THOMMESEN G. (1995) Symptoms of the musculoskeletal system and exposure to magnetic fields in an aluminium plant. Occup Environ Med, **52**(8): 524-527.

MOEN B.E., DRABLOS P.A., PEDERSEN S., SJOEN M. & THOMMESEN G. (1996) Absence of relation between sick leave caused by musculoskeletal disorders and exposure to magnetic fields in an aluminum plant. Bioelectromagnetics, **17**(1): 37-43.

MOHTAT N., COZENS F.L., HANCOCK-CHEN T., SCAIANO J.C., MCLEAN J. & KIM J. (1998) Magnetic field effects on the behavior of radicals in protein and DNA environments. Photochem Photobiol, **67**(1): 111-118.

MÖSE J.R. & FISCHER G. (1970) [Effect of electrostatic fields: results of further animal experiments]. Arch Hyg Bakteriol, **154**(4): 378-386.

MOURITSEN H., JANSSEN-BIENHOLD U., LIEDVOGEL M., FEENDERS G., STALLEICKEN J., DIRKS P. & WEILER R. (2004) Cryptochromes and neuronal-activity markers colocalize in the retina of migratory birds during magnetic orientation. Proc Natl Acad Sci USA, **101**(39): 14294-14299.

MÜLLER S. & HOTZ M. (1990) Human brainstem auditory evoked potentials (BAEP) before and after MR examinations. Magn Reson Med, **16**(3): 476-480.

MUNRO U., MUNRO J.A., PHILLIPS J.B., WILTSCHKO R. & WILTSCHKO W. (1997) Evidence for a magnetite-based navigational "map" in birds. Naturwissenschaften, **84** 26-28.

MUR J.M., MOULIN J.J., MEYER-BISCH C., MASSIN N., COULON J.P. & LOULERGUE J. (1987) Mortality of aluminium reduction plant workers in France. Int J Epidemiol, **16**(2): 257-264.

MUR J.M., WILD P., RAPP R., VAUTRIN J.P. & COULON J.P. (1998) Demographic evaluation of the fertility of aluminium industry workers: influence of exposure to heat and static magnetic fields. Hum Reprod, **13**(7): 2016-2019.

MURAKAMI J., TORII Y. & MASUDA K. (1992) Fetal development of mice following intrauterine exposure to a static magnetic field of 6.3 T. Magn Reson Imaging, **10**(3): 433-437.

MURAYAMA M. (1965) Orientation of sickled erythrocytes in a magnetic field. Nature, **206**(982): 420-422.

MYERS C., DUNCAN K.R., GOWLAND P.A., JOHNSON I.R. & BAKER P.N. (1998) Failure to detect intrauterine growth restriction following in utero exposure to MRI. Br J Radiol, **71**(845): 549-551.

NAKAGAWA M. (1978) [Changes of the cardiovascular system of rabbits subjected to static magnetic field of 600 Oe (author's transl)]. Sangyo Igaku, 20(2): 112-113.

NAKAGAWA M. (1984) Detection of electrophysiological responses in rabbits affected by short-term exposure to static magnetic field. Nippon Eiseigaku Zasshi, 38(6): 899-908.

NAKAGAWA M. & MATSUDA Y. (1988) A strong static-magnetic field alters operant responding by rats. Bioelectromagnetics, 9(1): 25-37.

NAKAHARA T., YAGUCHI H., YOSHIDA M. & MIYAKOSHI J. (2002) Effects of exposure of CHO-K1 cells to a 10-T static magnetic field. Radiology, 224(3): 817-822.

NAKAOKA Y., TAKEDA R. & SHIMIZU K. (2002) Orientation of Paramecium swimming in a DC magnetic field. Bioelectromagnetics, 23(8): 607-613.

NARRA V.R., HOWELL R.W., GODDU S.M. & RAO D.V. (1996) Effects of a 1.5-Tesla static magnetic field on spermatogenesis and embryogenesis in mice. Invest Radiol, 31(9): 586-590.

NEURATH P.W. (1968) High gradient magnetic field inhibits embryonic development of frogs. Nature, 219(161): 1358-1359.

NGO F.Q., BLUE J.W. & ROBERTS W.K. (1987) The effects of a static magnetic field on DNA synthesis and survival of mammalian cells irradiated with fast neutrons. Magn Reson Med, 5(4): 307-317.

NIKOL'SKAIA K.A., ESHCHENKO O.V. & SHPIN'KOVA V.N. (2000) [Magnetic field and alcohol addiction]. Biofizika, 45(5): 941-946.

NIKOLSKAIA K. & ECHENKO O. (2002) Alcohol addiction as the result of cognitive activity in altered natural magnetic field. Electromagnetic Biol Med, 21(1): 1-18.

NIKOLSKAIA K.A., YESHCHENKO O.V. & PRATUSEVICH V. (1999) The opioid system and magnetic field perception. Electro Magnetobiol, 18(3): 277-290.

NOBLE, D., MCKINLAY, A., REPACHOLI, M., & eds. (2005) Effects of static magnetic fields relevant to human health. Prog Biophys Mol Biol, 87(2-3).

NOLTE C.M., PITTMAN D.W., KALEVITCH B., HENDERSON R. & SMITH J.C. (1998) Magnetic field conditioned taste aversion in rats. Physiol Behav, **63**(4): 683-688.

NORIMURA T., IMADA H., KUNUGITA N., YOSHIDA N. & NIKAIDO M. (1993) Effects of strong magnetic fields on cell growth and radiation response of human T-lymphocytes in culture. J UOEH, **15**(2): 103-112.

NOSSOL B., BUSE G. & SILNY J. (1993) Influence of weak static and 50 Hz magnetic fields on the redox activity of cytochrome-C oxidase. Bioelectromagnetics, **14**(4): 361-372.

NRPB - NATIONAL RADIOLOGICAL PROTECTION BOARD (1993) Restrictions on human exposure to static and time varying electromagnetic fields and radiation: scientific basis and recommandations for the implementation of the Board's Statement. Docs NRPB, **4**(5).

OHKUBO C. & XU S. (1997) Acute effects of static magnetic fields on cutaneous microcirculation in rabbits. In Vivo, **11**(3): 221-225.

OKANO H., GMITROV J. & OHKUBO C. (1999) Biphasic effects of static magnetic fields on cutaneous microcirculation in rabbits. Bioelectromagnetics, **20**(3): 161-171.

OKANO H., MASUDA H. & OHKUBO C. (2005a) Decreased plasma levels of nitric oxide metabolites, angiotensin II, and aldosterone in spontaneously hypertensive rats exposed to 5 mT static magnetic field. Bioelectromagnetics, **26**(3): 161-172.

OKANO H., MASUDA H. & OHKUBO C. (2005b) Effects of 25 mT static magnetic field on blood pressure in reserpine-induced hypotensive Wistar-Kyoto rats. Bioelectromagnetics, **26**(1): 36-48.

OKANO H. & OHKUBO C. (2001) Modulatory effects of static magnetic fields on blood pressure in rabbits. Bioelectromagnetics, **22**(6): 408-418.

OKANO H. & OHKUBO C. (2003a) Anti-pressor effects of whole-body exposure to static magnetic field on pharmacologically induced hypertension in conscious rabbits. Bioelectromagnetics, **24** 139-147.

OKANO H. & OHKUBO C. (2003b) Effects of static magnetic fields on plasma levels of angiotensin II and aldosterone associated with arterial blood pressure in genetically hypertensive rats. Bioelectromagnetics, **24**(6): 403-412.

OKAZAKI M., KON K., MAEDA N. & SHIGA T. (1988) Distribution of erythrocyte in a model vessel exposed to inhomogeneous magnetic fields. Physiol Chem Phys Med NMR, **20**(1): 3-14.

OKAZAKI M., SEIYAMA A., KON K., MAEDA N. & SHIGA T. (1991) Boycott effect with vertical cylinder for paramagnetic red blood cells under the inhomogenous magnetic field. J Coll Interface Sci, **146**(2): 590-593.

OKAZAKI R., OOTSUYAMA A., UCHIDA S. & NORIMURA T. (2001) Effects of a 4.7 T static magnetic field on fetal development in ICR mice. J Radiat Res (Tokyo), **42**(3): 273-283.

OKONOGI H., NAKAGAWA M. & TSUJI Y. (1996) The effects of a 4.7 tesla static magnetic field on the frequency of micronucleated cells induced by mitomycin C. Tohoku J Exp Med, **180**(3): 209-215.

OKUNO K., FUJINAMI R., ANO T. & SHODA M. (2001) Disappearance of growth advantage in stationary phase (GASP) phenomenon under a high magnetic field. Bioelectrochemistry, **53**(2): 165-169.

OLCESE J. & HURLBUT E. (1989) Comparative studies on the retinal dopamine response to altered magnetic fields in rodents. Brain Res, **498**(1): 145-148.

OLCESE J. & REUSS S. (1986) Magnetic field effects on pineal gland melatonin synthesis: comparative studies on albino and pigmented rodents. Brain Res, **369**(1-2): 365-368.

OLCESE J., REUSS S., STEHLE J., STEINLECHNER S. & VOLLRATH L. (1988) Responses of the mammalian retina to experimental alteration of the ambient magnetic field. Brain Res, **448**(2): 325-330.

OLCESE J., REUSS S. & VOLLRATH L. (1985) Evidence for the involvement of the visual system in mediating magnetic field effects on pineal melatonin synthesis in the rat. Brain Res, **333**(2): 382-384.

ONODERA H., JIN Z., CHIDA S., SUZUKI Y., TAGO H. & ITOYAMA Y. (2003) Effects of 10-T static magnetic field on human peripheral blood immune cells. Radiat Res, 159(6): 775-779.

OSBAKKEN M., GRIFFITH J. & TACZANOWSKY P. (1986) A gross morphologic, histologic, hematologic, and blood chemistry study of adult and neonatal mice chronically exposed to high magnetic fields. Magn Reson Med, 3(4): 502-517.

OSSENKOPP K.P., INNIS N.K., PRATO F.S. & SESTINI E. (1986) Behavioral effects of exposure to nuclear magnetic resonance imaging: I. Open-field behavior and passive avoidance learning in rats. Magn Reson Imaging, 4(4): 275-280.

OSSENKOPP K.P., KAVALIERS M., PRATO F.S., TESKEY G.C., SESTINI E. & HIRST M. (1985) Exposure to nuclear magnetic resonance imaging procedure attenuates morphine-induced analgesia in mice. Life Sci, 37(16): 1507-1514.

OSUGA T. & TATSUOKA H. (1999) Effect of 1.5 T steady magnetic field on neuroconduction of a bullfrog sciatic nerve in a partially active state within several hours after extraction. Magn Reson Imaging, 17(5): 791-794.

PACINI S., ATERINI S., PACINI P., RUGGIERO C., GULISANO M. & RUGGIERO M. (1999a) Influence of static magnetic field on the antiproliferative effects of vitamin D on human breast cancer cells. Oncol Res, 11(6): 265-271.

PACINI S., VANNELLI G.B., BARNI T., RUGGIERO M., SARDI I., PACINI P. & GULISANO M. (1999b) Effect of 0.2 T static magnetic field on human neurons: remodeling and inhibition of signal transduction without genome instability. Neurosci Lett, 267(3): 185-188.

PAPADOPULOS M.A., HORLER I., GERBER H., RAHN B.A. & RAKOSI T. (1992) [The effect of static magnetic fields on osteoblast activity: an in- vitro study]. Fortschr Kieferorthop, 53(4): 218-222.

PAPATHEOFANIS F.J. (1990) Use of calcium channel antagonists as magnetoprotective agents. Radiat Res, 122(1): 24-28.

PAPATHEOFANIS F.J. & PAPATHEOFANIS B.J. (1989a) Acid and alkaline phosphatase activity in bone following intense magnetic field irradiation of short duration. Int J Radiat Biol, 55(6): 1033-1035.

PAPATHEOFANIS F.J. & PAPATHEOFANIS B.J. (1989b) Short-term effect of exposure to intense magnetic fields on hematologic indices of bone metabolism. Invest Radiol, 24(3): 221-223.

PARAFINIUK M., GORCZYNSKA E., GUTSCH A. & PARAFINIUK W. (1992) Effect of constant magnetic field on the liver of guinea pig. Electron microscopic studies. Folia Histochem Cytobiol, 30(3): 119-123.

PARK L. (2000) Voodoo science: the road from foolishness to fraud. New York, NY: Oxford University Press.

PATE K., BENGHUZZI H., TUCCI M., PUCKETT A. & CASON Z. (2003) Morphological evaluation of MRC-5 fibroblasts after stimulation with static magnetic field and pulsating electromagnetic field. Biomed Sci Instrum, 39 460-465.

PAUL F., ROATH S. & MELVILLE D. (1978) Differential blood cell separation using a high gradient magnetic field. Br J Haematol, 38(2): 273-280.

PETERSON H.P., VON WANGENHEIM K.H. & FEINENDEGEN L.E. (1992) Magnetic field exposure of marrow donor mice can increase the number of spleen colonies (CFU-S 7d) in marrow recipient mice. Radiat Environ Biophys, 31(1): 31-38.

PHILLIPS J.B. (1996) Magnetic navigation. J Theor Biol, 180 309-319.

PHILLIPS J.B., DEUTSCHLANDER M.E., FREAKE M.J. & BORLAND S.C. (2001) The role of extraocular photoreceptors in newt magnetic compass orientation: parallels between light-dependent magnetoreception and polarized light detection in vertebrates. J Exp Biol, 204(Pt 14): 2543-2552.

PHILLIPS J.B., FREAKE M.J., FISCHER J.H. & BORLAND C. (2002) Behavioral titration of a magnetic map coordinate. J Comp Physiol A Neuroethol Sens Neural Behav Physiol, 188(2): 157-160.

PIATTI E., CRISTINA A.M., BAFFONE W., FRATERNALE D., CITTERIO B., PIERA P.M., DACHA M., VETRANO F. & ACCORSI A. (2002) Antibacterial effect of a magnetic field on Serratia marcescens and related virulence to Hordeum vulgare and Rubus fruticosus callus cells. Comp Biochem Physiol B Biochem Mol Biol, 132(2): 359-365.

POLK C., POSTOW E. & EDS. (1996) Biological effects of electromagnetic fields. Boca Raton, FL: CRC Press.

POYNTON C.H., DICKE K.A., CULBERT S., FRANKEL L.S., JAGANNATH S. & READING C.L. (1983) Immunomagnetic removal of CALLA positive cells from human bone marrow. Lancet, 1(8323): 524.

PRASAD N., BUSHONG S.C., THORNBY J.I., BRYAN R.N., HAZLEWOOD C.F. & HARRELL J.E. (1984) Effect of nuclear magnetic resonance on chromosomes of mouse bone marrow cells. Magn Reson Imaging, 2(1): 37-39.

PRASAD N., WRIGHT D.A., FORD J.J. & THORNBY J.I. (1990) Safety of 4-T MR imaging: study of effects on developing frog embryos. Radiology, 174(1): 251-253.

PRASAD N., WRIGHT D.A. & FORSTER J.D. (1982) Effect of nuclear magnetic resonance on early stages of amphibian development. Magn Reson Imaging, 1(1): 35-38.

PRATO F.S., FRAPPIER J.R., SHIVERS R.R., KAVALIERS M., ZABEL P., DROST D. & LEE T.Y. (1990) Magnetic resonance imaging increases the blood-brain barrier permeability to 153-gadolinium diethylenetriaminepentaacetic acid in rats. Brain Res, 523(2): 301-304.

PRATO F.S., KAVALIERS M., CULLEN A.P. & THOMAS A.W. (1997) Light-dependent and -independent behavioral effects of extremely low frequency magnetic fields in a land snail are consistent with a parametric resonance mechanism. Bioelectromagnetics, 18(3): 284-291.

PRATO F.S., WILLS J.M., ROGER J., FRAPPIER H., DROST D.J., LEE T.Y., SHIVERS R.R. & ZABEL P. (1994) Blood-brain barrier permeability in rats is altered by exposure to magnetic fields associated with magnetic resonance imaging at 1.5 T. Microsc Res Tech, 27(6): 528-534.

PREECE A.W., WESNES K.A. & IWI G.R. (1998) The effect of a 50 Hz magnetic field on cognitive function in humans. Int J Radiat Biol, 74(4): 463-470.

PTITSYNA N.G., VILLORESI G., DORMAN L.I., IUCCI N. & TYASTO M.I. (1998) Natural and man-made low-frequency magnetic fields as a potential health hazard. Physics Uspekhi, 41 687-709.

RAMIREZ E., MONTEAGUDO J.L., GARCIA-GRACIA M. & DELGADO J.M. (1983) Oviposition and development of Drosophila modified by magnetic fields. Bioelectromagnetics, 4(4): 315-326.

RAYBOURN M.S. (1983) The effects of direct-current magnetic fields on turtle retinas in vitro. Science, 220(4598): 715-717.

RAYLMAN R.R., CLAVO A.C., CRAWFORD S.C., RECKER B. & WAHL R.L. (1997) Magnetically-enhanced radionuclide therapy (MERiT): in vitro evaluation. Int J Radiat Oncol Biol Phys, 37(5): 1201-1206.

RAYLMAN R.R., CLAVO A.C. & WAHL R.L. (1996) Exposure to strong static magnetic field slows the growth of human cancer cells in vitro. Bioelectromagnetics, 17(5): 358-363.

REINA F.G. & PASCUAL L.A. (2001) Influence of a stationary magnetic field on water relations in lettuce seeds. Part I: theoretical considerations. Bioelectromagnetics, 22(8): 589-595.

REINA F.G., PASCUAL L.A. & FUNDORA I.A. (2001) Influence of a stationary magnetic field on water relations in lettuce seeds. Part II: experimental results. Bioelectromagnetics, 22(8): 596-602.

RENO V.R. & BEISCHER D.E. (1966) Cardiac excitability in high magnetic fields. Aerosp Med, 37(12): 1229-1232.

REPACHOLI M.H. & CARDIS E. (1997) Criteria for health risk assessment. Rad Prot Dos, 72(3-4): 305-312.

REUSS S. & OLCESE J. (1986) Magnetic field effects on the rat pineal gland: role of retinal activation by light. Neurosci Lett, 64(1): 97-101.

REUSS S., SEMM P. & VOLLRATH L. (1983) Different types of magnetically sensitive cells in the rat pineal gland. Neurosci Lett, 40(1): 23-26.

RICHARDSON B.A., YAGA K., REITER R.J. & MORTON D.J. (1992) Pulsed static magnetic field effects on in-vitro pineal indoleamine metabolism. Biochim Biophys Acta, 1137(1): 59-64.

RITZ T., ADEM S. & SCHULTEN K. (2000) A model for photoreceptor-based magnetoreception in birds. Biophys J, 78(2): 707-718.

RITZ T., DOMMER D.H. & PHILLIPS J.B. (2002) Shedding light on vertebrate magnetoreception. Neuron, **34**(4): 503-506.

ROCKETTE H.E. & ARENA V.C. (1983) Mortality studies of aluminum reduction plant workers: potroom and carbon department. J Occup Med, **25**(7): 549-557.

ROCKWELL S. (1977) Influence of a 1400-gauss magnetic field on the radiosensitivity and recovery of EMT6 cells in vitro. Int J Radiat Biol Relat Stud Phys Chem Med, **31**(2): 153-160.

ROFSKY N.M., PIZZARELLO D.J., DUHANEY M.O., FALICK A.K., PRENDERGAST N. & WEINREB J.C. (1995) Effect of magnetic resonance exposure combined with gadopentetate dimeglumine on chromosomes in animal specimens. Acad Radiol, **2**(6): 492-496.

RØNNEBERG A. (1995) Mortality and cancer morbidity in workers from an aluminium smelter with prebaked carbon anodes--Part I: Exposure assessment. Occup Environ Med, **52**(4): 242-249.

RØNNEBERG A. & ANDERSEN A. (1995) Mortality and cancer morbidity in workers from an aluminium smelter with prebaked carbon anodes--Part II: Cancer morbidity. Occup Environ Med, **52**(4): 250-254.

RØNNEBERG A., HALDORSEN T., ROMUNDSTAD P. & ANDERSEN A. (1999) Occupational exposure and cancer incidence among workers from an aluminum smelter in western Norway. Scand J Work Environ Health, **25**(3): 207-214.

ROSEN A.D. (1992) Magnetic field influence on acetylcholine release at the neuromuscular junction. Am J Physiol, **262**(6 Pt 1): C1418-C1422.

ROSEN A.D. (1993) Membrane response to static magnetic fields: effect of exposure duration. Biochim Biophys Acta, **1148**(2): 317-320.

ROSEN A.D. (1994) Threshold and limits of magnetic field action at the presynaptic membrane. Biochim Biophys Acta, **1193**(1): 62-66.

ROSEN A.D. (1996) Inhibition of calcium channel activation in GH3 cells by static magnetic fields. Biochim Biophys Acta, **1282**(1): 149-155.

ROSEN A.D. (2003a) Effect of a 125 mT static magnetic field on the kinetics of voltage activated Na+ channels in GH3 cells. Bioelectromagnetics, **24**(7): 517-523.

ROSEN A.D. (2003b) Mechanism of action of moderate-intensity static magnetic fields on biological systems. Cell Biochem Biophys, **39**(2): 163-173.

ROSEN A.D. & LUBOWSKY J. (1987) Magnetic field influence on central nervous system function. Exp Neurol, **95**(3): 679-687.

ROSEN A.D. & LUBOWSKY J. (1990) Modification of spontaneous unit discharge in the lateral geniculate body by a magnetic field. Exp Neurol, **108**(3): 261-265.

ROSEN M.S. & ROSEN A.D. (1990) Magnetic field influence on paramecium motility. Life Sci, **46**(21): 1509-1515.

ROSSNER P. & MATEJKA M. (1977) Potential genetic risks from stationary magnetic field. J Hyg Epidemiol Microbiol Immunol, **21**(4): 465-467.

RUDOLPH K., WIRZ-JUSTICE A., KRAUCHI K. & FEER H. (1988) Static magnetic fields decrease nocturnal pineal cAMP in the rat. Brain Res, **446**(1): 159-160.

SABO J., MIROSSAY L., HOROVCAK L., SARISSKY M., MIROSSAY A. & MOJZIS J. (2002) Effects of static magnetic field on human leukemic cell line HL-60. Bioelectrochemistry, **56**(1-2): 227-231.

SACKS E., WORGUL B.V., MERRIAM G.R., JR. & HILAL S. (1986) The effects of nuclear magnetic resonance imaging on ocular tissues. Arch Ophthalmol, **104**(6): 890-893.

SAKHNINI L. & KHUZAIE R. (2001) Magnetic behavior of human erythrocytes at different hemoglobin states. Eur Biophys J, **30**(6): 467-470.

SAKURAI H., OKUNO K., KUBO A., NAKAMURA K. & SHODA M. (1999) Effect of a 7-tesla homogeneous magnetic field on mammalian cells. Bioelectrochem Bioenerg, **49**(1): 57-63.

SALERNO S., LO C.A., CACCAMO N., D'ANNA C., DE MARIA M., LAGALLA R., SCOLA L. & CARDINALE A.E. (1999) Static magnetic fields generated by a 0.5 T MRI unit affects in vitro expression of activation markers and interleukin release in human peripheral blood mononuclear cells (PBMC). Int J Radiat Biol, **75**(4): 457-463.

SANTINI M.T., CAMETTI C., STRAFACE E., GRANDOLFO M. & INDOVINA P.L. (1994) A static magnetic field does not affect the dielectric properties of chick embryo myoblast membranes. Int J Radiat Biol, **65**(2): 277-284.

SATO K., YAMAGUCHI H., MIYAMOTO H. & KINOUCHI Y. (1992) Growth of human cultured cells exposed to a non-homogeneous static magnetic field generated by Sm-Co magnets. Biochim Biophys Acta, **1136**(3): 231-238.

SATO T., YAMADA Y., SAIJO S., HORI T., HIROSE R., TANAKA N., SAZAKI G., NAKAJIMA K., IGARASHI N., TANAKA M. & MATSUURA Y. (2000) Enhancement in the perfection of orthorhombic lysozyme crystals grown in a high magnetic field (10 T). Acta Crystallogr D Biol Crystallogr, **56** (Pt 8) 1079-1083.

SATOH M., TSUJI Y., WATANABE Y., OKONOGI H., SUZUKI Y., NAKAGAWA M. & SHIMIZU H. (1996) Metallothionein content increased in the liver of mice exposed to magnetic fields. Arch Toxicol, **70**(5): 315-318.

SATOW Y., MATSUNAMI K., KAWASHIMA T., SATAKE H. & HUDA K. (2001) A strong constant magnetic field affects muscle tension development in bullfrog neuromuscular preparations. Bioelectromagnetics, **22**(1): 53-59.

SCHENCK J.F. (1992) Health and physiological effects of human exposure to whole-body four- tesla magnetic fields during MRI. Ann N Y Acad Sci, **649** 285-301.

SCHENCK J.F. (2000) Safety of strong, static magnetic fields. J Magn Reson Imaging, **12**(1): 2-19.

SCHENCK J.F. (2005) Physical interactions of static magnetic fields with living tissues. Prog Biophys Mol Biol, **87**(2-3): 185-204.

SCHENCK J.F., DUMOULIN C.L., REDINGTON R.W., KRESSEL H.Y., ELLIOTT R.T. & MCDOUGALL I.L. (1992) Human exposure to 4.0-Tesla magnetic fields in a whole-body scanner. Med Phys, **19**(4): 1089-1098.

SCHIFFER I.B., SCHREIBER W.G., GRAF R., SCHREIBER E.M., JUNG D., ROSE D.M., HEHN M., GEBHARD S., SAGEMULLER J., SPIESS H.W., OESCH F., THELEN M. & HENGSTLER J.G. (2003) No influence of magnetic fields on cell cycle progression using conditions relevant for patients during MRI. Bioelectromagnetics, **24**(4): 241-250.

SCHMIDT F., MANNSAKER T. & LOVLIE R. (1999) [Creatinine and calcium in urine and blood after brief exposure to magnetic fields]. Tidsskr Nor Laegeforen, **119**(4): 491-494.

SCHMITT F., STEHLING M.K. & TURNER R. (1998) Echo-planar imaging. Theory, technique and application. New York, NY: Springer.

SCHNEEWEISS F.H., SHARAN R.N. & FEINENDEGEN L.E. (1995) Change of ADP-ribosylation in human kidney T1-cells by various external stimuli. Indian J Biochem Biophys, **32**(3): 119-124.

SCHREIBER W.G., TEICHMANN E.M., SCHIFFER I., HAST J., AKBARI W., GEORGI H., GRAF R., HEHN M., SPIEBETA H.W., THELEN M., OESCH F. & HENGSTLER J.G. (2001) Lack of mutagenic and co-mutagenic effects of magnetic fields during magnetic resonance imaging. J Magn Reson Imaging, **14**(6): 779-788.

SCHULTEN K. (1982) Magnetic field effects in chemistry and biology. In: Festkörperprobleme (Advanced Solid State Physics), vol. 22 (ed. Treusch, J.), pp. 61-83. Braunschweig: Vieweg.

SCHWARTZ J.L. (1978) Influence of a constant magnetic field on nervous tissues: I. Nerve conduction velocity studies. IEEE Trans Biomed Eng, **25**(5): 467-473.

SCHWARTZ J.L. (1979) Influence of a constant magnetic field on nervous tissues: II. Voltage-clamp studies. IEEE Trans Biomed Eng, **26** 238-243.

SEGAL N.A., TODA Y., HUSTON J., SAEKI Y., SHIMIZU M., FUCHS H., SHIMAOKA Y., HOLCOMB R. & MCLEAN M.J. (2001) Two configurations of static magnetic fields for treating rheumatoid arthritis of the knee: a double-blind clinical trial. Arch Phys Med Rehabil, **82**(10): 1453-1460.

SEMM P., SCHNEIDER T. & VOLLRATH L. (1980) Effects of an earth-strength magnetic field on electrical activity of pineal cells. Nature, **288**(5791): 607-608.

SHELLOCK F.G. & CRUES J.V. (1987) Temperature, heart rate, and blood pressure changes associated with clinical MR imaging at 1.5 T. Radiology, 163(1): 259-262.

SHELLOCK F.G., SCHAEFER D.J. & CRUES J.V. (1989) Exposure to a 1.5-T static magnetic field does not alter body and skin temperatures in man. Magn Reson Med, 11(3): 371-375.

SHELLOCK F.G., SCHAEFER D.J. & GORDON C.J. (1986) Effect of a 1.5 T static magnetic field on body temperature of man. Magn Reson Med, 3(4): 644-647.

SHIGA T., OKAZAKI O., SEIYAMA A. & MAEDA N. (1993) Paramagnetic attraction of erythrocyte flow due to inhomogeneous magnetic field. Bioelectrochem Bioenerg, 30 181-188.

SHIVERS R.R., KAVALIERS M., TESKEY G.C., PRATO F.S. & PELLETIER R.M. (1987) Magnetic resonance imaging temporarily alters blood-brain barrier permeability in the rat. Neurosci Lett, 76(1): 25-31.

SHORT W.O., GOODWILL L., TAYLOR C.W., JOB C., ARTHUR M.E. & CRESS A.E. (1992) Alteration of human tumor cell adhesion by high-strength static magnetic fields. Invest Radiol, 27(10): 836-840.

SHUVALOVA L.A., OSTROVSKAIA M.V., SOSUNOV E.A. & LEDNEV V.V. (1991) [The effect of a weak magnetic field in the paramagnetic resonance mode on the rate of the calmodulin-dependent phosphorylation of myosin in solution]. Dokl Akad Nauk SSSR, 317(1): 227-230.

SIKOV M.R., MAHLUM D.D., MONTGOMERY L.D. & DECKER J.R. (1979) Development of mice after intrauterine exposure to direct-current magnetic fields. In: Biological effects of extremely low frequency electromagnetic fields (eds. Phillips, R. D., Gillis, M. F., Kaune, W. T. & Mahlum, D. D.), pp. 462-473. Springfield, VA: U.S. Department of Energy, National Technical Information Service.

SIMON J.H. & SZUMOWSKI J. (1992) Proton (fat/water) chemical shift imaging in medical magnetic resonance imaging. Current status. Invest Radiol, 27(10): 865-874.

SKOTTE J.H. & HJOLLUND H.I. (1997) Exposure of welders and other metal workers to ELF magnetic fields. Bioelectromagnetics, 18(7): 470-477.

SKYBERG K., HANSTEEN I.L. & VISTNES A.I. (1993) Chromosome aberrations in lymphocytes of high-voltage laboratory cable splicers exposed to electromagnetic fields. Scand J Work Environ Health, **19**(1): 29-34.

SMIRNOVA N.P., KLIMOVSKAIA L.D. & D'IAKONOV A.S. (1982) [Significance of magnetic field parameters for altering brain evoked bioelectrical activity]. Kosm Biol Aviakosm Med, **16**(4): 61-63.

SNYDER D.J., JAHNG J.W., SMITH J.C. & HOUPT T.A. (2000) c-Fos induction in visceral and vestibular nuclei of the rat brain stem by a 9.4 T magnetic field. Neuroreport, **11**(12): 2681-2685.

SONNIER H., KOLOMYTKIN O. & MARINO A. (2003) Action potentials from human neuroblastoma cells in magnetic fields. Neurosci Lett, **337**(3): 163-166.

SONNIER H., KOLOMYTKIN O.V. & MARINO A.A. (2000) Resting potential of excitable neuroblastoma cells in weak magnetic fields. Cell Mol Life Sci, **57**(3): 514-520.

SPINELLI J.J., BAND P.R., SVIRCHEV L.M. & GALLAGHER R.P. (1991) Mortality and cancer incidence in aluminum reduction plant workers. J Occup Med, **33**(11): 1150-1155.

STANFORD LINEAR ACCELERATOR CENTER (1970) Limits on human exposure to static magnetic fields. Palo Alto, CA: Stanford Linear Accelerator Center.

STANSELL M.J., WINTERS W.D., DOE R.H. & DART B.K. (2001) Increased antibiotic resistance of E. coli exposed to static magnetic fields. Bioelectromagnetics, **22**(2): 129-137.

STASIUK G.A. (1974) [Effect of a steady magnetic field on Mycobacterium tuberculosis]. Probl Tuberk, **0**(7): 75-77.

STEGEMANN S., ALTMAN K.I., MUHLENSIEPEN H. & FEINENDEGEN L.E. (1993) Influence of a stationary magnetic field on acetylcholinesterase in murine bone marrow cells. Radiat Environ Biophys, **32**(1): 65-72.

STEHLE J., REUSS S., SCHRODER H., HENSCHEL M. & VOLLRATH L. (1988) Magnetic field effects on pineal N-acetyltransferase activity and melatonin content in the gerbil--role of pigmentation and sex. Physiol Behav, **44**(1): 91-94.

STEPANIAN R.S., BARSEGIAN A.A., ALAVERDIAN Z., OGANESIAN G.G., MARKOSIAN L.S. & AIRAPETIAN S.N. (2000) [The effect of magnetic fields on the growth and division of the lon mutant of Escherichia coli K-12]. Radiats Biol Radioecol, **40**(3): 319-322.

STEYN P.F., RAMEY D.W., KIRSCHVINK J. & UHRIG J. (2000) Effect of a static magnetic field on blood flow to the metacarpus in horses. J Am Vet Med Assoc, **217**(6): 874-877.

STICK C., HINKELMANN K., EGGERT P. & WENDHAUSEN H. (1991) [Do strong static magnetic fields in NMR tomography modify tissue perfusion?]. Rofo Fortschr Geb Rontgenstr Neuen Bildgeb Verfahr, **154**(3): 326-331.

STOJAN L., SPERBER D. & DRANSFELD K. (1990) Influence of high steady magnetic fields on the electrical activity of the electric fish Apteronotus. Z Naturforsch [C], **45**(3-4): 303-305.

STRICKMAN D., TIMBERLAKE B., ESTRADA-FRACO J., WEISSMAN M., FENIMORE P.W. & NOVAK R.J. (2000) Effects of magnetic fields on mosquitoes. J Am Mosq Control Assoc, **16**(2): 131-137.

STUCHLY M.A. (1986) Human exposure to static and time-varying magnetic fields. Health Phys, **51**(2): 215-225.

STUCHLY M.A. & DAWSON T.W. (2000) Interaction of low frequency electric and magnetic fields with the human body. Proc IEEE, **88** 643-646.

STUCHLY M.A. & LECUYER D.W. (1987) Survey of static magnetic fields around magnetic resonance imaging devices. Health Phys, **53**(3): 321-324.

SUD V.K. & SEKHON G.S. (1989) Blood flow through the human arterial system in the presence of a steady magnetic field. Phys Med Biol, **34**(7): 795-805.

SUD V.K., SURI P.K. & MISHRA R.K. (1978) Laminar flow of blood in an elastic tube in the presence of a magnetic field. Stud Biophys, **69** 175-186.

SUNDARAM N.M., ASHOK M. & KALKURA S.N. (2002) Observation of cholesterol nucleation in a magnetic field. Acta Crystallogr D Biol Crystallogr, **58**(Pt 10 Pt 1): 1711-1714.

SUOMI R. & KOCEJA D.M. (2001) Effect of magnetic insoles on postural sway measures in men and women during a static balance test. Percept Mot Skills, **92**(2): 469-476.

SUTTER B.C., BILLAUDEL B., SUTTER-DUB M.T. & BELLOSSI A. (1987) Effects of constant magnetic fields on the B-cells and insulin target cells in the rat. Aviat Space Environ Med, **58**(6): 537-540.

SUZUKI Y., IKEHATA M., NAKAMURA K., NISHIOKA M., ASANUMA K., KOANA T. & SHIMIZU H. (2001) Induction of micronuclei in mice exposed to static magnetic fields. Mutagenesis, **16**(6): 499-501.

SWANSON J. (1994) Measurement of static magnetic fields in homes in the UK and their implication for epidemiological studies of exposure to alternating magnetic fields. J Radiol Prot, **14**(1): 67-75.

SWEETLAND J., KERTESZ A., PRATO F.S. & NANTAU K. (1987) The effect of magnetic resonance imaging on human cognition. Magn Reson Imaging, **5**(2): 129-135.

TABLADO L., PEREZ-SANCHEZ F., NUNEZ J., NUNEZ M. & SOLER C. (1998) Effects of exposure to static magnetic fields on the morphology and morphometry of mouse epididymal sperm. Bioelectromagnetics, **19**(6): 377-383.

TABLADO L., PEREZ-SANCHEZ F. & SOLER C. (1996) Is sperm motility maturation affected by static magnetic fields? Environ Health Perspect, **104**(11): 1212-1216.

TABLADO L., SOLER C., NUNEZ M., NUNEZ J. & PEREZ-SANCHEZ F. (2000) Development of mouse testis and epididymis following intrauterine exposure to a static magnetic field. Bioelectromagnetics, **21**(1): 19-24.

TAKATSUJI T., SASAKI M.S. & TAKEKOSHI H. (1989) Effect of static magnetic field on the induction of chromosome aberrations by 4.9 MeV protons and 23 MeV alpha particles. J Radiat Res (Tokyo), **30**(3): 238-246.

TAKESHIGE C. & SATO M. (1996) Comparisons of pain relief mechanisms between needling to the muscle, static magnetic field, external qigong and needling to the acupuncture point. Acupunct Electrother Res, **21**(2): 119-131.

TAMAKI T., YOSHIOKA T. & NAKANO S. (1987) Effect of magnetic field on the contractility and glycogen content in neuromuscular preparation. Tokai J Exp Clin Med, **12**(1): 55-59.

TAOKA S., PADMAKUMAR R., GRISSOM C.B. & BANERJEE R. (1997) Magnetic field effects on coenzyme B12-dependent enzymes: validation of ethanolamine ammonia lyase results and extension to human methylmalonyl CoA mutase. Bioelectromagnetics, **18**(7): 506-513.

TARABAN M.B. & LESHINA T.V. (1997) Magnetic field dependence of electron trabsfer and the role of electron spin in heme enzymes: horseradish peroxidase. J Am Chem Soc, **119** 5768-5769.

TAUSCH-TREML R., SCHERER H., GEWIESE B. & ZIESSOW D. (1989) [Effect of static magnetic fields on the acoustic action potential of the cochlea in guinea pigs]. Naturwissenschaften, **76**(3): 114-117.

TEICHMANN E.M., HENGSTLER J.G., SCHREIBER W.G., AKBARI W., GEORGI H., HEHN M., SCHIFFER I., OESCH F., SPIESS H.W. & THELEN M. (2000) [Possible mutagenic effects of magnetic fields]. Rofo Fortschr Geb Rontgenstr Neuen Bildgeb Verfahr, **172**(11): 934-939.

TENFORDE T.S. (1985) Mechanisms for biological effects of magnetic fields. In: Biological effects and dosimetry of static and ELF electromagnetic fields (eds. Grandolfo, M., Michaelson, S. M. & Rindi, A.), pp. 71-92. New York, London: Plenum Press.

TENFORDE T.S. (2005) Magnetically induced electric fields and currents in the circulatory system. Prog Biophys Mol Biol, **87**(2-3): 279-288.

TENFORDE T.S. & BUDINGER T.F. (1986) Biological effects and physical safety aspects of NMR imaging and in vivo spectroscopy. In: NMR in medicine: Instrumentation and clinical applications (eds. Thomas, S. R. & Dixon, R. L.), pp. 493-548. New York: American Association of Physicists in Medicine.

TENFORDE T.S., GAFFEY C.T., MOYER B.R. & BUDINGER T.F. (1983) Cardiovascular alterations in Macaca monkeys exposed to stationary magnetic fields: experimental observations and theoretical analysis. Bioelectromagnetics, **4**(1): 1-9.

TENFORDE T.S. & LIBURDY R.P. (1988) Magnetite deformation of phospholipid bilayers - effects on liposome shape and solute permeability at prephase transition temperatures. J Theor Biol, **133** 385-396.

TENFORDE T.S. & SHIFRINE M. (1984) Assessment of the immune responsiveness of mice exposed to a 1.5-Tesla stationary magnetic field. Bioelectromagnetics, **5**(4): 443-446.

TENGKU B.S., JOSEPH B.K., HARBROW D., TAVERNE A.A. & SYMONS A.L. (2000) Effect of a static magnetic field on orthodontic tooth movement in the rat. Eur J Orthod, **22**(5): 475-487.

TEODORI L., GRABAREK J., SMOLEWSKI P., GHIBELLI L., BERGAMASCHI A., DE NICOLA M. & DARZYNKIEWICZ Z. (2002) Exposure of cells to static magnetic field accelerates loss of integrity of plasma membrane during apoptosis. Cytometry, **49**(3): 113-118.

TESKEY G.C., OSSENKOPP K.P., PRATO F.S. & SESTINI E. (1987) Survivability and long-term stress reactivity levels following repeated exposure to nuclear magnetic resonance imaging procedures in rats. Physiol Chem Phys Med NMR, **19**(1): 43-49.

TESTORF M.F., AKE O.P., IWASAKA M. & UENO S. (2002) Melanophore aggregation in strong static magnetic fields. Bioelectromagnetics, **23**(6): 444-449.

THOMAS A.W., DROST D.J. & PRATO F.S. (2001) Human subjects exposed to a specific pulsed (200 microT) magnetic field: effects on normal standing balance. Neurosci Lett, **297**(2): 121-124.

TILL U., TIMMEL C.R., BROCKLEHURST B. & HORE P.J. (1998) The influence of very small magnetic fields on radical recombination reactions in the limit of slow recombination. Chem Phys Lett, **298** 7-14.

TIMMEL C.R., CINTOLESI F., BROCKLEHURST B. & HORE P.J. (2001) Model calculations of magnetic field effects on the recombination reactions of radicals with anisotropic hyperfine interactions. Chem Phys Lett, **334** 387-395.

TIMMEL C.R., TILL U., BROCKLEHURST B., MCLAUCHLAN K.A. & HORE P.J. (1998) Effects of weak magnetic fields on free radical recombination reactions. Molecular Physics, **95**(1): 71-89.

TKACH E.V., ABILOVA A.N. & GAZALIEVA S. (1987) [Characteristics of the effect of a constant electromagnetic field on reparative processes in spinal cord injuries]. Zh Nevropatol Psikhiatr Im S S Korsakova, **89**(5): 41-44.

TOFANI S., BARONE D., BERARDELLI M., BERNO E., CINTORINO M., FOGLIA L., OSSOLA P., RONCHETTO F., TOSO E. & EANDI M. (2003) Static and ELF magnetic fields enhance the in vivo anti-tumor efficacy of cis-platin against lewis lung carcinoma, but not of cyclophosphamide against B16 melanotic melanoma. Pharmacol Res, **48**(1): 83-90.

TOFANI S., BARONE D., CINTORINO M., DE SANTI M.M., FERRARA A., ORLASSINO R., OSSOLA P., PEROGLIO F., ROLFO K. & RONCHETTO F. (2001) Static and ELF magnetic fields induce tumor growth inhibition and apoptosis. Bioelectromagnetics, **22**(6): 419-428.

TOGAWA T., OKAI O. & OSHIMA M. (1967) Observation of blood flow E.M.F. in externally applied strong magnetic field by surface electrodes. Med Biol Eng, **5**(2): 169-170.

TRABULSI R., PAWLOWSKI B. & WIERASZKO A. (1996) The influence of steady magnetic fields on the mouse hippocampal evoked potentials in vitro. Brain Res, **728**(1): 135-139.

TRZECIAK H.I., GRZESIK J., BORTEL M., KUSKA R., DUDA D., MICHNIK J. & MALECKI A. (1993) Behavioral effects of long-term exposure to magnetic fields in rats. Bioelectromagnetics, **14**(4): 287-297.

TSUCHIYA K., OKUNO K., ANO T., TANAKA K., TAKAHASHI H. & SHODA M. (1999) High magnetic field enhances stationary phase-specific transcription activity of Escherichia coli. Bioelectrochem Bioenerg, **48**(2): 383-387.

TSUJI Y., NAKAGAWA M. & SUZUKI Y. (1996) Five-tesla static magnetic fields suppress food and water consumption and weight gain in mice. Ind Health, **34**(4): 347-357.

TURIEVA-DZODZIKOVA M.E., SALBIEV K.D. & KOKABADZE S.A. (1995) [The tissue basophils of the rat mesentery under the influence of a permanent magnetic field]. Morfologiia, 108(1): 46-49.

TUSCHL H., NEUBAUER G., SCHMID G., WEBER E. & WINKER N. (2000) Occupational exposure to static, ELF, VF and VLF magnetic fields and immune parameters. Int J Occup Med Environ Health, 13(1): 39-50.

TYNDALL D.A. (1990) MRI effects on the teratogenicity of x-irradiation in the C57BL/6J mouse. Magn Reson Imaging, 8(4): 423-433.

TYNDALL D.A. (1993) MRI effects on craniofacial size and crown-rump length in C57BL/6J mice in 1.5T fields. Oral Surg Oral Med Oral Pathol, 76(5): 655-660.

TYNDALL D.A. & SULIK K.K. (1991) Effects of magnetic resonance imaging on eye development in the C57BL/6J mouse. Teratology, 43(3): 263-275.

UENO S., HARADA K. & SHIOKAWA K. (1984) The embryonic development of frogs under strong DC magnetic fields. IEEE Trans Magnet, Mag, 20(5): 1663-1665.

UENO S., IWASAKA M. & SHIOKAWA K. (1990) Early embryonic development of Xenopus laevis under static magnetic fields up to 6.34 T. J Appl Phys, 67(9): 5841-5843.

UENO S., IWASAKA M. & SHIOKAWA K. (1994) Early embryonic development of frogs under intense magnetic fields up to 8 T. J Appl Phys, 75(10): 7165-7167.

VAINSHTEIN M., SUZINA N., KUDRYASHOVA E. & ARISKINA E. (2002) New magnet-sensitive structures in bacterial and archaeal cells. Biol Cell, 94(1): 29-35.

VALBERG P.A., KAVET R. & RAFFERTY C.N. (1997) Can low-level 50/60 Hz electric and magnetic fields cause biological effects? Radiat Res, 148(1): 2-21.

VALLBONA C., HAZLEWOOD C.F. & JURIDA G. (1997) Response of pain to static magnetic fields in postpolio patients: a double-blind pilot study. Arch Phys Med Rehabil, 78(11): 1200-1203.

VALLES J.M., JR., LIN K., DENEGRE J.M. & MOWRY K.L. (1997) Stable magnetic field gradient levitation of Xenopus laevis: toward low-gravity simulation. Biophys J, **73**(2): 1130-1133.

VALLES J.M., JR., WASSERMAN S.R., SCHWEIDENBACK C., EDWARDSON J., DENEGRE J.M. & MOWRY K.L. (2002) Processes that occur before second cleavage determine third cleavage orientation in Xenopus. Exp Cell Res, **274**(1): 112-118.

VAN DEVENTER T.E., SAUNDERS R. & REPACHOLI M.H. (2005) WHO health risk assessment process for static fields. Prog Biophys Mol Biol, **87**(2-3): 355-363.

VOGL T., KRIMMEL K., FUCHS A. & LISSNER J. (1988) Influence of magnetic resonance imaging on human body core and intravascular temperature. Med Phys, **15**(4): 562-566.

VOGL T., LISSNER J., SEIDERER M., KRIMMEL K. & SANDNER H. (1986) [Effect of types of field used in nuclear magnetic resonance tomography on core and surface temperature in the human body. Results of in vitro and in vivo experiments]. ROFO Fortschr Geb Rontgenstr Nuklearmed, **144**(5): 591-596.

VOGL T.J., PAULUS W., FUCHS A., KRAFCZYK S. & LISSNER J. (1991) Influence of magnetic resonance imaging on evoked potentials and nerve conduction velocities in humans. Invest Radiol, **26**(5): 432-437.

VOLKOW N.D., WANG G.J., FOWLER J.S., ROONEY W.D., FELDER C.A., LEE J.H., FRANCESCHI D., MAYNARD L., SCHLYER D.J., PAN J.W., GATLEY S.J. & SPRINGER JR C.S. (2000) Resting brain metabolic activity in a 4 tesla magnetic field. Magn Reson Med, **44**(5): 701-705.

VON KLITZING L. (1987) [Effect of static NMR magnetic fields on the processing of biological signals in man]. Rontgenpraxis, **40**(9): 321-323.

VON KLITZING L. (1989) Static magnetic fields increase the power intensity of EEG of man. Brain Res, **483**(1): 201-203.

VON KLITZING L. & TESSMANN G. (1989) [Effect of a static 0.2 T magnetic field on the EEG power spectrum in periodic median nerve stimulation]. EEG EMG Z Elektroenzephalogr Elektromyogr Verwandte Geb, **20**(1): 50-53.

WALLECZEK J. (1995) Magnetokinetic effects on radical pairs: a paradigm for magnetic field interactions with biological systems at lower than thermal energy. Electromagnetic Fields, **250** 395-420.

WATANABE Y., NAKAGAWA M. & MIYAKOSHI Y. (1997) Enhancement of lipid peroxidation in the liver of mice exposed to magnetic fields. Ind Health, **35**(2): 285-290.

WEIKL A., MOSHAGE W., HENTSCHEL D., SCHITTENHELM R. & BACHMANN K. (1989) [ECG changes caused by the effect of static magnetic fields of nuclear magnetic resonance tomography using magnets with a field power of 0.5 to 4.0 Telsa]. Z Kardiol, **78**(9): 578-586.

WEINTRAUB M.I., WOLFE G.I., BAROHN R.A., COLE S.P., PARRY G.J., HAYAT G., COHEN J.A., PAGE J.C., BROMBERG M.B. & SCHWARTZ S.L. (2003) Static magnetic field therapy for symptomatic diabetic neuropathy: a randomized, double-blind, placebo-controlled trial. Arch Phys Med Rehabil, **84**(5): 736-746.

WEISS J., HERRICK R.C., TABER K.H., CONTANT C. & PLISHKER G.A. (1992) Bio-effects of high magnetic fields: a study using a simple animal model. Magn Reson Imaging, **10**(4): 689-694.

WELKER H.A., SEMM P., WILLIG R.P., COMMENTZ J.C., WILTSCHKO W. & VOLLRATH L. (1983) Effects of an artificial magnetic field on serotonin N- acetyltransferase activity and melatonin content of the rat pineal gland. Exp Brain Res, **50**(2-3): 426-432.

WHITAKER J.M. & ADDERLY B. (1998) The pain relief breakthrough: the power of magnets to relieve backaches, arthritis, menstrual cramps, carpal tunnel syndrome, sports injuries, and more. New York, NY: Little, Brown, Boston.

WHO - WORLD HEALTH ORGANIZATION (1984) Extremely low frequency (ELF) fields. Geneva: World Health Organization (Environmental Health Criteria 35).

WHO - WORLD HEALTH ORGANIZATION (1987) Magnetic fields. Geneva: World Health Organization (Environmental Health Criteria 69).

WHO - WORLD HEALTH ORGANIZATION (1990) Revised guidelines for the preparation of Environmental Health Criteria monographs. Geneva: World Health Organization (PCS/90.69).

WHO - WORLD HEALTH ORGANIZATION (1993) Electromagnetic fields (300 Hz to 300 GHz). Geneva: World Health Organization (Environmental Health Criteria 137).

WIDDER K.J., SENYEI A.E. & SEARS B. (1982) Experimental methods in cancer therapeutics. J Pharm Sci, **71**(4): 379-387.

WIERASZKO A. (2000) Dantrolene modulates the influence of steady magnetic fields on hippocampal evoked potentials in vitro. Bioelectromagnetics, **21**(3): 175-182.

WIKSWO J.P. & BARACH J.P. (1980) An estimate of the steady magnetic field strength required to influence nerve conduction. IEEE Trans Biomed Eng, **27**(12): 722-723.

WILLIS R.J. & BROOKS W.M. (1984) Potential hazards of NMR imaging. No evidence of the possible effects of static and changing magnetic fields on cardiac function of the rat and guinea pig. Magn Reson Imaging, **2**(2): 89-95.

WILTSCHKO W., TRAUDT J., GUNTURKUN O., PRIOR H. & WILTSCHKO R. (2002) Lateralization of magnetic compass orientation in a migratory bird. Nature, **419**(6906): 467-470.

WILTSCHKO W. & WILTSCHKO R. (2002) Magnetic compass orientation in birds and its physiological basis. Naturwissenschaften, **89** 445-452.

WINKLHOFER M., HOLTKAMP-ROTZLER E., HANZLIK M., FLEISSNER G. & PETERSEN N. (2001) Clusters of superparamagnetic magnetite particles in the upper beak skin of homing pigeons: evidence of a magnetoreceptor? Eur J Mineral, **13** 659-669.

WINTHER F.O., RASMUSSEN K., TVETE O., HALVORSEN U. & HAUGSDAL B. (1999) Static magnetic field and the inner ear. A functional study of hearing and vestibular function in man after exposure to a static magnetic field. Scand Audiol, **28**(1): 57-59.

WISKIRCHEN J., GROENEWAELLER E.F., KEHLBACH R., HEINZELMANN F., WITTAU M., RODEMANN H.P., CLAUSSEN C.D. & DUDA S.H. (1999) Long-term effects of repetitive exposure to a static magnetic field (1.5 T) on proliferation of human fetal lung fibroblasts. Magn Reson Med, **41**(3): 464-468.

WITHERS H.R., MASON K.A. & DAVIS C.A. (1985) MR effect on murine spermatogenesis. Radiology, **156**(3): 741-742.

WOLFF S., CROOKS L.E., BROWN P., HOWARD R. & PAINTER R.B. (1980) Tests for DNA and chromosomal damage induced by nuclear magnetic resonance imaging. Radiology, **136**(3): 707-710.

WOLFF S., JAMES T.L., YOUNG G.B., MARGULIS A.R., BODYCOTE J. & AFZAL V. (1985) Magnetic resonance imaging: absence of in vitro cytogenetic damage. Radiology, **155**(1): 163-165.

XU S., OKANO H. & OHKUBO C. (1998) Subchronic effects of static magnetic fields on cutaneous microcirculation in rabbits. In Vivo, **12**(4): 383-389.

XU S., TOMITA N., OHATA R., YAN Q. & IKADA Y. (2001) Static magnetic field effects on bone formation of rats with an ischemic bone model. Biomed Mater Eng, **11**(3): 257-263.

YAGA K., REITER R.J., MANCHESTER L.C., NIEVES H., SUN J.H. & CHEN L.D. (1993) Pineal sensitivity to pulsed static magnetic fields changes during the photoperiod. Brain Res Bull, **30**(1-2): 153-156.

YAMAGUCHI H., HOSOKAWA K., SODA A., MIYAMOTO H. & KINOUCHI Y. (1993) Effects of seven months' exposure to a static 0.2 T magnetic field on growth and glycolytic activity of human gingival fibroblasts. Biochim Biophys Acta, **1156**(3): 302-306.

YAMAZAKI E., MATSUBARA S. & YAMADA I. (1993) Effect of Gd-DTPA and/or magnetic field and radiofrequency exposure on sister chromatid exchange in human peripheral lymphocytes. Acta Radiol, **34**(6): 607-611.

YAN Q.C., TOMITA N. & IKADA Y. (1998) Effects of static magnetic field on bone formation of rat femurs. Med Eng Phys, **20**(6): 397-402.

YANO A., HIDAKA E., FUJIWARA K. & IIMOTO M. (2001) Induction of primary root curvature in radish seedlings in a static magnetic field. Bioelectromagnetics, **22**(3): 194-199.

YIP Y.P., CAPRIOTTI C., NORBASH S.G., TALAGALA S.L. & YIP J.W. (1994a) Effects of MR exposure on cell proliferation and migration of chick motoneurons. J Magn Reson Imaging, **4**(6): 799-804.

YIP Y.P., CAPRIOTTI C., TALAGALA S.L. & YIP J.W. (1994b) Effects of MR exposure at 1.5 T on early embryonic development of the chick. J Magn Reson Imaging, 4(5): 742-748.

YIP Y.P., CAPRIOTTI C. & YIP J.W. (1995) Effects of MR exposure on axonal outgrowth in the sympathetic nervous system of the chick. J Magn Reson Imaging, 5(4): 457-462.

YOST M.G. & LIBURDY R.P. (1992) Time-varying and static magnetic fields act in combination to alter calcium signal transduction in the lymphocyte. FEBS Lett, 296(2): 117-122.

ZHADIN M.N. (2001) Review of russian literature on biological action of DC and low- frequency AC magnetic fields. Bioelectromagnetics, 22(1): 27-45.

ZHANG Q.M., TOKIWA M., DOI T., NAKAHARA T., CHANG P.W., NAKAMURA N., HORI M., MIYAKOSHI J. & YONEI S. (2003) Strong static magnetic field and the induction of mutations through elevated production of reactive oxygen species in Escherichia coli soxR. Int J Radiat Biol, 79(4): 281-286.

ZHANG S., WEI W., ZHANG J., MAO Y. & LIU S. (2002) Effect of static magnetic field on growth of Escherichia coli and relative response model of series piezoelectric quartz crystal. Analyst, 127(3): 373-377.

ZHERNOVOI A.I., SKORIK V.I., CHIRUKHIN V.A. & SHARSHINA L.M. (2001) Effect of stationary magnetic field on in vivo oxygen binding by blood. Bull Exp Biol Med, 131(2): 121-123.

ZIMMERMANN B. & HENTSCHEL D. (1987) [Effect of a static magnetic field (3.5 T) on the reproductive behavior of mice, on the embryo and fetal development and on selected hematologic parameters]. Digitale Bilddiagn, 7(4): 155-161.

ZMYSLONY M., PALUS J., JAJTE J., DZIUBALTOWSKA E. & RAJKOWSKA E. (2000) DNA damage in rat lymphocytes treated in vitro with iron cations and exposed to 7 mT magnetic fields (static or 50 Hz). Mutat Res, 453(1): 89-96.

Blood-brain barrier
A functional concept developed to explain why many substances that are transported by blood readily enter other tissues, but do not enter the brain. The 'barrier' functions as if it were a continuous membrane lining the vasculature of the brain. These brain capillary endothelial cells form a nearly continuous barrier to entry of substances into the brain from the vasculature.

Calcium efflux/influx
The release/uptake of calcium ions from a sample into a surrounding solution.

Cancer
Diseases characterized by the uncontrolled and abnormal division of eukaryotic cells and by the spread of the disease (metastasis) to disparate sites in the organism.

Carcinogens
Natural and artificial agents, mostly chemicals and types of radiation, that increase the frequency with which cells become cancerous.

Case-control study
An investigation into the extent to which a group of persons with a specific disease (the cases) and comparable persons who do not have the disease (the controls) differ with respect to exposure to putative risk factors.

Cell cycle
The cyclical process of growth and cellular reproduction in unicellular and multicellular eukaryotes. The cycle includes nuclear division, or mitosis, and cell division, or cytokinesis.

Chromosomal mutation (aberration)
The variation from the wild-type condition in either chromosome number or chromosome structure.

Chromosome
The genetic material of the cell, complexed with protein and organized into a number of linear structures. It literally means 'coloured body,' because the threadlike structures are visible under the microscope only after they are stained with dyes.

Chronic exposure
Exposure lasting for very long periods, e.g. significant periods of the working life.

Cohort study
An investigation involving the identification of a group of individuals (the cohort) about whom certain exposure information is collected, followed by ascertainment of the occurrence of diseases at later times. For each individual, information on exposure can be related to subsequent disease experience.

Coil
Arrangement of current carrying wires for the purpose of producing a magnetic field. Some common types: Helmholtz coils, Merritt coils.

Confidence interval (CI)
An interval calculated from data when making inferences about an unknown parameter. In hypothetical repetitions of the study, the interval will include the parameter in question on a specified percentage of occasions (e.g. 95% for a 95% confidence interval).

Conductivity, electrical
The scalar or vector quantity which, when multiplied by the electric field strength, yields the conduction current density. It is the reciprocal of resistivity. Expressed in siemens per meter ($S\ m^{-1}$).

Continuous wave
A wave whose successive oscillations are identical under steady-state conditions.

Current density
A vector of which the integral over a given surface is equal to the current flowing through the surface. The mean density in a linear conductor is equal to the current divided by the cross-sectional area of the conductor. Expressed in ampere per square meter ($A\ m^{-2}$).

DC
Abbreviation for 'direct current', but also used to indicate constancy of fields, see 'Static field.'

Diamagnetic
A weakly magnetic material with relative permeability slightly less than one.

Dielectric constant
See permittivity.

Direct effect
A biological effect resulting from direct interaction of EMF with biological structures.

Dizziness
Dizziness may be experienced as lightheadedness, feeling like you might faint, being unsteady, loss of balance, or vertigo (a feeling that you or the room is spinning or moving).

Dosimeter
An instrument that can be worn on the body of a person for measuring exposure over time.

Dosimetry
Measurement, or determination by calculation, of internal electric field strength or induced current density, of the specific energy absorption, or specific energy absorption rate distribution, in humans or animals exposed to electromagnetic fields.

DNA (deoxyribonucleic acid)
This polymeric molecule (consisting of deoxyribonucleotide building blocks that in a double-stranded, double-helical form) is the genetic material of most organisms.

ECG
An electrocardiogram (ECG) is a test that records the electrical activity of the heart. An ECG is used to measure the rate and regularity of heartbeats, as well as the size and position of the chambers, the presence of any damage to the heart, and the effects of drugs or devices (such as a pacemaker) used to regulate the heart.

Electric field strength
The force (E) on a stationary unit positive charge at a point in an electric field. Measured in volt per meter ($V\ m^{-1}$).

Electromagnetic energy
The energy stored in an electromagnetic field. Expressed in joule (J).

Electromagnetic fields or EMF
The combination of electric and magnetic fields in the environment. This term is often confused with 'electromagnetic radiation' and can therefore be misleading when used with extremely low frequencies for which the radiation is barely detectable.

Electrostatic fields
Electric static fields produced by fixed potential differences.

ELF
Extremely low frequency (in the range of 1 - 300 Hz) electromagnetic fields.

Enzyme
A protein that facilitates a biochemical reaction in a cell.

Exposure dose
The amount of a chemical or physical agent in the environment that a person comes into contact with over a period of time.

Exposure, long-term
This term indicates exposure during a major part of the lifetime of the involved biological system. It may, therefore, vary from a few weeks to many years in duration.

Exposure assessment
The evaluation of a person's exposure by measurements, modelling, information about sources or other means.

Exposure metric
A single number that summarizes exposure to an electric and/or magnetic field. The metric is usually determined by a combination of the instrument's signal processing and the data analysis performed after the measurement.

Expression (genetic)
The process by which the information in a gene is used to create proteins.

Ferromagnetic
Strongly magnetic materials with relative permeabilities that are non-linear functions of the applied magnetic field.

Field characteristics
Detailed physical properties of electric or magnetic fields such as the magnitude, frequency spectrum, polarization, modulation, etc.

Free radical
An unchanged atomic or molecular species with an unpaired electron. In the context of this book, spin-correlated free radicals form the basis for a proposed mechanism by which magnetic fields may interact with biological tissue. Not to be confused with freely diffusing free radicals that are not systematically affected by magnetic fields.

Frequency
The number of sinusoidal cycles completed by electromagnetic waves in 1 second. Expressed in hertz (Hz).

Gauss (G)
Older unit of magnetic flux density. 1 gauss = 10^{-4} tesla (T).

General public
Those persons who do not fall under the definition of workers.

Geomagnetic field
Magnetic field originating from the Earth (including the atmosphere). Predominantly a static magnetic field, but includes some oscillating components and transients.

Gradient magnetic field
A magnetic field that is not spatially uniform. The rate at which the magnetic field changes as a function of location, which is measured in units of tesla per meter (T m^{-1}).

Heart rate
The measurement of the number of heartbeats per minute.

High-voltage DC lines
High voltage direct current lines operating at up to 500 kV, usually for the transmission of electricity over long distances.

Indirect effect
Health effects resulting from impairment of functioning of biomedical equipment caused by electromagnetic interference from external sources.

Magnetite
Magnetite, also known as lodestone, is a magnetic mineral form of iron oxide. Biogenic magnetite form the basis for a proposed mechanism by which magnetic fields influence biological systems.

Magnet
An object that has a (static) magnetic field.

Magnetic field
An vector quantity, H, specifies a magnetic field at any point in space, and is expressed in ampere per meter (A m^{-1}). See also magnetic flux density.

Magnetophosphenes
The sensation of flashes of light caused by induced electric currents stimulating the retina.

Magnetostatic fields
Static fields established by permanent magnets and by steady currents.

Magnetic flux density
A vector field quantity, B, that results in a force that acts on a moving charge or charges, and is expressed in tesla (T). The magnetic flux density is often called the magnetic field, because the two terms differ only by a proportionality factor in vacuum (air).

Magnetic Resonance Imaging (MRI)
A diagnostic imaging technology that exploits the tendency of nuclei with magnetic moments (typically protons) to precess about static magnetic fields at frequencies proportional to the local value of the static magnetic field. Resonant radiofrequency fields excite these nuclei and are later received from relaxing nuclei, effectively reporting their locations. Magnetic field gradients are used to spatially encode the region of interest.

Magnetic Resonance Spectroscopy (MRS)
MRS uses principals similar to those used in MRI. However, uniform static magnetic fields are used without magnetic field gradients in MRS. The molecular environment near the relaxing nuclei cause differences in received frequencies. Frequency components of the resulting spectra provide a chemical analysis of the region of interest. MRS may be done *in vivo* in MR scanners. Most MRS is done *in vitro* on machines that accept only small chemical samples.

Microwaves
Electromagnetic radiation with the frequency range of 300 MHz - 300 GHz.

Mutagen
A substance that is able to cause a mutation.

Mutation
Any detectable and heritable change in the genetic material not caused by genetic recombination.

Non-ionizing Radiation (NIR)
Includes all radiations and fields of the electromagnetic spectrum that do not normally have sufficient energy to produce ionization in matter. These are characterized by energy per photon less than about 12 eV, which is

equivalent to wavelengths greater than 100 nm or frequencies lower than 3×10^{15} Hz.

Occupational exposure
All exposure to EMF experienced by individuals in the course of performing their work.

Odds ratio (OR)
The ratio of the odds of disease occurrence in a group with exposure to a factor to the odds in an unexposed group. Within each group, the odds are the ratio of the numbers of diseased and non-diseased individuals.

PAH
Polycyclic aromatic hydrocarbon.

Paramagnetic
A weakly magnetic material with relative permeability slightly greater than one.

Permeability
The scalar or tensor quantity whose product by the magnetic field strength is the magnetic flux density. Note: For isotropic media, the permeability is a scalar; for anisotropic media, a matrix. Synonym: absolute permeability. If the permeability of a material or medium is divided by the permeability of vacuum (magnetic constant) μ_0, then the result is termed relative permeability (μ). Unit: henry per meter (H m^{-1}).

Permittivity
A constant defining the influence of an isotropic medium on the forces of attraction or repulsion between electrified bodies, and expressed in farad per meter (F m^{-1}). Relative permittivity is the permittivity of a material or medium divided by the permittivity of vacuum, ϵ_0.

Phosphenes
Weak visual sensations that occur in response to magnetic fields or by direct electrostimulation. The effect is believed to result from the interaction of the induced current with electrically excitable cells in the retina.

Power density
In radio wave propagation, the power crossing a unit area normal to the direction of wave propagation. Expressed in watt per square meter (W m^{-2}).

Public exposure
All exposure to EMF experienced by members of the general public, excluding occupational exposure and exposure during medical procedures.

Plasma membrane
Lipid bilayer that surrounds the cytoplasm of both animal and plant cells.

Protein
One of a group of high-molecular weight, nitrogen-containing, organic compounds of complex shape and composition.

Radiofrequency (RF)
Electromagnetic energy with frequencies in the range 3 kHz - 300 GHz.

Relative permeability
(Absolute) permeability (q.v.) divided by the permeability in vacuum. A value near one signifies that the material is only weakly magnetized by an external field.

Relative risk (RR)
The ratio of the disease rate in the group under study to that in a comparison group, with any required adjustments for confounding factors such as age. For rare diseases, the relative risk is practically the same as the odds ratio.

Ribonucleic acid (RNA)
A usually single-stranded polymeric molecule consisting of ribonucleotide building blocks. RNA is chemically very similar to DNA. The three major types of RNA in cells are ribosomal RNA (rRNA), transfer RNA (tRNA), and messenger RNA (mRNA), each of which performs an essential role in protein synthesis (translation). In some viruses, RNA (rather than DNA) is the genetic material.

Root mean square (rms)
Certain electrical effects are proportional to the square root of the mean of the square of a periodic function (over one period). This value is known as the effective or root-mean-square (rms) value, since it is derived by first squaring the function, determining the mean value of the squares obtained, and taking the square root of that mean value. Often used for averaging the magnitude of time-varying electric and magnetic fields.

S.I.
Abbreviation for the International System of units.

Static field
A field that does not vary with time. In most environments, electric and magnetic fields change with time, but their frequency spectrum has a component at 0 Hz. This 'quasi-static' component of the field can be measured by averaging the oscillating signal over the sample time.

Systolic and diastolic blood pressure
Blood pressure is a measurement of the force applied to the walls of the arteries as the heart pumps blood through the body. Blood pressure readings are usually given as two numbers: for example, 110 over 70 (written as 110/70). The first number is the systolic blood pressure reading, and it represents the maximum pressure exerted when the heart contracts. The second number is the diastolic blood pressure reading, and it represents the pressure in the arteries when the heart is at rest.

Tesla (T)
International System unit of magnetic flux density. 1 tesla = 10000 gauss (G).

Time-weighted average (TWA)
A weighted average of exposure measurements taken over a period of time, with the weighting factor equal to the time interval between measurements. When the measurements are made with a monitor with a fixed sampling rate, the TWA is equal to the arithmetic mean of the measurements.

Transients
Brief bursts of high-frequency fields, usually resulting from mechanical switching of AC electricity.

Voxels
Cubic cells with sides of 1 - 10 mm used to represent animal and human tissues in dosimetry models.

Waveform
A single component of the field measured as a function of time by an instrument with a response time much faster than the field's frequency of oscillation. The term also refers to the shape of the wave as displayed on a graph or oscilloscope trace.

Wavelength
The distance between two successive points of a periodic wave in the direction of propagation, at which the oscillation has the same phase.

Workers
Those people who can be exposed to electric, magnetic or electromagnetic fields in the course of their professional duties, who have been informed about the possible risks associated with such exposure, and have been trained how to reduce these risks.

13. RESUME ET RECOMMANDATIONS POUR LES ETUDES ULTERIEURES

13.1 Résumé

13.1.1 Sources naturelles et anthropogéniques

Des champs électriques statiques sont présents à l'état naturel dans l'atmosphère. Sous les nuages d'orage ils peuvent atteindre une valeur de 3 kVm^{-1}, mais par beau temps, leur valeur se situe normalement entre 1 et 100 V m^{-1}. En dehors de cela, la cause la plus commune d'exposition à des champs électrostatiques est la séparation des charges provoquée par les frottements. Par exemple, en marchant sur un tapis non conducteur, on peut faire naître, par accumulation de charges électriques, des potentiels de plusieurs kilovolts capables d'engendrer des champs électrostatiques locaux allant jusqu'à 500 kV par mètre. L'intensité du champ électrostatique créé par les lignes de transport de courant continu peut atteindre 20 kVm^{-1} ; elle peut aller jusqu'à 300 kV m^{-1} à l'intérieur des trains à traction électrique par courant continu et à 30 cm d'un système de visualisation (VDU), on enregistre des champs électriques de 10 à 20 kV m^{-1}.

A la surface de la Terre, le champ magnétique terrestre varie entre 35 et 70 µT et il joue un rôle dans l'orientation et la migration de certaines espèces animales. Chaque fois qu'on utilise des courants continus, par exemple pour certains moyens de transport , diverses opérations industrielles comme la production d'aluminium ou le soudage au gaz, on produit des champs magnétostatiques. On a enregistré des valeurs de la densité de flux magnétique allant jusqu'à 2 mT à l'intérieur des trains à traction électrique et dans les systèmes à lévitation magnétique (MagLev) en cours de développement. Dans les ateliers où s'opère la réduction électrolytique de l'alumine, le personnel est exposé à des champs encore plus intenses (jusqu'à 60 mT environ) et dans un rayon de 1 cm autour des câbles de soudage à l'arc, le champ est d'environ 5 mT.

L'arrivée des supraconducteurs dans les années 1970 à 1980 a facilité l'utilisation de champs magnétiques beaucoup plus intenses pour le diagnostic médical grâce à la mise au point de techniques comme l'imagerie par résonance magnétique (IRM) , la spectroscopie par résonance magnétique (SRM) [2] ou encore la résonance magnétique nucléaire (RMN) dans le domaine de la recherche. On estime que l'on a pratiqué jusqu'ici quelque 200 millions d'IRM dans le monde. Le champ

---

[2] Dans tout le texte, il n'est question que de l'IRM , mais l'exposition au champ généré par les dispositifs de SRM est du même ordre.

magnétostatique engendré par un appareil d'IRM est dû aux aimants permanents, aux aimants supraconducteurs et à leurs combinaisons ; il est de l'ordre de 0,2 à 3 T dans le cas des appareils habituellement utilisés dans la pratique clinique. En recherche, on a recours à des champs plus intenses, pouvant aller jusqu'à 9,4 T, pour l'imagerie du corps entier. Le champ parasite généré par les aimants utilisés en IRM est bien défini et il est réduit au minimum avec les appareils muni d'un blindage approprié. En ce qui concerne l'exposition de l'opérateur au niveau de la console de commande, on a généralement une densité de flux magnétique d'environ 0,5 mT, mais cette valeur peut être dépassée. Cela étant, l'exposition professionnelle peut atteindre ou dépasser 1 T lors du montage et de l'essai de ces appareils ou encore lors d'actes médicaux pratiqués pendant une IRM interventionnelle. Dans certaines recherches en physique ou lors de la mise en oeuvre de techniques nécessitant des énergies élevées, on utilise également des supraconducteurs et le personnel peut alors être exposé régulièrement et longuement à des champs susceptibles d'atteindre 1,5 T.

13.1.2 Mécanismes d'interaction

Les données expérimentales on permis d'établir l'existence de trois types d'interaction physique entre les champs magnétostatiques et les systèmes biologiques, à savoir :

1) Les interactions électrodynamiques avec les courants de conduction ionique. Ces interactions entre un champ magnétostatique et un courant ionique sont dues aux forces de Laplace-Lorentz qui s'exercent sur les charges en mouvement. Ces effets font apparaître des potentiels (potentiels d'écoulement) et des courants électriques. Chez l'Homme et l'animal, les potentiels d'écoulement sont généralement liés à la contraction ventriculaire et à l'éjection du sang dans l'aorte. L'interaction de Laplace-Lorentz engendre également une force magnétohydrodynamique qui s'oppose à l'écoulement du sang. On a calculé qu'en présence d'un champ de 15 T, l'écoulement du sang dans l'aorte pouvait être réduit dans une proportion pouvant aller jusqu'à 10 %.

2) Les effets magnétomécaniques, et notamment l'orientation des structures présentant une anisotropie magnétique dans un champ uniforme et le déplacement des matériaux paramagnétiques et ferromagnétiques dans un gradient de champ magnétique. Les interactions dues aux forces et aux couples qui s'exercent sur les objets métalliques endogènes ou exogènes constituent un point extrêmement important.

3)   Les effets sur les états de spin électronique des intermédiaires
réactionnels. Les effets chimiques et biologiques des champs
magnétiques sont depuis longtemps envisagés dans le cadre de la
chimie des paires de radicaux à spins corrélés. Plusieurs types de
réactions chimiques organiques sont sensibles aux champs
magnétostatiques d'une intensité comprise entre 10 et 100 mT en
raison de l'effet que ces champs exercent sur les états de spin
des intermédiaires réactionnels. Une paire de radicaux à spins
corrélés peut se recombiner et empêcher la réaction de se
produire lorsque les deux conditions suivantes sont respectées:
a) la paire formée, qui se trouve à l'état triplet, doit passer à l'état
singulet sous l'effet d'un certain d'un mécanisme ; b) les radicaux
doivent être à nouveau en interaction physique pour pouvoir se
recombiner. L'étape a) peut être sensible à l'action d'un champ
magnétique. La plupart des recherches concernent la possibilité
d'utiliser les effets des champs magnétiques sur les paires de
radicaux pour étudier les réactions enzymatiques. Il ne semble
toutefois pas qu'il puisse y avoir d'effets ayant des conséquences
d'ordre physiologique sur les fonctions cellulaires ni d'ailleurs
d'effets mutagènes à long terme qui découleraient des
modifications produites par les champs magnétiques sur la
concentration ou le flux des radicaux libres.

Dosimétrie

Pour bien comprendre les effets biologiques des champs électriques ou
magnétiques, il faut s'intéresser aux champs qui influent directement sur
les cellules des différentes parties de l'organisme et des tissus. On peut
dans ce cas définir la dose au moyen d'une fonction appropriée de
l'intensité du champ électrique ou magnétique au point d'interaction. La
dosimétrie a pour principal objet d'établir la relation qui existe entre entre
les champs extérieurs non perturbés et les champs internes. A cet égard,
les études informatiques utilisant des modèles voxélisés d'organismes
humains et animaux, de même que l'étude expérimentale de l'exposition ,
jouent un rôle important.

Les interactions entre un champ magnétostatique et un tissu donné
impliquent vraisemblablement comme paramètres les propriétés
physiques suivantes du champ:

le vecteur champ magnétique, le gradient du champ et/ou le produit de ces
grandeurs, qui est une force. Certaines interactions plus importantes
résultent de déplacements qui se produisent dans un champ ou un gradient
de champ, en raison par exemple de mouvements du corps ou du courant
sanguin.

Les paramètres dosimétriques appropriés sont choisis en fonction du mécanisme physique qui conditionne le problème de sécurité en cause. Il est clair qu'aucun objet ferromagnétique ne doit se trouver à proximité de l'aimant. Il est donc impératif de vérifier qu'il n'y a aucun objet de ce genre ni d'implants qui pourraient entrer en mouvement sous l'action des forces ou des couples exercés. Il est bon de mesurer la valeur maximale du vecteur induction magnétique ainsi que celle de la force magnétique. On peut cartographier le champ de manière à pouvoir déterminer son intensité en divers points du voisinage de l'aimant où le personnel pourrait être exposé , mais le port de dosimètres personnels est peut-être plus utile.

Les mouvements du corps ou de certaines parties du corps, par exemples des yeux ou de la tête, qui se produisent dans un gradient de champ magnétostatique vont également donner naissance à un champ et à un courant électriques pendant la durée de ces mouvements. Les calculs dosimétriques montrent que des mouvements normaux induisent un champ électrique notable à proximité ou à l'intérieur d'un champ d'intensité supérieure à 2-3 T et leur présence pourrait expliquer les nombreux cas de vertiges ou de phosphènes magnétiques occasionnels subis par des malades, des volontaires ou des personnels lors de mouvements dans le champ magnétique.

Les sources d'exposition sont multiples. Les appareils d'imagerie par résonance magnétique (IRM) en sont l'une des plus généreuses. Au cours de la dernière décennie, on s'est attaché à faire en sorte que ces appareils travaillent avec des champs très intenses. Avec l'appareillage le plus couramment utilisé dans la pratique clinique, le champ central est de 1,5 T, mais on accepte maintenant d'utiliser en routine des dispositifs travaillant avec un champ de 3,0 T et en 2004, plus de 100 de ces appareils étaient en usage dans le monde. On met actuellement au point pour la recherche en imagerie clinique des appareils qui utilisent un champ de 4 à 9,4 T. A mesure que l'intensité du champ d'un appareil d'IRM augmente, il en va de même des divers types d'interactions susceptibles de se produire entre ce champ et les tissus. Cette tendance à utiliser des champs intenses, rend d'autant plus importante la connaissance des interactions entre les champs électromagnétiques engendrés par les appareils d'IRM et l'organisme humain.

13.1.3 Etudes in vitro

Les études *in vitro* fournissent des données qui sont utiles pour élucider les mécanismes d'interaction et déterminer quelles sortes d'effets seraient à étudier *in vivo*, mais sans une confirmation par des études *in vivo*, elles sont insuffisantes pour permettre de mettre en évidence les effets sanitaires.

Un certain nombre d'effets biologiques dus aux champs magnétostatiques ont été étudiés *in vitro*. On les a étudiés à différents niveaux d'organisation : systèmes acellulaires constitués de membranes ou d'enzymes isolées ou impliquant certaines réactions biochimiques ou encore divers modèles cellulaires constitués de cellules bactériennes ou mammaliennes. Les points d'aboutissement des interactions étudiées étaient les suivants :

orientation cellulaire , activité métabolique cellulaire, physiologie des membranes cellulaires, expression des gènes , croissance cellulaire et génotoxicité. Sur tous ces points, on a fait état de résultats positifs ou négatifs, mais dans la plupart des cas, ils n'ont pas été reproduits.Les effets observés sont plutôt variés et ont été constatés après exposition à une large gamme de densités de flux magnétique. Il apparaît qu'un champ magnétostatique peut avoir plusieurs effets biologiques à des intensités inférieures à 1 T et de l'ordre du mT. Pour quelques-uns de ces effets, l'existence d'un seuil a été indiquée, mais selon d'autres études, la réponse ne serait pas linéaire et ne comporterait pas de seuil bien défini.

Au dessus de 1 T , on constate systématiquement un effet du champ magnétostatique sur l'orientation des cellules, mais la signification de cet effet *in vivo* reste discutable. Quelques études donnent à penser que l'association d'un champ magnétostatique et d'autres agents comme par exemple des substances chimiques génotoxiques pourrait peut-être avoir des effets synergiques, aussi bien protecteurs que stimulants. Les données actuelles sont insuffisantes et doivent être confirmées pour que l'on puisse en tirer des conclusions définitives en ce qui concerne la santé humaine.
Outre leurs relations complexes avec des paramètres physiques tels que l'intensité, la durée, la répétition ou le gradient de l'exposition, les variables biologiques jouent manifestement un rôle important dans les effets exercés par les champs magnétostatiques. On a ainsi montré que des variables comme le type de cellule, l'activation cellulaire et d'autres états physiologiques présents lors de l'exposition pouvaient influencer les résultats expérimentaux. Les mécanismes à la base de ces effets ne sont pas connus, mais il pourrait y avoir des effets sur les radicaux et les ions .Des études *in vitro* fournissent certaines indications sur ce point.

Pour autant qu'elles mettent en évidence des effets biologiques, les très rares études portant sur les signaux IRM et autres champs associés n'en révèlent aucun qui soit différent de ceux que produisent à eux seuls les champs magnétostatiques.

Dans l'ensemble, l'expérimentation *in vitro* ne permet pas de se faire une idée claire des effets spécifiques exercés par les champs magnétostatiques et de ce fait, elle ne permet pas de conclure à la possibilité d'effets nocifs sur la santé.

13.1.4 Etudes sur l'animal

Il n'y a guère eu d'études consacrées aux effets des champs électrostatiques sur l'animal; aucun signe d'effets sanitaires indésirables n'a été observé autres que ceux qui résultent des sensations liées à la présence de charges électriques superficielles.

S'agissant des effets des champs magnétostatiques, un grand nombre d'études ont été effectuées sur l'animal. La plupart de celles qui sont jugées utiles en ce qui concerne la santé humaine portent sur des champs beaucoup plus intenses que le champ magnétique terrestre. Certaines d'entre elles portent notamment sur l'exposition à des champs dont l'intensité est de l'ordre du millitesla, c'est-à-dire comparable à une exposition relativement élevée en milieu industriel. Plus récemment, l'avènement des technologies utilisant des aimants supraconducteurs et de l'IRM a suscité des études sur les effets comportementaux, physiologiques et génésiques pour des densités de flux magnétique approximativement égales ou supérieures à 1 T. Toutefois, rares sont celles qui examinent les effets chroniques possibles de l'exposition, notamment d'éventuels effets cancérogènes.

Les réactions les plus régulièrement observées lors des études neurocomportementales incitent à penser que les mouvements d'un rongeur de laboratoire dans un champ magnétostatique égal ou supérieur à 4 T peut provoquer des sensations désagréables qui déterminent une aversion et des reflexes d'évitement conditionnés. On estime que ces observations cadrent bien avec des effets magnétohydrodynamiques sur l'endolymphe de l'appareil vestibulaire. Les autres résultats sont variables.

On est fondé à penser que plusieurs espèces de vertébrés et d'invertébrés sont capables de s'orienter en utilisant des champs magnétostatiques d'intensité aussi faible que celle du champ magnétique terrestre, mais on estime que ces comportements sont sans aucun rapport avec d'éventuels effets sur la santé humaine.

Il est largement prouvé que l'exposition à des champs d'intensité supérieure à environ 1 T

(0,1 T dans le cas des gros animaux) engendre des potentiels d'écoulement dans le voisinage du coeur et des gros vaisseaux , mais les conséquences physiologiques de ce phénomène ne sont pas clairement établies. Des porcs exposés plusieurs heures dans la région du coeur à une densité de flux magnétique très élevée dont la valeur pouvait atteindre 8 T n'ont présenté aucun effet cardiovasculaire. Chez le lapin, une exposition de brève ou de longue durée à des champs dont l'intensité allait de celle du champ terrestre à des valeurs de l'ordre du millitesla, auraient provoqué des effets sur l'appareil cardiovasculaire, mais les données ne sont pas très probantes.

Une équipe a obtenu des résultats qui donnent à penser qu'un champ magnétique de l'ordre du mT pourrait inhiber une élévation précoce de la tension artérielle par le truchement du système de régulation hormonale. Selon cette même équipe, un champ magnétostatique de faible intensité (jusqu' à 0,2 T) pourrait , grâce à des effets localisés sur le courant sanguin, apporter une amélioration de la microcirculation. Par ailleurs, selon une autre équipe, pour des valeurs de la densité de flux magnétique allant jusqu'à 10 T, il pourrait y avoir réduction du courant sanguin et de la température cutanés. Dans tous ces cas cependant, les points d'aboutissement des effets biologiques sont plutôt labiles, avec une situation qui a pu être compliquée par des interventions pharmacologiques - notamment une anesthésie dans certains cas - et par l'immobilisation des sujets. Dans l'ensemble, il est difficile d'aboutir à des conclusions définitives sans que ces résultats soient reproduits de façon indépendante.

Il existe plusieurs études qui décrivent les effets possibles d'une exposition à un champ magnétique sur les éléments figurés du sang et le système hématopoïétique. Toutefois, leurs résultats sont ambigus, ce qui limite les conclusions que l'on peut en tirer. Les données dont on dispose au sujet des effets produits par une exposition à un champ magnétostatique sur les constituants ioniques et enzymatiques du sérum émanent essentiellement d'un seul laboratoire. Il faut que ces résultats soient confirmés par des laboratoires indépendants avant que l'on puisse en tirer des conclusions.

En ce qui concerne les effets sur le système endocrine, plusieurs études effectuées par un laboratoire tendent à montrer que l'exposition à un champ magnétostatique peut affecter la synthèse épiphysaire et notamment la teneur en mélatonine. Toutefois, lors d'études effectuées dans d'autres laboratoires, cet effet n'a pas pu être mis en évidence. Avant de pouvoir tirer des conclusions définitives quant à un effet suppresseur des champs magnétostatiques sur la synthèse de la mélatonine, la confirmation de cet effet par d'autres recherches est nécessaire. D'une façon générale et à part le cas de l'épiphyse, peu de travaux ont été consacrés à l'étude des effets des champs magnétostatiques sur le système endocrine. Aucun effet ne semble avoir été systématiquement observé.

Les effets génésiques et développementaux d'une exposition au champ généré par les appareils d'IRM sont une considération très importante pour les malades comme pour le personnel soignant. On ne possède à cet égard que quelques bonnes études portant sur des champs magnétostatiques d'intensité supérieure à 1 T. Les études par IRM ne pas informatives en soi car l'effet du champ statique ne peut pas être distingué des effets éventuellement produits par les champs de radiofréquence et les champs à gradient pulsé en général. Ces points doivent être examinés sans délai pour que l'on puisse évaluer le risque sanitaire lié à ce type d'exposition.

En ce qui concerne la génotoxicité et les effets cancérogènes, les études sur l'animal sont, dans l'ensemble, si peu nombreuses que l'on ne peut en tirer aucune conclusion définitive.

13.1.5 Etudes en laboratoire sur des sujets humains

Un champ électrostatique ne pénètre pas à l'intérieur des corps conducteurs, comme l'organisme humain ; le champ provoque l'apparition de charges électriques superficielles et il est toujours dirigé normalement à la surface du corps. Lorsque la densité de la charge superficielle est suffisamment grande, elle devient perceptible par son interaction avec le système pileux ou encore par d'autres effets comme des décharges électriques sous forme d'étincelles (microchocs). Le seuil de perception individuel dépend de divers facteurs et peut se situer entre 10 et 45 kV m^{-1}. Le seuil de sensation désagréable est sans doute également variable, mais il n'a pas été étudié de façon systématique. Des microchocs douloureux peuvent se produire lorsqu'une personne bien isolée du sol touche un objet qui est à la terre ou lorsque une personne " à la terre" touche un corps conducteur bien isolé du sol; toutefois, la valeur-seuil du champ électrostatique dépend du degré d'isolation et de divers autres facteurs.

L'expérimentation sur des sujets humains porte sur des points tels que la fonction nerveuse périphérique, l'activité cérébrale, les fonctions neurocomportementales et cognitives, la perception sensorielle , la fonction cardiaque , la tension artérielle, la fréquence cardiaque, les taux sériques de protéines et d'hormones, la température centrale et cutanée et les effets thérapeutiques. On a travaillé avec des niveaux d'exposition allant jusqu'à 8 T et les études ont porté sur des champs purement statiques ainsi que sur les champs engendrés par les appareils d'IRM. Les durées d'exposition allaient de quelques secondes à neuf heures , mais elles étaient généralement inférieures à une heure. Les données disponibles sont limitées et ce, pour plusieurs raisons; en général, les échantillons prélevés sur les patients ou des volontaires en bonne santé étaient ceux qu'il était commode d'obtenir et le nombre de sujets était faible.

D'après les résultats obtenus, il ne semble pas que l'exposition à un champ magnétostatique ait un effet sur les réactions neurophysiologiques ni sur les fonctions cognitives de volontaires immobiles, mais ces résultats ne permettent pas non plus d'exclure l'existence de tels effets. Des travailleurs, des patients et des volontaires qui effectuaient des mouvements dans un champ statique de plus de 2 T environ, ont ressenti des vertiges et des nausées qui dépendaient de la dose. Selon une étude, on a constaté chez des personnes qui se tenaient à proximité d'un appareil d'IRM de 1,5 T, une diminution de la coordination oeil-main et une perte de sensibilité aux contrastes en vision de près. L'apparition de ces effets dépend vraisemblablement du gradient du champ et des mouvements effectués par le sujet. Certaines études font état de petites variations dans la tension artérielle et la fréquence cardiaque, mais qui restent cependant dans les limites physiologiques normales. Rien n'indique que les champs magnétostatiques aient des effets sur d'autres aspects de la physiologie du système cardiovasculaire, ni sur les protéines ou hormones sériques. Jusqu'à une valeur de 8 T, il ne semble pas que ces champs provoquent des variations de température chez les sujets humains.

A noter toutefois que la plupart des études étaient de faible envergure, utilisaient des échantillons commodes à obtenir et portaient souvent sur des groupes de sujets non comparables. Il n'est donc pas possible de tirer la moindre conclusion concernant les effets très divers examinés dans le présent rapport.

13.1.6 Etudes épidémiologiques

Les études épidémiologiques qui ont été effectuées concernent presque exclusivement des travailleurs exposés à des champs magnétostatiques engendrés par des appareils alimentés en courant continu de forte intensité. La plupart de ces travailleurs étaient exposés à des champs magnétostatiques allant jusqu'à plusieurs dizaines de mT; il s'agissait de soudeurs, de fondeurs d'aluminium ou de travailleurs employés dans diverses installations industrielles effectuant des opérations de séparation chimique dans de grandes cuves d'électrolyse.Il est cependant possible que ces activités aient exposé les travailleurs à toutes sortes de fumées et d'aérosols potentiellement toxiques constituant autant de facteurs de confusion. Les effets étudiés chez ces travailleurs étaient les suivants: cancers, anomalies hématologiques et leurs conséquences, fréquence des aberrations chromosomiques, conséquences sur le plan génésique et troubles musculosquelettiques. En outre, quelques études ont porté sur la fécondité et l'issue de la grossesse d'opératrices d'appareils IRM ayant pu être exposées à des champs magnétostatiques relativement intenses allant jusqu'à 1 mT environ. Deux de ces études ont examiné l'issue de la grossesse de volontaires en bonne santé ayant subi des examens par IRM pendant la gestation.

Il a été fait état d'un risque accru de cancers de diverses localisations, par exemple de cancers du poumon, du pancréas ou encore d'affections hématologiques malignes, mais il n'y a guère de concordance entre les résultats des différentes études. Les rares études épidémiologiques publiées jusqu'ici laissent un certain nombre de questions sans réponse eu égard à la possibilité d'un risque accru de cancer en cas d'exposition à des champs magnétostatiques. L'évaluation de l'exposition laisse à désirer et comme certaines études n'ont porté que sur un nombre de sujets très restreint, elles ne peuvent , dans le cas de maladies aussi rares, n'observer de risque que lorsque celui-ci est très élevé. On est d'autant plus fondé à douter de la capacité de ces investigations à fournir des informations utiles qu'on manque de preuves indubitables au sujet d'autres facteurs cancérogènes mieux connus qui étaient également présents sur certains des lieux de travail étudiés. D'autres effets sanitaires non néoplasiques ont été également envisagés, mais de façon encore plus sporadique. La plupart de ces travaux portent sur des effectifs très faibles et présentent nombre d'insuffisances sur le plan méthodologique. On n'a pas suffisamment étudié d'autres situations ou des travailleurs - par exemple des opérateurs IRM - pourraient être exposés à des champs intenses. Les données actuelles sont insuffisantes pour permettre une évaluation d'ordre sanitaire.

13.1.7 Evaluation du risque sanitaire

Champs électrostatiques

On ne dispose pas d'études sur l'exposition à des champs électrostatiques dont on puisse tirer une conclusion quant à l'existence d'effets chroniques ou retardés. Selon le Centre international de recherche sur le cancer (CIRC, 2002) les données sont insuffisantes pour permettre de se prononcer sur la cancérogénicité des champs électrostatiques.

Peu d'études ont été consacrées aux effets aigus d'une exposition à un champ électrostatique. Dans l'ensemble, les résultats obtenus indiquent qu'il n'y a d'autre effet aigu indésirable que celui qui est lié à la perception directe du champ et à la sensation désagréable produite par les microchocs électriques.

Champs magnétostatiques

En ce qui concerne les effets chroniques ou retardés, les données fournies par les études épidémiologiques et les travaux de laboratoire sont insuffisantes pour permettre de tirer la moindre conclusion. Le CIRC (CIRC, 2002) estime ne pas avoir de preuves suffisantes, ni de données valables tirées de l'expérimentation animale, pour conclure que l'exposition à un champ magnétostatique a des effets cancérogènes chez l'Homme. Il n'est donc pas possible, à l'heure actuelle, d'affecter les champs magnétostatiques à une classe quelconque de cancérogénicité.

Une exposition de brève durée à un champ magnétostatique de l'ordre du tesla et au gradient de champ associé provoque un certain nombre d'effets aigus.

Des réactions de nature cardiovasculaire - modification de la tension artérielle et de la fréquence cardiaque - ont parfois été observées chez des volontaires humains ainsi que lors d'études sur l'animal. Toutefois, pour des expositions à des champs allant jusqu'à 8 T, elles sont restées dans les limites physiologiques normales.

Bien que ce point n'ait pas été vérifié expérimentalement, il est important de noter que le calcul permet de conclure à l'existence possible de trois effets dus aux potentiels d'écoulement induits : une légère modification de la fréquence cardiaque (dont on peut considérer qu'elle est sans conséquence pathologique), la production d'extrasystoles (qui pourrait être plus importante sur le plan physiologique) et un risque accru d'arythmie par réentrée (susceptible de déboucher sur une fibrillation ventriculaire). On pense que pour les deux premiers effets, le seuil se situe au-delà de 8 T. Dans le cas du troisième, la valeur du seuil est encore difficile à déterminer en raison de la complexité de la modélisation. Environ 5 à 10 personnes sur 10 000 sont particulièrement sensibles à une arythmie par réentrée et ces personnes peuvent présenter un risque plus important en cas d'exposition à un champ magnétostatique ou à un gradient de champ.

Toutefois, les données disponibles présentent de telles insuffisances que dans leur ensemble, elles ne permettent pas de tirer de conclusions définitives quant aux effets des champs magnétostatiques sur les paramètres physiologiques évoqués plus haut.

Lorsqu'un sujet effectue des mouvements dans un gradient de champ statique, il peut éprouver une sensation de vertige , des nausées, parfois des phosphènes et un goût métallique au niveau de la cavité buccale si l'intensité du champ statique dépasse environ 2 à 4 T. Même s'ils sont passagers, ces effets peuvent être indésirables pour le sujet. S'ajoutant à une éventuelle perte de coordination oeil-main , ces effets peuvent perturber l'exécution de tâches délicates (interventions chirurgicales par ex.) et donc menacer la sécurité.

On a fait état d'autres effets sur les réactions physiologiques, mais il est difficile d'en tirer des conclusions définitives tant que ces résultats n'auront pas été reproduits de façon indépendante.

13.1.8 Recommandations à l'intention des autorités nationales

Il est recommandé aux autorités nationales de mettre en oeuvre des programmes en vue de protéger la population et les travailleurs contre tout effet nocif des champs statiques. Toutefois, comme le principal effet d'un champ électrostatique est la sensation désagréable provoquée par les décharges électriques qu'il provoque dans les tissus de l'organisme, ce programme de protection pourrait consister simplement à indiquer dans quels cas on risque de se trouver exposé à un champ électrostatique intense et comment éviter ce genre de situation. Dans le cas des champs magnétostatiques, il est nécessaire d'établir un programme de protection contre les effets aigus dont ils sont reconnus responsables. Comme les informations dont on dispose actuellement au sujet de leurs effets chroniques ou retardés sont insuffisantes, il pourrait être nécessaire de prendre certaines mesures de précaution analogues à celles qu'a élaborées l'OMS (www.who.int/emf) afin de limiter l'exposition de la population et des travailleurs.

Les autorités nationales devraient adopter des normes fondées sur des données scientifiques solides afin de limiter l'exposition de la population aux champs magnétostatiques. La fixation de normes à visée sanitaire constitue la mesure de protection primordiale pour la population et les travailleurs. Il existe des normes internationales applicables aux champs magnétostatiques (CIPRNI, 1994) qui sont exposées à l'appendice 1. L'OMS recommande cependant de revoir ces normes à la lumière des données les plus récentes publiées dans la littérature scientifique.

Les autorités nationales devraient établir des programmes - ou compléter les programmes existants - en vue d'assurer une protection contre les effets éventuels des champs magnétostatiques. En ce qui concerne les mesures de protection à mettre en oeuvre dans le cadre de l'usage industriel et scientifique des champs magnétiques, on peut distinguer les mesures d'ordre technique, le respect d'une certaine distance par rapport à l'appareillage et les mesures administratives. La protection contre les dangers secondaires résultant d'interférences magnétiques avec des équipements de secours , l'appareillage électronique médical ou encore avec des implants chirurgicaux ou dentaires est un domaine d'une importance toute particulière, compte tenu des effets indésirables possibles des champs magnétostatiques. En raison des forces mécaniques susceptibles de s'exercer sur les implants ferromagnétiques et les objets non fixés dans une installation où règnent des champs intenses, des précautions doivent être prises.

Les autorités nationales doivent envisager de soumettre à une autorisation préalable les installations d'IRM afin de faire en sorte que les mesures de précaution soient effectivement prises. Dans ce cas, les installations d'IRM dont l'intensité du champ dépasse la norme nationale ou est supérieure à 2 T devraient également satisfaire à des exigences supplémentaires. Il s'agit en l'occurrence des informations à fournir au sujet des malades, du personnel et de tout incident ou lésion imputable à la présence de champs magnétiques intenses.

Les autorités nationales doivent financer des recherches visant combler les lacunes importantes qui subsistent au sujet de la sécurité des personnes exposées à des champs magnétostatiques. Les futures recherches à entreprendre sont indiquées dans la suite du présent document (voir plus loin) et également exposées sur le site Internet de l'OMS (voir www.who.int/emf). Les chercheurs doivent recevoir un financement qui leur permette d'effectuer les études recommandées dans le programme de recherche de l'OMS.

Il faut que les autorités nationales apportent un appui financier aux installations d'IRM pour leur permettre de recueillir, sur l'exposition de leur personnel et de leurs patients aux champs magnétostatiques, des informations qui seront mises à la disposition des futures études épidémiologiques. Elles devront également financer l'établissement de banques de données où seront rassemblées des informations sur les travailleurs qui subissent une exposition de longue durée, comme c'est le cas du personnel employé à la fabrication des appareils d'IRM et d'appareillages utilisant également des aimants de forte puissance ou qui travaille sur des technologies nouvelles comme les trains à lévitation magnétique.

13.2   Recommandations en vue des études futures

La mise en évidence des lacunes qui subsistent dans nos connaissances est un élément essentiel de l'évaluation de ce risque sanitaire et on trouvera ci-après des recommandations en vue des recherches futures.

13.2.1 Champs électrostatiques

Il ne semble pas qu'il y ait grand intérêt à poursuivre la recherche sur les effets sanitaires éventuels des champs électrostatiques. Aucune des études effectuées à ce jour n'indique l'existence d'effets indésirables, si ce n'est la possibilité d'un stress en cas d'exposition prolongée à des microchocs électriques. Dans ces conditions, il n'y a pas lieu de recommander d'autres recherches sur les effets biologiques des champs électrostatiques.Par ailleurs, les occasions d'exposition importante à de tels champs sur les lieux de travail ou de vie restent limitées et ne justifient donc pas d'études épidémiologiques.

13.2.2 Champs magnétostatiques

En règle générale, les recherches menées jusqu'ici ne l'ont pas été de façon systématique et ont souvent été effectuées en l'absence de méthodologie appropriée et d'information sur l'exposition. Des programmes de recherche coordonnés sont recommandés en vue d'une meilleure systématisation de la recherche. Il faudrait également étudier l'incidence de paramètres physiques tels que l'intensité, la durée et le gradient sur l'issue biologique de l'exposition.

13.2.2.1 Etudes théoriques et études sur modèles informatiques

La dosimétrie informatique permet de relier le champ magnétostatique extérieur aux champs électriques et aux courants induits internes qui sont engendrés par les mouvements des tissus vivants dans ce champ. Cet outil théorique permet de caractériser le champ au niveau d'un organe ou d'un tissu donné. Il existe quatre fantômes anthropomorphes voxélisés à haute résolution , anatomiquement réalistes, qui représentent des adultes de sexe masculin. Ces fantômes sont largement utilisés pour l'étude des champs électromagnétiques variables dans le temps. Par contre, très peu de travaux ont été effectués sur les champs magnétostatiques et on estime qu'il est important de poursuivre la recherche au moyen de ces modèles. Il importe en outre de travailler sur des fantômes de tailles diverses et sur des fantômes anthropomorphes féminins modélisant notamment des femmes enceintes porteuses de foetus à différents âges. On pourrait également effectuer des études sur des fantômes de femelles gravides pour faciliter l'interprétation des études sur le développement au moyen de tels modèles (**priorité moyenne**).

Il faudrait mettre au point un fantôme anthropomorphe modélisant la tête et les épaules et l'utiliser pour étudier les champs et les courants électriques ainsi que les phosphènes ou vertiges auxquels ils semblent associés. Ce genre de modèle pourrait également être utilisé pour étudier les champs et courants engendrés par les mouvements de la tête et des yeux dans un champ magnétostatique. Ce dernier point est jugé particulièrement important en IRM interventionnelle, lorsque la réduction des mouvements de la tête des chirurgiens et autres personnels cliniques peut contraindre à une augmentation des mouvements oculaires. Il faudrait également simuler les grands mouvements effectués par le personnel autour de l'appareil (**priorité élevée**).

On estime important de procéder à des calculs basés sur une modélisation détaillée du myocarde et des pathologies cardiaques courantes. Cette modélisation devrait prendre en compte la microarchitecture du coeur ainsi que les petits vaisseaux du myocarde où seraient susceptibles d'apparaître des champs et des courants capables d'influer sur la génération du rythme par le noeud sinusal et sur la propagation de l'onde de dépolarisation. En outre, il est nécessaire de déterminer par le calcul l'intensité et la distribution spatiale des courants induits dans le myocarde par l'exposition à un champ et à un gradient de champ. Il faudrait étudier un grand nombre d'orientations par rapport à la direction du vecteur champ, ce qui permettrait une comparaison avec les courants dont le calcul a montré qu'ils produisent des effets cardiaques. Il est recommandé de s'appuyer sur des études expérimentales et des expériences en laboratoire (**priorité élevée**).

On hésite encore, pour le moment, à soumettre les femmes enceintes à des examens IRM à haute intensité, mais il faut admettre que cette situation pourrait changer. Il serait donc souhaitable de procéder à des études par modélisation sur les courants induits au niveau du foetus par les mouvements de la mère ou du foetus lui-même dans un champ de forte intensité. Ces calculs (de même que des travaux similaires sur les gradients de champ et les champs de radiofréquence) permettraient d'évaluer la probabilité d'effets éventuels sur le foetus (**priorité élevée**).

13.2.2.2   *Etudes in vitro*

Les champs magnétostatiques peuvent interagir avec les systèmes biologiques de différentes manières, encore que les effets à conséquence sanitaire les plus probables soient imputables à l'action du champ sur les molécules chargées et sur la vitesse des réactions biochimiques.

Il est nécessaire de poursuivre les études sur les cibles des effets biologiques des champs magnétostatiques et sur leur mécanisme. Il est notamment recommandé d'étudier les effets de champs d'une intensité de 0,01 à 10 T sur l'interaction entre les ions (par ex. les ions Ca^{2+} et Mg^{2+}) et les enzymes et sur la formation de paires de radicaux libres. Sans se cacher la difficulté du problème, il vaut la peine de rechercher s'il y a encore d'autres réactions enzymatiques dont le mécanisme repose sur la formation de paires de radicaux, en se servant pour cela de modèles qui puissent être également valables en santé humaine. On pourrait également se concentrer sur des espèces radicalaires toxiques, comme le radical superoxyde, dont on sait qu'elles produisent des lésions et sont formées selon des mécanismes impliquant des radicaux libres (**priorité moyenne**).

S'agissant de la cancérogénicité éventuelle des champs magnétostatiques, les études faisant état d'un effet co-mutagène sur diverses cellules sont particulièrement intéressantes. Il faudrait effectuer des recherches de ce genre sur des cellules primaires humaines et les étendre à la transformation cellulaire et aux systèmes génétiquement modifiés (**priorité élevée**).

Dans certaines conditions d'exposition, les champs magnétostatiques pourraient affecter l'expression des gènes et les fonctions correspondantes dans les cellules humaines et mammaliennes, mais on ne dispose que de peu de données à ce sujet. Les techniques de la génomique et de la protéomique devraient être appliquées à des cellules primaires humaines afin de rechercher, par la présence éventuelle de marqueurs, la trace d'effets de ces champs susceptibles d'avoir un retentissement sur la santé humaine (**priorité faible**).

13.2.2.3   Expérimentation animale

On peut étudier sur des modèles animaux les effets d'une exposition chronique aux champs magnétostatiques. En l'absence d'informations précises sur le pouvoir cancérogène de ces champs, des études de longue durée (notamment sur toute la durée de la vie) sont recommandées. On pourrait travailler à la fois sur des animaux normaux et sur des animaux génétiquement modifiés. Par exemple, si l'on considère que la multiplication des radicaux libres pourrait augmenter le risque de cancérisation, on pourrait utiliser comme modèle des souris privées du gène de la superoxyde-dismutase. Ce modèle présente une sensibilité fortement accrue aux tumeurs et autres pathologies liées à la formation de radicaux libres. L'utilisation de biopuces permet de déterminer et de quantifier sans peine les effets des différents paramètres de l'exposition sur le génome et le protéome (**priorité élevée**).

Il faut étudier étudier de façon systématique la possibilité d'un risque accru d'anomalies du développement et d'effets tératogènes. Il est possible que pendant sa phase de développement, l'encéphale soit particulièrement sensible aux effets de courants induits par les mouvements : les effets d'orientation sont très importants pour guider la croissance normale des dendrites neuronales. Il n'est pas exclu qu'une exposition relativement

305

brève puisse entraîner des modifications persistantes. L'étude des paramètres neurocomportementaux peut permettre d'explorer de façon rapide et sensible les effets d'une exposition sur les fonctions du cerveau en phase de développement, aussi est-il recommandé d'entreprendre de telles études. Il serait également utile de relever systématiquement, pendant cette phase de développement, la présence éventuelle de modifications morphologiques subtiles dans des régions déterminées de l'encéphale comme le cortex et l'hippocampe. On devrait également envisager d'utiliser des modèles transgéniques appropriés (**priorité élevée**).

Même si certaines données indiquent que l'exposition d'animaux (et d'êtres humains) à des champs d'environ 2 T n'entraîne aucun effet physiologique, il serait utile de connaître les effets de champs plus intenses. On pourrait donc étudier avec fruit sur l'animal les effets d'une exposition à des champs dont l'intensité atteint ou dépasse 10 T (**priorité moyenne**).

Divers autres points d'aboutissement de l'effet des champs magnétostatiques ont été étudiés, mais les résultats obtenus jusqu'ici ne donnent que des informations limitées. Entreprendre une série d'études portant chacune sur l'un de ces points ne serait pas très économique, mais il serait peut-être intéressant de procéder à une expérimentation animale générale couvrant différents points (**faible priorité**).

13.2.2.4   *Expérimentation sur des sujets humains*

Les effets des champs magnétiques sur le comportement et les fonctions cognitives doivent être étudiés plus avant, même si les données disponibles n'indiquent pas l'existence d'un risque particulier pour certains aspects précis des fonctions cognitives et ne permettent guère de savoir quels paramètres seraient à étudier en laboratoire. Faute d'orientation claire, on pourrait éventuellement étudier les effets d'une exposition sur les résultats d'une batterie de tests psychotechniques, comportant notamment des tests classiques d'attention, de temps de réaction et de mémorisation, ne serait-ce que pour procéder à une première sélection dans l'attente de travaux plus pointus. Ce travail expérimental pourrait commencer par des études sur des volontaires (**priorité moyenne**).

Avec la généralisation des examens IRM au cours desquels le personnel technique se trouve à proximité immédiate des malades et des électroaimants, comme c'est le cas en IRM interventionnelle, il devient nécessaire de procéder à des études complémentaires sur la coordination de la tête et des yeux ainsi que sur les fonctions cognitives et comportementales en présence d'un gradient de champ. On estime qu'il serait d'un grand intérêt d'étudier de manière plus approfondie les mécanismes et l'intensité des troubles vestibulaires provoqués par les champs, notamment les vertiges, car il est de plus en plus probable que le personnel médical va être amené à effectuer des tâches longues et complexes dans un champ magnétique (**priorité élevée**).

De même, il serait utile de poursuivre les études sur la fonction cardiaque ainsi que sur les effets qui pourraient s'exercer sur l'appareil cardiovasculaire. Il pourrait également être nécessaire d'étendre ces études à des champs de plus de 3 T afin d'évaluer les autres types de risque qui pourraient s'ajouter à ceux qui existent dans la pratique clinique habituelle (**faible priorité**).

13.2.2.5 Etudes épidémiologiques

Un certain nombre de catégories de travailleurs sont fortement exposées à des champs magnétostatiques, comme par exemple les techniciens d'IRM, les ouvriers des fonderies d'aluminium et certains employés de l'industrie des transports (métro, trains à sustentation magnétique, trains de banlieue et métro léger). Dans le cas de maladies chroniques rares comme le cancer, il est nécessaire d'effectuer des études de faisabilité afin d'identifier les groupes fortement exposés dont on pourrait s'assurer la participation à des études épidémiologiques. Des études de faisabilité sont également nécessaires pour déterminer si ces métiers impliquent d'autres types d'exposition. Si l'on parvient à identifier un nombre suffisant de travailleurs, le mieux serait probablement d'envisager des études cas-témoins imbriquées, car il faut obtenir des données détaillées sur l'exposition et sur les facteurs de confusion importants comme la présence de rayonnements ionisants. Il faudra vraisemblablement organiser des études collectives internationales de manière à disposer d'un nombre suffisant de sujets (**priorité élevée**).

Dans le cas des autres conséquences sanitaires plus courantes à courte période de latence on peut également identifier et suivre longitudinalement les groupes professionnels concernés, par exemple les travailleurs des industries qui fabriquent des appareils d'IRM. Des informations sur un certain nombre d'effets sanitaires pourraient d'ailleurs déjà être tirées des examens médicaux systématiques subis par ces personnels, mais elles ne sauraient être utilisées que si des données analogues concernant des groupes non exposés comparables sont également disponibles. Une enquête sanitaire portant sur des chirurgiens, des infirmières et autres personnels utilisant l'IRM interventionnelle permettrait d'obtenir des renseignements utiles sur le niveau, la durée et la fréquence de l'exposition des travailleurs aux champs magnétostatiques de ces appareils. De même, les dossiers médicaux que possèdent certains hôpitaux pourraient aussi permettre d'obtenir des données sur des personnes exposées mais dont la pathologie s'est ultérieurement révélée bénigne (**priorité élevée**).

On estime qu'il y aurait également avantage à effectuer une étude prospective sur les risques en cas d'exposition à des champs magnétostatiques pendant la grossesse et à suivre également l'issue de la grossesse chez les femmes qui ont dû subir des examens par IRM (**priorité élevée**).

L'expérience tirée de l'étude d'autres fréquences montre qu'il peut être très difficile d'obtenir une estimation fiable de l'exposition aux champs électromagnétiques qui puisse être utilisée pour des études épidémiologiques et leur substituer d'autres variables comme le nature du travail effectué ou la distance à telle ou telle source ne permet pas toujours une évaluation précise. Il est donc nécessaire d'utiliser un appareillage spécial pour mesurer l'exposition. Des dosimètres personnels relativement peu encombrants se sont révélés très utiles pour les travaux sur les champs électriques de très basse fréquence, aussi l'usage de dosimètres personnels améliorerait-il grandement l'évaluation de l'exposition aux fins des études épidémiologiques. Il conviendrait de procéder à la validation numérique et expérimentale de ces dosimètres. Il faudrait enregistrer l'intensité du champ magnétique, le gradient du champ, la durée de l'exposition et, dans la mesure du possible, la vitesse de variation du champ due aux mouvements (**priorité élevée**).

Tableau 1. Recommandations en vue de la recherche

Mécanismes d'interaction
Chimie des réactions mettant en jeu des paires de radicaux (0,1-10 T)
Effets co-mutagènes sur cellules humaines

Etudes théoriques et informatiques
Etudes dosimétriques sur fantômes voxélisés (homme/ femme/ femme enceinte)
Courants intraoculaires induits
Potentiels d'écoulement myocardiques

Etudes *in vitro*
Mécanismes d'interaction : réactions mettant en jeu des paires de radicaux et activité enzymatique
Influence des paramètres physiques (intensité, durée, répétition, gradient de champ magnétostatique)

Mutagénicité et transformation cellulaire sur cellules humaines primaires
Expression des gènes dans des cellules primaires humaines

Expérimentation animale
Cancer
Effets sur le développement et effets neurocomportementaux
Fonction cardiaque (~ 20 T)

Expérimentation sur des volontaires
Fonction vestibulaire, coordination de la tête et des yeux
Fonctions cognitives et comportement
Effets cardiovasculaires

Etudes épidémiologiques
Etude de faisabilité portant sur les sources d'exposition, les facteurs de confusion et le nombre de sujets exposés
Etude cas-témoins imbriquée portant sur des pathologies chroniques comme le cancer (si réalisable)
Issue de la grossesse après exposition professionnelle ou examen IRM
Etude de cohorte sur les effets à court terme dans les professions fortement exposées

---

14 КРАТКИЙ ОБЗОР И РЕКОМЕНДАЦИИ К ДАЛЬНЕЙШИМ ИССЛЕДОВАНИЯМ

14.1 Краткий обзор

14.1.1 Природные и техногенные источники постоянных полей[3]

В природе электрические поля присутствуют в атмосфере. Напряженность электрического поля может достигать 3 кВ м$^{-1}$ под грозовыми тучами, однако при хорошей погоде она может изменяться в пределах от 1 до 100 В м$^{-1}$. В других случаях основным источником воздействия электрических полей на человека является разделение зарядов в результате трения. Например, шарканье по непроводящему ковру может привести к накоплению электрического потенциала порядка нескольких киловольт и возникновению локальных полей до 500 кВ м$^{-1}$. При передаче постоянного электрического тока (ПЭТ) создаются электрические поля напряженностью до 20 кВ м$^{-1}$. В электропоездах, работающих на постоянном токе, регистрируются поля до 300 В м$^{-1}$. При работе мониторов компьютеров создаются электростатические поля порядка 10-20 кВ м$^{-1}$ на расстоянии 30 см.

Геомагнитное поле Земли изменяется в диапазоне 35-70 мкТл вблизи земной поверхности. Некоторые виды животных ориентируются в пространстве по силовым линиям магнитного поля. Техногенные магнитные поля создаются в местах, где используются источники постоянного тока, например в системах транспорта, работающих на электричестве, в промышленных процессах, таких как производство алюминия или электросварка, и, как правило, выше природных магнитных полей. Так, например, внутри электропоездов и поездов на магнитной подушке создаются постоянные магнитные поля до 2 мТл. Профессиональные рабочие, как правило, подвергаются воздействию более сильных полей, например, при электролитическом восстановлении алюминия создаются поля около 60 мТл, а электрическая дуга при сварке создает магнитное поле порядка 5 мТл на расстоянии 1 см от сварочного кабеля.

Примечание переводчика:

[3] В этом документе рассматриваются не изменяющиеся во времени электрические или магнитные поля, т.е. с частотой 0 Гц.

Создание сверхпроводников в 1970-80-х гг. способствовало применению более сильных магнитных полей в медицинской диагностике в результате разработки методов исследования, использующих магнитно-резонансное изображение (МРИ) и спектроскопию (МРС)[4], и ядерно-магнитный резонанс (ЯМР). По имеющимся оценкам, к настоящему времени во всем мире было проведено около 200 миллионов МРИ исследований. В повседневных клинических исследованиях магнитные поля МРИ-сканеров, составляющие порядка 0,2 – 3 Тл, создаются постоянными магнитами, сверхпроводящими магнитами и их комбинацией. В исследовательских целях при сканировании всего тела пациента создаются поля, достигающие 9,4 Тл. Величина магнитных полей вокруг магнитов, используемых в МРИ исследованиях, может быть легко оценена, что позволит снизить воздействие на персонал путем использования магнитов с защитой. Как правило, на рабочем месте оператора величина магнитного поля составляет 0,5 мТл. Однако, во время сборки и тестирования такого оборудования или при проведении медицинских процедур, когда пациент и медицинский персонал находятся внутри магнита, воздействие на персонал может достигать 1 Тл и выше. В некоторых физических исследованиях и в высокоэнергетических технологиях могут использоваться сверхпроводники, в результате чего рабочие могут регулярно в течение длительных периодов времени подвергаться воздействию полей порядка 1,5 Тл.

14.1.2 Механизмы взаимодействия

Различают следующие три типа физического взаимодействия постоянных магнитных полей с биологическими системами, установленные на основе экспериментальных данных:

(1)   Электродинамическое взаимодействие токами проводимости (например, с текущим раствором электролита). Магнитное поле в результате возникновения силы Лоренца действует на движущиеся носители электрического заряда. Это приводит к индукции электрического потенциала (так называемого «потенциала потока») и тока. «Потенциалы потока» у животных и человека обычно связаны с сокращением сердечных желудочков и выбросом крови в аорту. Лоренцево взаимодействие также приводит к возникновению магнитно-гидродинамической силы, направленной противоположно кровотоку. Считается, что снижение кровотока в аорте достигает 10% при действии магнитного поля 15 Тл.

---

[4] В этом документе рассматривается метод МРИ, уровни воздействия при обследовании МРС практически такие же.

(2) Магнитно-механические эффекты, включая ориентацию магнитно-анизотропных структур в однородных полях и смещение парамагнитных и ферромагнитных материалов в градиентах магнитного поля. Особое внимание в механизмах взаимодействия представляет возникновение сил и вращающих моментов, действующих на эндогенные и экзогенные металлические предметы.

(3) Эффекты воздействия на состояние электронного спина промежуточных продуктов реакции. Химия спин-коррелированных пар радикалов в течение длительного периода времени рассматривалась в химии и биологии как проявление эффектов магнитного поля. Постоянные магнитные поля в диапазоне от 10 до 100 мТл могут. влиять на протекание некоторых органических химических реакций в результате воздействия на состояние электронного спина промежуточных продуктов реакции. Спин-коррелированная пара радикалов может рекомбинироваться и препятствовать образованию продуктов реакции в следующих условиях: (а) пара, образованная в триплетном состоянии, должна перейти в синглетное состояние посредством какого-либо механизма и (б) радикалы должны быть расположены близко, чтобы рекомбинировать. Условие (а) очень чувствительно к воздействию магнитного поля. Наибольшее число исследований было направлено на применение таких эффектов с целью изучения реакций энзимов. Однако индуцированное магнитным полем изменение концентраций или потоков свободных радикалов возможно не приводит к физиологическим последствиям для клеточных функций или отдаленным мутагенным эффектам.

Дозиметрия

Для понимания биологических эффектов воздействия электрических и магнитных полей необходимо рассматривать поля, непосредственно воздействующие на клетки различных частей тела и тканей. Доза может быть определена как соответствующая функция электрических и магнитных полей в точке взаимодействия. Установление взаимосвязи между внешними невозмущенными полями и внутренними полями является основной задачей дозиметрии. Важными аспектами дозиметрических исследований являются как расчетные методы с использованием воксельных моделей, так и экспериментальные исследования воздействия полей.

Действие магнитного поля на биологические ткани, вероятно, зависит от физических характеристик поля, таких как вектор магнитной индукции, градиент магнитного поля и/или производная этих параметров, которая обычно называется «производная сил». Некоторые из сильных взаимодействий характеризуются движением через силовые параметры, например перемещение тела или кровоток в магнитном поле.

Соответствующие дозиметрические параметры зависят от физических механизмов, приводящих к возникновению неблагоприятных эффектов для здоровья. Очевидно, что ферромагнитные предметы не должны находиться вблизи магнита. Поэтому настоятельно рекомендуется проводить скрининг на присутствие таких предметов и имплантатов, которые могут перемещаться в результате приложения сил или возникновения вращающих моментов. Необходимо также проводить измерения максимального значения вектора магнитной индукции и производной магнитной силы. Для оценки этих параметров в различных локализациях около магнита, где воздействию может подвергаться персонал, могут быть использованы карты полей, однако индивидуальная дозиметрия является преимущественной.

Движение всего или частей тела, например глаз или головы, в градиенте магнитного поля приведет к индукции электрического поля и тока во время движения. Дозиметрические расчеты показали, что величина таких индуцированных электрических полей становится значительной при нормальном движении вокруг или внутри магнитных полей более 2-3 Тл. Это может являться причиной индивидуальных свидетельств о появлении головокружения и порой о возникновении вспышек света в глазах у пациентов, добровольцев и персонала во время перемещения в магнитном поле.

Источники действия постоянных магнитных полей на человека многочисленны и разнообразны. В последнее время одним из наиболее часто встречающихся источников воздействия является МРИ оборудование. В последнее десятилетие были приложены значительные усилия, дающие возможность использовать МРИ-системы при очень сильных полях. В повседневной клинической практике применяются МРИ-системы с величиной поля в центре магнита около 1,5 Тл. Однако, в настоящее время для проведения рутинных клинических исследований разрешены системы с магнитным полем порядка 3,0 Тл; в результате, к 2004 году по всему миру применялось более 100 таких систем. Кроме этого, для медицинских целей разрабатывается исследовательское оборудование с магнитным полем порядка 4 – 9,4 Тл. Так как величина поля МРИ-систем постоянно увеличивается, это приводит к различным взаимодействиям полей с биологическими тканями. Таким образом, в результате возрастающей тенденции к использованию более сильных полей понимание механизмов взаимодействия электромагнитных полей, генерируемых МРИ-системами, с телом человека становится все более значимым.

14.1.3 Исследования in vitro

Результаты *in vitro* исследований ценны для понимания механизмов взаимодействия и оценки возможных эффектов, которые могут исследоваться *in vivo*. Однако они не являются достаточными для оценки эффектов для здоровья человека без подтверждения результатов в исследованиях *in vivo*.

В опытах *in vitro* были обнаружены некоторые биологические эффекты воздействия постоянных магнитных полей. В качестве объектов исследования рассматривались различные уровни организации: системы, изолированные от клетки, включающие мембраны, энзимы биохимических реакций, и различные клеточные модели на бактериях и клетках млекопитающих. В опытах изучались такие биологические эффекты, как ориентация клеток, метаболическая активность клеток, физиология клеточных мембран, экспрессия генов, клеточный рост и генотоксичность.

В исследованиях наблюдались как положительные, так и отрицательные реакции, однако большая часть наблюдений не была продублирована. Наблюдаемые эффекты характеризовались разнообразием и обнаруживались после воздействия постоянных магнитных полей в широком диапазоне. Было обнаружено, что магнитные поля могут неблагоприятно действовать на некоторые системы при интенсивностях ниже 1 Тл, обычно в диапазоне мТл. В одних исследованиях для некоторых эффектов был обнаружен порог, однако в других исследованиях наблюдалась нелинейная зависимость «доза-эффект» без видимого порога.

Для магнитных полей выше 1 Тл были получены согласованные данные по эффектам их действия на ориентацию клеток, однако значимость этих эффектов *in vivo* не ясна. Анализ некоторых исследований предполагает, что комбинированные эффекты действия постоянных магнитных полей и других агентов, таких как генотоксические вещества, могут привести к синергетическим эффектам, как защитным, так и стимулирующим. В настоящее время информация, полученная в опытах *in vitro,* является противоречивой и нуждается в подтверждении до принятия каких-либо выводов, касающихся эффектов воздействия на здоровье человека.

Эффект воздействия постоянных магнитных полей зависит не только от физических параметров, таких как интенсивность, длительность, повторяемость и градиент воздействия, но и от биологических. Показано, что тип клетки, клеточная активация и другие физиологические условия во время воздействия поля существенно влияют на результат эксперимента. Механизмы этих эффектов до сих пор неизвестны, но они могут быть обусловлены эффектами действия постоянного магнитного поля на радикалы и ионы. Вероятная роль такого действия была подтверждена в некоторых исследованиях *in vitro*.

Результаты некоторых исследований, направленных на изучение воздействия МРИ-сигнала и других комбинированных полей, показали, что биологические эффекты действия комбинированных полей не отличаются от эффектов действия только постоянного магнитного поля, если такие эффекты могут существовать.

В целом исследования *in vitro* не дают ясной картины специфического воздействия магнитных полей. Таким образом, они не указывают на возможное неблагоприятное воздействие на здоровье человека.

14.1.4 Исследования на лабораторных животных

Результаты нескольких исследований эффектов воздействия электрических полей на лабораторных животных не свидетельствовали о неблагоприятном воздействии, за исключением эффектов, связанных с ощущением поверхностного электрического заряда.

Большое количество исследований на животных проводилось с целью изучения эффектов воздействия постоянного магнитного поля. В большинстве этих исследований, которые рассматриваются по отношению к здоровью человека, изучалось воздействие полей, значительно превышающих природные геомагнитные поля. Несколько исследований были выполнены в мТл-диапазоне магнитной индукции, сравнимом с относительно высоким промышленным воздействием. В последнее время в связи с развитием технологии сверхпроводящих магнитов и МРИ-систем проводилось изучение воздействия полей, превышающих 1 Тл, на поведение, физиологическое состояние и репродуктивную функцию. В некоторых исследованиях изучались возможные эффекты хронического воздействия, в частности, в отношении канцерогенеза.

Наиболее согласованные результаты исследований были получены относительно нейроповеденческих реакций. А именно, перемещение лабораторных грызунов в постоянном магнитном поле порядка 4 Тл и выше было агрессивным и характеризовалось как проявление отвращения и избегания. Эти эффекты, вероятно, связаны с магнитно-гидродинамическими эффектами воздействия на лимфатическую систему вестибулярного аппарата. В отношении других возможных причин данные противоречивы.

Считается, что некоторые позвоночные и беспозвоночные виды могут использовать магнитные поля на уровнях, близких к геомагнитному полю, с целью ориентации в окружающей среде, однако считается, что такие эффекты не являются существенными для здоровья.

В исследованиях было подтверждено, что действие магнитных полей выше 1 Тл (0,1 Тл для крупных животных) индуцирует «потенциал потока» около сердца и основных кровеносных сосудов, однако физиологические последствия такого воздействия до сих пор остаются неясными. Воздействие сильных полей (до 8 Тл) в области сердца в течение нескольких часов не привело к возникновению сердечно-сосудистых эффектов у свиней. Кратковременное и длительное воздействие полей в диапазоне от геомагнитных уровней до нескольких мТл приводило к неблагоприятному воздействию на сердечно-сосудистую систему у кроликов, однако наблюдаемая зависимость не была значимой.

Результаты одной группы исследователей показали, что магнитные поля мТл-диапазона могут угнетать повышение артериального давления посредством действия на гормональную регуляторную систему. Эта же группа показала, что постоянные поля малой интенсивности (порядка 0,2 Тл) могут индуцировать локальные эффекты в кровотоке, что может привести к улучшению микроциркуляции. Дополнительно, другая группа исследователей показала, что воздействие магнитных полей порядка 10 Тл может привести к снижению подкожного кровотока и температуры. Однако, во всех этих случаях изучаемые параметры были очень изменчивы, что, вероятно, обусловлено фармакологическими действиями, включающими анестезию и иммобилизацию. В целом, без проведения независимых повторных исследований сложно прийти к какому-либо выводу.

Несколько исследований были посвящены изучению возможных эффектов воздействия магнитного поля на клетки крови и гемопоэтическую систему. Однако, результаты этих исследований сомнительны, что ограничивает их использование. В лабораторных опытах были обнаружены эффекты действия магнитных полей на энзимные и ионные компоненты плазмы крови. Однако, эти результаты должны быть подтверждены независимыми лабораторными исследованиями с целью принятия заключения.

Результаты опытов, проведенных в одной лаборатории в отношении воздействия на эндокринную систему, показали, что магнитные поля могут неблагоприятно влиять на функции шишковидного тела и содержание мелатонина. Однако исследования, проведенные в других лабораториях, не смогли подтвердить эти результаты. Угнетение выработки мелатонина в результате воздействия постоянных магнитных полей должно быть подтверждено в дальнейших исследованиях с целью принятия заключения. Кроме этого, было проведено только несколько исследований, касающихся воздействия магнитных полей на другие органы эндокринной системы (кроме шишковидного тела), однако согласованных результатов получено не было.

Важными вопросами в изучении воздействия МРИ-систем на пациентов и медицинский персонал являются репродуктивность и развитие. В этом направлении было проведено только несколько хороших исследований, в которых рассматривались магнитные поля выше 1 Тл. МРИ-исследования сами по себе не являются информативными, поскольку эффект воздействия постоянного поля не может быть отличим от возможного эффекта воздействия радиочастотного поля и импульсного магнитного поля. Таким образом, для оценки риска для здоровья человека необходимо проведение дальнейших исследований.

Проведено небольшое число исследований на лабораторных животных с целью изучения генотоксичности и рака, на основе результатов которых сложно прийти к какому-либо выводу.

14.1.5 Лабораторные исследования на человеке

Электрические поля не проникают в электропроводящие предметы, такие как тело человека. Поле создает электрический заряд на поверхности тела и направлено перпендикулярно поверхности тела. Достаточно большой заряд на поверхности тела может ощущаться по его взаимодействию с волосами и по другим эффектам, таким как искровые электрические разряды (микроразряды). Порог ощущения у человека зависит от многих факторов и может изменяться в диапазоне 10-45 кВ м$^{-1}$. Порог раздражения, вероятно, изменяется в таком же диапазоне, однако он систематически не изучался. Болевые микроразряды могут появляться в тех случаях, когда человек, хорошо изолированный от земли, прикасается к заземленному объекту, или наоборот, когда заземленный человек прикасается к проводящему материалу, который не заземлен. Однако, величина порога электрического поля будет изменяться в зависимости от степени изоляции и других факторов.

В экспериментальных исследованиях на человеке изучалось воздействие магнитных полей на периферическую нервную систему, мозговую активность, нейроповеденческую и когнитивную функции, сенсорное ощущение, сердечную функцию, артериальное давление, сердцебиение, гормональный уровень и уровень протеинов в плазме, температуру тела и кожи, терапевтические эффекты. Уровни магнитного поля изменялись в широком диапазоне (до 8 Тл). При этом изучались эффекты воздействия постоянных полей и полей, создаваемых МРИ-системами. Время воздействия изменялось от нескольких секунд до 9 часов, однако, в большинстве случаев воздействие длилось менее часа. Результаты этих исследований имеют ограниченное применение, т.к. изучались больные или добровольцы с хорошим состоянием здоровья, кроме того, исследования проводились в небольших группах обследуемых.

Результаты проведенных исследований не указывают на неблагоприятное воздействие постоянных магнитных полей на нейрофизиологические реакции и когнитивную функцию, однако они не исключают возникновения этих эффектов. Обнаружена дозовая зависимость тяжести возникновения головокружения и тошноты у профессионалов, пациентов и добровольцев в результате перемещения в магнитных полях выше 2 Тл. В одном исследовании было показано, что при действии полей МРИ-систем порядка 1,5 Тл снижается визуальная координация рук и восприятие контрастов. Возникновение этих эффектов, вероятно, зависит от градиента поля и перемещения человека в магнитном поле. В других исследованиях наблюдались незначительные изменения артериального давления и сердцебиения, но они находились в пределах физиологической изменчивости. Не было обнаружено эффектов воздействия постоянных магнитных полей на другие аспекты сердечно-сосудистой физиологии, концентрацию протеинов в плазме и гормональный фон. Воздействие магнитных полей в диапазоне до 8 Тл не привело к изменению температуры тела у человека.

Однако следует отметить, что большинство исследований проводилось в группах с небольшим количеством человек и часто включало несопоставимый контроль. Таким образом, выводы, касающиеся воздействия магнитных полей на функционирование различных систем человека, в настоящем документе не приводятся.

14.1.6 Эпидемиологические исследования

Эпидемиологические исследования проводились в основном на профессиональных рабочих, которые подвергались воздействию магнитных полей, генерируемых оборудованием, использующим большой постоянный ток. Основная доля персонала, включающая сварщиков, плавильщиков алюминия и рабочих промышленных производств, в которых используются большие электролитические ванны для химических процессов разделения, подвергалась воздействию магнитных полей в промежуточном диапазоне до нескольких десятков мТл. Однако, для таких процессов характерно воздействие и других потенциально опасных паров и аэрозолей, что может привести к искажению результатов исследований и некорректным выводам. В эпидемиологических исследованиях изучались частота возникновения онкологических заболеваний, гематологические изменения, частота хромосомных аббераций, репродуктивные эффекты, расстройства скелетно-мышечной системы. Дополнительно, в некоторых исследованиях изучалось состояние репродуктивной функции и исходы беременностей у женщин-операторов МРИ-систем, которые могли подвергаться воздействию относительно высоких магнитных полей, достигающих 1 Тл. Два исследования были направлены на изучение исходов беременности у здоровых женщин-добровольцев, которые проходили МРИ-обследования во время беременности.

В результате проведенных исследований был обнаружен повышенный риск возникновения рака различных типов, например, рака легких, рака поджелудочной железы и гематологических злокачественных заболеваний, однако результаты этих исследований не согласованы. Небольшое количество эпидемиологических исследований, опубликованных к настоящему времени, оставляет много нерешенных вопросов о возможности повышенного риска возникновения рака в результате воздействия постоянных магнитных полей. Дозиметрические оценки воздействия в этих исследованиях были ненадежными, а число участников в нескольких исследованиях было незначительным. Таким образом, в этих исследованиях невозможно было обнаружить риск для таких редких заболеваний. Невозможность этих исследований предоставить ценную информацию об эффектах воздействия магнитных полей подтверждается отсутствием данных о возникновении других, наиболее установленных канцерогенных факторов, характерных для некоторых типов рабочего процесса. Нераковые эффекты воздействия магнитных полей на здоровье человека исследовались еще реже. Большинство эпидемиологических исследований проводилось на небольших выборках и характеризовалось множеством методических ограничений. К сожалению, не оценивались эффекты для других условий работы, характеризующихся потенциально высокими полями, например, у операторов МРИ-систем. В настоящее время данные, необходимые для оценки риска, рассматриваются как неадекватные.

14.1.7 Оценка риска для здоровья человека

Постоянные электрические поля

В настоящее время невозможно прийти к заключению относительно хронических или отдаленных эффектов воздействия электрических полей. Международное агентство по исследованию рака (МАИР) (IARC, 2002) указало на недостаточность оценок канцерогенности постоянных электрических полей.

Результаты нескольких исследований острых эффектов воздействия электрических полей предполагают, что единственно возможные эффекты для здоровья человека непосредственно связаны с ощущением полей и дискомфорта от электрических микроразрядов.

Постоянные магнитные поля

В отношении хронических и отдаленных эффектов имеющиеся результаты лабораторных и эпидемиологических исследований не позволяют сделать четких обоснованных выводов. МАИР (IARC, 2002) указывает на неадекватность результатов исследований на человеке канцерогенности постоянных магнитных полей и отсутствие значимых данных в исследованиях на животных. Таким образом, в настоящее время постоянные магнитные поля не могут быть классифицированы как обладающие возможным канцерогенным воздействием на здоровье человека.

Исследования кратковременного воздействия магнитных полей и градиентов полей в тесла-диапазоне свидетельствуют о возникновении некоторых острых эффектов.

Реакции со стороны сердечно-сосудистой системы, такие как изменение артериального давления и пульса, изредка наблюдались у добровольцев и в исследованиях на животных. Однако, эти изменения находились в пределах нормального физиологического функционирования при воздействии магнитных полей до 8 Тл.

Теоретические исследования предполагают, что в результате индукции «потенциала потока» возможно развитие следующих трех возможных эффектов: незначительное изменение скорости сердцебиения (которое, как предполагается, не приводит к отрицательным последствиям для здоровья), индукция эктопического ритма (которая может быть более физиологически значимой) и повышение вероятности возникновения первичной аритмии (возможно приводящей к фибрилляции желудочков). Однако, эти эффекты должны быть подтверждены в эксперименте. Для первых двух эффектов предполагается наличие порога, превышающего 8 Тл, для последнего эффекта величину порога оценить достаточно сложно из-за трудностей моделирования. Возможно, 5-10 человек из 10000 особенно уязвимы к возникновению аритмии, и риск для таких людей может быть повышен при воздействии постоянных магнитных полей и градиентов полей.

Ограничения имеющихся данных таковы, что на их основе в целом невозможно прийти к четкому выводу об эффектах воздействия постоянных магнитных полей на системы и функции, изучавшиеся в исследованиях.

Результаты исследований показали, что физическое перемещение в градиенте магнитного поля, превышающего 2-4 Тл, может привести к ощущению головокружения и тошноты, а также металлического привкуса во рту. Несмотря на то, что такие эффекты кратковременны, они могут неблагоприятно действовать на здоровье человека. Принимая во внимание возможные эффекты на визуальную координацию рук, магнитные поля могут в целом влиять на качество и выполнение тонкой работы, выполняемой специалистами (например, хирургами), и, таким образом, воздействовать на безопасность пациента и специалиста.

Дополнительно были опубликованы результаты исследований воздействия магнитных полей для других физиологических реакций, однако без независимого повторения таких исследований невозможно прийти к надежным выводам.

14.1.8 Рекомендации для национальных органов власти

Национальным органам власти рекомендуется выполнять программы, направленные на защиту населения и персонала от любого неблагоприятного воздействия постоянных электрических и магнитных полей. Однако, принимая во внимание, что основным эффектом влияния электрических полей является ощущение дискомфорта от электрических микроразрядов на поверхности тела, программа защиты может быть направлена на информирование людей о ситуациях, которые могут привести к воздействию сильных электрических полей, и каким образом их можно избежать. Для постоянных магнитных полей необходима программа защиты от возникновения острых эффектов, обнаруженных в исследованиях.

По причине недостатка информации о хронических и отдаленных эффектах Всемирной Организацией Здравоохранения (ВОЗ, www.who.int/emf) разрабатываются предупредительные меры, основанные на анализе «затраты – польза», которые могут быть необходимы для снижения воздействия на профессионалов и население.

Национальным органам власти следует адаптировать стандарты, основанные на результатах надежных научных исследований, которые ограничивают воздействие постоянных магнитных полей на человека. Выполнение стандартов, основанных на эффектах для здоровья человека, обеспечивает основную защиту для персонала и населения. Международные стандарты разработаны для постоянных магнитных полей (ICNIRP, 1994) и описаны в Приложении 1 к документу на английском языке. Однако, ВОЗ рекомендует провести пересмотр существующих стандартов в свете новых научных данных.

Национальным органам власти следует установить или дополнить существующие программы, которые обеспечивают безопасность населения и персонала от возможных неблагоприятных эффектов воздействия магнитных полей. Защитные меры в отношении промышленного и научно-исследовательского использования магнитных полей могут быть подразделены на несколько категорий: контроль технологического процесса, защита расстоянием, административный контроль. Защитные меры от дополнительного вреда в результате магнитной интерференции с аварийным или медицинским электронным оборудованием, а также для хирургических или зубных имплантатов являются областью особого внимания в связи с возможными неблагоприятными эффектами воздействия постоянных магнитных полей на здоровье человека. В связи с тем, что при помещении ферромагнитных имплантатов и свободно перемещающихся объектов в сильное магнитное поле, создаваемое, например, МРИ оборудованием, возникают механические силы, действующие на эти объекты, необходимо применение предупредительных мер.

Национальным органам власти следует рассматривать необходимость проведения лицензирования МРИ-оборудования с целью обеспечения выполнения защитных мер. Это также позволит установить дополнительное оборудование для МРИ-систем, в которых создаются поля, превышающие национальные стандарты или уровень 2 Тл. Такие рекомендации включают предоставление информации о пациентах, персонале и любых случаях возникновения инцидентов или причинения вреда в результате воздействия сильных магнитных полей.

Национальным органам власти следует финансировать исследования с целью заполнения пробелов в знаниях, необходимых для обеспечения безопасности людей, подвергающихся воздействию магнитных полей. Рекомендации к дальнейшим исследованиям будут рассмотрены в данном документе (см. ниже) и размещены на веб-сайте ВОЗ www.who.int/emf. Финансовую поддержку следует оказывать исследованиям, рекомендованным ВОЗ.

Национальным органам власти следует финансировать МРИ лаборатории с целью сбора информации о воздействии магнитных полей на персонал и пациентов при МРИ исследованиях, необходимой для проведения эпидемиологических исследований. Кроме этого, необходимо оказывать финансовую поддержку созданию и поддержанию баз данных, содержащих информацию о дополнительном воздействии сильных полей на персонал, которые, например, создаются при производстве МРИ- или подобных магнитов, а также новых технологий, таких как электропоезда на магнитных подушках.

14.2 Рекомендации к дальнейшим исследованиям

Определение пробелов в наших знаниях о возможном неблагоприятном воздействии постоянных электрических и магнитных полей на здоровье человека является существенной частью процесса оценки риска для здоровья человека. В связи с этим разработаны рекомендации к дальнейшим исследованиям.

14.2.1 Постоянные электрические поля

Считается, что продолжение исследований относительно эффектов воздействия электрических полей на здоровье человека не является результативным. Имеющиеся результаты исследований не свидетельствуют о возникновении неблагоприятных последствий для здоровья человека, за исключением возможного возникновения стресса в результате длительного действия микроразрядов. Таким образом, продолжение исследований биологических эффектов воздействия электрических полей не рекомендуется. Кроме того, воздействие сильных полей на рабочих местах или в среде обитания маловероятно и, таким образом, не может служить основанием к проведению эпидемиологических исследований.

14.2.2 Постоянные магнитные поля

К настоящему времени исследования в этой области не являлись систематичными и, как правило, выполнялись без соответствующей методологии и данных о воздействии. Поэтому рекомендуется проведение координированной исследовательской программы, основанной на системном подходе. Кроме этого, необходимо провести изучение значимости влияния таких физических параметров на биологический ответ, как интенсивность, продолжительность и градиент воздействия.

В результате обсуждения ограничений существующих исследований, рекомендуется проведение дальнейших исследований, затрагивающих эпидемиологические исследования, исследования на добровольцах, исследования на животных и *in vitro*, а также изучение механизмов взаимодействия и теоретическое моделирование. В таблице 1 представлен обзор предлагаемых рекомендаций.

14.2.2.1   Теоретические исследования и моделирование

Методы расчетной дозиметрии позволяют оценить связь между величиной внешнего магнитного поля и внутренними электрическими полями и индуцированными токами, вызванными движением живой объекта в поле. Такие теоретические методы позволяют охарактеризовать поля в определенных органах и тканях. В настоящее время разработано 4 воксельных фантома взрослого человека с высоким разрешением, наиболее реалистично описывающие его анатомическое строение. Эти фантомы широко используются в исследованиях электромагнитных полей, изменяющихся во времени. Однако исследованию постоянных полей уделялось мало внимания, таким образом, необходимо проведение дальнейших исследований с использованием этих фантомов. В частности, приоритетными направлениями являются исследования с фантомами различного размера, фантомом женщины, а также фантомами беременной женщины на различных стадиях беременности. Подобные исследования могут быть проведены на фантомах беременных животных с целью интерпретации результатов теоретических расчетов (**Промежуточный приоритет**).

Необходимо разработать фантом головы-и-плеч очень высокого разрешения с целью исследования связи электрических полей и токов с такими наблюдаемыми реакциями, как головокружение и вспышки света в глазах. Подобная модель может быть применена для исследования полей и токов, индуцируемых движением головы и глаз в магнитном поле. Это особенно важно при проведении медицинских МРИ-процедур, при которых снижение подвижности головы (хирургами и другим медицинским персоналом) компенсируется повышенной подвижностью глаз. Кроме этого необходимо смоделировать перемещение персонала в зоне воздействия МРИ-магнита (**Высокий приоритет**).

Рассматривается необходимость выполнения расчетов на основе детализированных моделей сердца и типичных сердечных патологий. В таких моделях должна рассматриваться микроархитектура сердца и кровеносные артерии и сосуды, в которых могут индуцироваться электрические поля и токи, влияющие на ритм, генерирующийся кардиостимулятором, а также на распространение деполяризации к клеткам сердечной мышцы. Кроме этого, необходимо провести расчеты для оценки величины и пространственного распределения токов, индуцируемых в сердце, в результате действия полей или градиентов полей. Необходимо изучить эффекты при различных ориентациях сердца к полю. Это бы позволило провести сопоставление с расчетными значениями токов, индуцирующих сердечные эффекты. Рекомендуется проводить экспериментальные и лабораторные исследования с целью поддержки теоретических расчетов (**Высокий приоритет**).

Несмотря на то, что в настоящее время предпочитают не проводить МРИ-исследования для беременных женщин, предполагается, что ситуация может измениться в будущем. Таким образом, рекомендуется провести моделирование токов, индуцированных в плоде, в результате движения матери или внутриутробного движения плода в магнитном поле. Эти расчеты (и подобные исследования с градиентами поля и радиочастотными полями) позволят оценить вероятность возникновения возможных эффектов у плода (**Высокий приоритет**).

14.2.2.2   *Исследования in vitro*

Постоянные магнитные поля могут взаимодействовать с биологическими системами по различным механизмам, однако наиболее вероятными механизмами, приводящими к возникновению эффектов для здоровья, являются индуцированные полем эффекты на заряженные молекулы и изменение скорости биохимических реакций.

Рекомендуется проведение дальнейших исследований, направленных на изучение возможных механизмов и мишеней биологических эффектов магнитных полей. Рекомендуется исследовать влияние постоянных магнитных полей 0,01 – 1 Тл на взаимодействие ионов (например, Ca^{2+} или Mg^{2+}) с энзимами и формирование пар радикалов. Несмотря на сложность выполнения таких исследований, необходимо продолжить поиск других энзимных реакций, которые протекают по механизму образования пар радикалов, в моделях, значимых для здоровья человека. Рекомендуется сконцентрировать усилия на изучение токсичных радикалов, например, супероксидов, которые обладают разрушительным действием и образуются по механизму свободных радикалов (**Промежуточный приоритет**).

Особый интерес о возможном канцерогенном действии магнитных полей представляют собой результаты исследований ко-мутагенных эффектов в различных клетках. Такое исследование следует провести и на клетках-предшественниках у человека и расширить исследования, включая модели на здоровых клетках, трансформированных в раковые клетки, или на генетически модифицированных клетках (**Высокий приоритет**).

При определенных условиях магнитные поля могут влиять на экспрессию генов и соответствующие функции в клетках человека и млекопитающих, однако в этом направлении информации недостаточно. Исследования с использованием методов геномики и протеомики следует проводить на клетках-предшественниках у человека с целью поиска возможных молекулярных маркеров воздействия постоянных полей на здоровье человека (**Низкий приоритет**).

14.2.2.3 *Исследования на лабораторных животных*

Эффекты длительного воздействия магнитных полей могут быть изучены в моделях на животных. В случае отсутствия специфической информации о потенциально возможном канцерогенном действии магнитных полей рекомендуется проводить длительные исследования (включая исследования в течение всей жизни животных). В исследованиях могут рассматриваться как нормальные, так и генетически-модифицированные животные. Например, если одним из возможных путей возникновения рака предполагается увеличение концентрации свободных радикалов, то может быть исследована модель на мышах с отсутствием гена супероксид дисмутазы. В такой модели существенно повышается уязвимость к раку и другим заболеваниям, связанным с образованием свободных радикалов. Использование технологий геномики и протеомики позволяет легко оценить эффекты влияния различных параметров воздействия (**Высокий приоритет**).

Возможность повышенного риска возникновения отклонений в развитии и тератогенных эффектов должна быть изучена на систематической основе. Развивающийся мозг может быть особенно уязвим к электрическим токам, индуцированным движением в магнитном поле: ориентационные эффекты важны для направления нормального роста дендритов нейронов. Возможно, что относительно коротким воздействием могут быть индуцированы продолжительные изменения. Изучение нервно-поведенческих параметров позволяет провести быстрый и чувствительный анализ возможных эффектов воздействия на развивающиеся мозговые функции, и такие исследования рекомендуются. Ценными являются исследования, позволяющие определить тонкие морфологические изменения, которые происходят во время развития определенных участков головного мозга, как, например, кора головного мозга. Может быть рассмотрена возможность проведения исследований с использованием соответствующих трансгенных моделей (**Высокий приоритет**).

Несмотря на то, что результаты исследований не свидетельствуют о возникновении электрофизиологических эффектов при воздействии полей порядка 2 Тл на животных и человека, полезно провести исследование эффектов воздействия более сильных полей. Таким образом, изучение эффектов воздействия полей до 10 Тл и выше в моделях на животных являлось бы полезным (**Промежуточный приоритет**).

Разнообразие реакций других систем и функций, исследовавшихся на животных, представляют только ограниченную информацию. Хотя проведение серии одиночных исследований в каждом из направлений может быть дорогостоящим, более расширенное исследование, касающееся изучения различных направлений, может оказаться целесообразным (**Низкий приоритет**).

14.2.2.4   *Экспериментальные исследования на человеке*

Рекомендуется продолжать исследования воздействия постоянных магнитных полей на когнитивную способность и поведение несмотря на то, что имеющиеся данные не свидетельствуют о риске для специфичных аспектов мышления и не выделяют возможные влияющие параметры, которые должны быть проверены в лабораторных условиях. Поскольку нет ясности в каких направлениях необходимо проводить исследования, одним из возможных направлений может являться исследование воздействия магнитного поля на выполнение комплекса интеллектуальных задач, которые включают стандартные тесты на внимательность, время реагирования и запоминания. Такое направление можно рассматривать как первоначальный скрининг с целью проведения последующего сфокусированного исследования. Первоначальные исследования могут быть проведены на добровольцах как часть экспериментальных исследований (**Промежуточный приоритет**).

В связи с расширяющимся применением МРИ исследований, при которых персонал находится в непосредственной близости или внутри магнита, необходимо проведение дополнительных исследований по координации глаз и головы, мыслительных способностей и поведения в градиенте поля. Особый интерес представляет проведение дальнейших исследований о механизмах возникновения и интенсивности индуцированных полем дисфункций вестибулярного аппарата, включая головокружение. Это связано с растущей вероятностью того, что персонал будет выполнять сложные задачи в зоне действия магнитного поля более длительные периоды времени (**Высокий приоритет**).

Таким же образом является полезным проведение дополнительных исследований сердечной функции и эффектов для сердечно-сосудистой системы. Такие исследования могут быть проведены при действии полей выше 3 Тл с целью оценки потенциального риска воздействий, превышающих уровни воздействия рутинных клинических исследований (**Низкий приоритет**).

14.2.2.5   *Эпидемиологические исследования*

Существует несколько категорий профессиональных работников, для которых характерно повышенное воздействие магнитных полей. К ним, например, относятся техники МРИ-систем, работники заводов по плавлению алюминия, работники некоторых видов транспорта (метро, поезда на магнитной подушке, электропоезда, троллейбусы, трамваи). При исследовании редких хронических заболеваний, таких как рак, необходимо проведение пилотных исследований с целью определения групп персонала с высоким (максимальным) воздействием, которые определенно примут участие в эпидемиологических исследованиях. Проведение пилотных исследований также необходимо для определения других типов воздействия в изучаемых группах. В случае, если будет сформирована большая группа работников, то проведение исследования методом «случай-контроль» будет наиболее подходящим, поскольку необходимо получить информацию об уровнях воздействия и о важных мешающих факторах, таких, как, например, ионизирующее излучение. С целью формирования больших выборок предпочтительно проводить совместные международные исследования (**Высокий приоритет**).

Для изучения других типичных эффектов воздействия полей на здоровье человека, имеющих короткие латентные периоды, может быть сформирована выборка профессиональных работников с наблюдением в течение длительного периода времени (когортные исследования). Например, группа рабочих предприятий, где производится МРИ-оборудование. Информация о состоянии здоровья может быть напрямую доступна из результатов рутинных медицинских обследований этих работников. Однако, эти данные могут быть использованы в анализе только в том случае, если подобная информация о состоянии здоровья будет доступна и для группы сравнения, не находящейся в условиях воздействия. Медицинский осмотр хирургов, медицинских сестер и других сотрудников, работающих внутри МРИ-магнитов, может позволить получить полезную информацию об уровнях, продолжительности и частоты воздействия постоянных полей этих систем на персонал. Кроме того, в архивах клиник могут храниться записи об историях болезней пациентов, что позволит получить и анализировать данные о людях, которые подвергались воздействию магнитных полей и состояние здоровья которых в последствии улучшилось (**Высокий приоритет**).

Предполагается, что полезная информация может быть получена при проведении проспективного исследования рисков во время беременности, связанных с профессиональным воздействием постоянных магнитных полей, а также при наблюдении за исходами беременностей у женщин, которые проходили МРИ исследования во время беременности (**Высокий приоритет**).

Опыт исследования полей других частот показал, что получение надежной информации об уровнях воздействия электромагнитных полей в эпидемиологических исследованиях является очень сложной задачей. А использование таких параметров, как характер работы, расстояние от источника воздействия не всегда позволяет получить надежные оценки уровней облучения. Таким образом, требуется проведение инструментальных измерений с целью надежной оценки доз. Применение небольших индивидуальных дозиметров показало их ценность в исследованиях крайне низкочастотных полей. Таким образом, использование индивидуальных дозиметров позволит существенно улучшить оценки доз необходимых для эпидемиологических исследований. С целью оценки надежности доз необходимо провести валидацию расчетных и измеренных значений. Для оценки доз следует записывать такие параметры, как величина магнитного поля, градиент магнитного поля, и, в идеальном случае, скорость изменения магнитного поля в результате движения.

Таблица 1. Рекомендации к дальнейшим исследованиям

Механизмы взаимодействия

Химия реакций пар радикалов (0,1 – 1 Тл)

Комутагенные эффекты с использованием клеток человека

Теоретические исследования и моделирование

Дозиметрические исследования с использованием воксельных фантомов мужчины/женщины/беременной женщины

Индуцированные токи в глазе

«Потенциал потока» в сердце

Исследования in vitro

Механизмы взаимодействия: реакции пар радикалов и активность энзимов

Влияние физических параметров (интенсивность, повторность, продолжительность, градиент магнитного поля)

Мутагенность и трансформация в клетках-предшественниках у человека

Экспрессия генов в клетках человека

Лабораторные исследования на животных

Рак

Эффекты развития и нейроповеденческие эффекты

Сердечно-сосудистая система (около 20 Тл)

Лабораторные исследования на человеке

Вестибулярный аппарат, координация головы и глаз

Когнитивная функция и поведение

Сердечно-сосудистые эффекты

Эпидемиологические исследования

Пилотное исследование источников воздействия, мешающих факторов, количества облученных

Изучение методом «случай – контроль» возникновения хронических заболеваний, например, рака (если выполнимо))

Исходы беременностей в связи с профессиональным воздействием и в результате МРИ исследований

Когортное исследование ранних эффектов в группе профессиональных работников с высокими уровнями воздействия полей

15 RESUMEN Y RECOMENDACIONES PARA MAYORES ESTUDIOS

15.1 Resumen

15.1.1 Fuentes naturales y artificiales

Los campos electrostáticos ocurren naturalmente en la atmósfera. Valores de hasta 3 kV m^{-1} pueden ocurrir bajo nubes de tormentas, de otro lado en condiciones de clima agradable están en el rango de 1-100 V m^{-1}. Por otro lado, la causa más común de la exposición humana es la separación carga como resultado de la fricción. Por ejemplo, caminando sobre alfombras no conductivas, potenciales de carga de varios kilovoltios pueden ser acumulados, generando campos locales de hasta 500 kV m^{-1}. La transmisión de la energía de corriente directa (DC) puede producir campos electrostáticos de hasta 20 kV m^{-1}, sistemas de ferrocarril utilizando DC pueden generar campos de hasta 300 V m^{-1} dentro del tren, y las unidades de monitoreo visual (VDU) crean campos eléctricos de alrededor de 10-20 kV m^{-1} a una distancia de 30 cm.

El campo geomagnético varía sobre la superficie de la Tierra entre 35-70 µT y esta implicado en la orientación y el comportamiento migratorio de ciertas especies de animales. Los campos magnetostáticos artificiales son generados donde quiera que las corrientes de DC sean utilizadas, tales como en algunos sistemas de transportes energizados por la electricidad, procesos industriales tales como producción de aluminio y en la soldadura a gas. Densidades de flujo magnético de hasta 2 mT han sido reportadas dentro de los trenes eléctricos y en los sistemas de levitación magnética (MagLev) en desarrollo. Los trabajadores están expuestos a grandes campos en la reducción electrolítica del aluminio de hasta alrededor de 60 mT, y en la soldadura con arcos eléctricos se producen alrededor de 5 mT a 1 cm de los cables eléctricos.

El advenimiento de los superconductores en los 1970 y 80 facilitó el uso de campos magnéticos mucho más grandes en el diagnóstico médico a través del desarrollo de la imaginología (MRI) y espectroscopia (MRS)[1] por resonancia magnética y la resonancia magnética nuclear (NMR) para investigación. Se estima que alrededor de 200 millones de escaneos de MRI han sido realizadas en todo el mundo. El campo magnetostático de los escaners de MRI es generado por los magnetos permanentes, los magnetos superconductivos y las combinaciones de ellos en el rango de 0.2-3 T para los sistemas de uso clínico rutinario. En las aplicaciones para investigación campos magnéticos más grandes de hasta

---

[1] Este documento se refiere totalmente a MRI; exposiciones experimentadas

9.4 T son utilizados en el escaneo de todo del cuerpo del paciente. Los campos magnéticos dispersos alrededor de los magnetos para los estudios de MRI están bien definidos y pueden ser minimizados en las versiones con protectores de magneto. Con respecto a la exposición, en la consola del operador la densidad del flujo magnético es típicamente 0.5 mT, pero podría ser superior. Sin embargo, exposición ocupacional hasta y más de 1 T puede ocurrir durante la construcción y pruebas de estos dispositivos y durante los procedimientos médicos realizados para MRI intervencional. Varias investigaciones en física y tecnologías de alta energía también emplean superconductores donde los trabajadores pueden ser expuestos regularmente y por más largos periodos a campos tan altos como 1.5 T.

15.1.2 Mecanismos de Interacción

Las siguientes tres clases de interacciones físicas de los campos magnetostáticos con los sistemas biológicos han sido bien establecidas sobre la base de datos experimentales:

(1)   Interacciones electrodinámicas con corrientes de conducción iónica. Las corrientes iónicas interactúan con los campos magnetostáticos como resultado de las fuerzas de Lorentz ejercidas sobre los portadores de carga en movimiento. Estos efectos conducen a la inducción de los potenciales (de flujo) eléctricos y las corrientes. Los potenciales de flujo son asociados generalmente con la contracción ventricular y la eyección de sangre en la aorta en animales y seres humanos. La interacción de Lorentz resulta también en una fuerza magnetohidrodinámica en oposición al flujo de la sangre. La reducción del flujo de sangre aórtica ha sido predicha llegar alrededor del 10% para 15 T.

(2)   Efectos magnetomecánicos, incluyen la orientación de las estructuras magnéticamente anisotrópicas en campos uniformes y en la translación de los materiales paramagnéticos y ferromagnéticos en las gradientes del campo magnético. Las fuerzas y torques sobre objetos endógenos y exógenos metálicos representan el mecanismo de interacción de mayor preocupación.

(3)   Efectos sobre los estados del spin electrónico de las reacciones intermedias. La química del par radical correlacionado con el spin ha sido por mucho tiempo una consideración para los efectos de campo magnético en química y biología. Varias clases de reacciones químicas orgánicas pueden ser influenciadas por campos magnetostáticos en el rango de 10 a 100 mT como resultado de los efectos sobre los estados del spin electrónico de las reacciones intermedias. El par radical correlacionado con el spin podría recombinarse y evitar la formación del producto de reacción si se cumplen dos condiciones: (a) El par, formado

en un triple estado, tiene que ser convertido en un único estado por algún mecanismo y (b) los radicales tienen que reunirse físicamente otra vez para recombinarse. El paso (a) puede ser sensible al campo magnético. Se ha realizado bastante investigación sobre el uso de los efectos del campo magnético del par radical como una herramienta para estudiar las reacciones de las enzimas. Sin embargo, no parece existir la posibilidad de efectos de consecuencia fisiológica sobre las funciones celulares o efectos mutagénicos de largo plazo provenientes de los cambios inducidos por el campo magnético en las concentraciones o flujos de radicales libres.

Dosimetría

Para comprender los efectos biológicos de los campos eléctricos y magnéticos es importante considerar los campos que directamente influyen sobre las células en diferentes partes del cuerpo y los tejidos. Una dosis puede ser definida como una función apropiada de los campos eléctricos y magnéticos en el punto de interacción. El establecimiento de la relación entre los campos externos no perturbados y los campos internos es el objetivo principal de la dosimetría. Los estudios computacionales que usan modelos de seres humanos y animales a basados en voxels, así como los estudios experimentales de exposición son aspectos importantes de la dosimetría.

Las interacciones del tejido con los campos magnetostáticos probablemente están relacionada con las propiedades físicas del campo que incluyen: el vector del campo magnético, la gradiente del campo magnético, y/o el producto de aquellas magnitudes con frecuencia llamado el "producto fuerza". Algunas de las grandes interacciones son caracterizadas por el movimiento a través de las magnitudes del campo tales como el movimiento del cuerpo o el flujo de sangre.

Los parámetros dosimétricos apropiados dependen del mecanismo físico para el efecto motivo de la preocupación de seguridad. Claramente, los objetos ferromagnéticos tienen que ser restringidos de la vecindad del magneto. La búsqueda tales objetos y de implantes que pueden moverse debido a las fuerzas o torques es imperativo. Las mediciones del vector de inducción magnética pico, y el producto pico de la fuerza magnética son apropiados. Mapas del campo pueden ser utilizadas para estimar estos en varias ubicaciones cercanas de los magnetos donde los trabajadores podrían estar expuestos, pero la dosimetría personal podría ser más útil.

El movimiento de todo o parte del cuerpo, por ej. los ojos y la cabeza, en la gradiente del campo magnetostático también inducirá un campo eléctrico y corriente durante el periodo de movimiento. El cálculo dosimétrico sugiere que tales campos eléctricos inducidos estarán substancialmente durante movimiento normal alrededor o dentro de campos > 2-3 T, y podría tomarse en cuenta para los numerosos reportes anecdóticos de vértigo y ocasionalmente los fosfenos magnéticos experimentados por pacientes, voluntarios y trabajadores durante el movimiento en el campo.

Existen muchas fuentes de exposición. Una de las más prolíficas exposiciones es aquella concerniente al equipo para imaginología por resonancia magnética (MRI). En la década pasada, ha existido un esfuerzo coordinado para permitir que el MRI opere en intensidades muy altas del campo. El sistema más común en uso clínico actual tiene un campo central de 1.5 T, sin embargo sistemas de 3.0 T ahora son aceptados para trabajo clínico rutinario y para el 2004 más de 100 sistemas estarán operando en todo el mundo. Sistemas para investigación de 4-9.4 T están siendo desarrollados ahora para imaginología clínica. Conforme la intensidad del campo del sistema de MRI se incrementa así pasa con el potencial para las interacciones tejido/campo de una variedad de tipos. Comprender las interacciones entre los campos electromagnéticos generados por los sistemas de MRI y el cuerpo humano ha llegado a ser más significativo con este empuje hacia altas intensidades de campo.

15.1.3 Estudios in vitro

Los resultados de los estudios in vitro son útiles para dilucidar los mecanismos de interacción, y para indicar los tipos de efectos que podrían ser investigados in vivo, pero no son suficientes para identificar los efectos a la salud sin evidencia corroborativa de los estudios in vivo.

Un número de diferentes efectos biológicos de los campos magnetostáticos han sido explorados in vitro. Los diferentes niveles de organización fueron investigados: sistemas de células libres, empleando membranas aisladas, enzimas o reacciones bioquímicas, y varios modelos de células, utilizando bacterias y células de mamíferos. Los criterios de valoración estudiados fueron la orientación celular, la actividad metabólica celular, fisiología de la membrana celular, la expresión del gen, el crecimiento celular y la genotoxicidad.

Para todos estos criterios de valoración, descubrimientos positivos y negativos han sido reportados. Sin embargo, la mayoría de datos no fueron replicados. Los efectos observados son muy diversos y fueron encontrados después de la exposición a un amplio rango de densidades de flujo magnético. Existe la evidencia que los campos magnetostáticos pueden afectar varios criterios de valoración en intensidades más bajas de 1 T, en el rango de los mT. Umbrales para algunos de los efectos fueron reportados, pero otros estudios indicaron una respuesta no lineal sin claros valores de umbral.

Los efectos de los campos magnetostáticos sobre la orientación de la célula han sido consistentemente encontrados por encima de 1 T, pero su relevancia in vivo es cuestionable. Pocos estudios sugieren que los efectos combinados del campo magnetostático con otros agentes tales como los químicos genotóxicos parecerían producir efectos sinergísticos tanto protectores como estimulantes. La presente información es inadecuada y necesita ser confirmada antes de que puedan sacarse conclusiones firmes sobre la salud humana.

Además, de la posible dependencia complicada respecto de los parámetros físicos tales como intensidad, duración, recurrencia y gradientes de exposición, las variables biológicas parecen ser importantes para los efectos de los campos magnetostáticos. Las variables tales como el tipo de célula, la activación de la célula, y otras condiciones fisiológicas durante la exposición mostraron afectar el resultado de los experimentos. Los mecanismos para estos efectos no son conocidos, pero efectos sobre los radicales y los iones podrían estar involucrados. Estudios in vitro proporcionan alguna evidencia para esto.

Los muy pocos estudios que emplean señales de MRI u otros campos combinados no muestran ningún efecto biológico diferente de aquellos causados por los campos magnetostáticos solos, si los hubiera.

En general, los experimentos in vitro no presentan un cuadro claro de los efectos específicos de los campos magnetostáticos, y a causa de ello tampoco no indican posibles efectos adversos a la salud.

15.1.4 Estudios en animales

Pocos estudios en animales han sido realizados sobre los efectos de los campos electrostáticos a la salud; ninguna evidencia de efectos adversos a la salud ha sido notada diferente de aquellos asociados con la percepción de la carga eléctrica superficial.

Un gran número de estudios en animales sobre los efectos de los campos magnetostáticos han sido realizados. Muchos de ellos considerados relevantes para la salud humana han examinado los efectos de los campos considerablemente más grandes que el campo geomagnético natural. Un número de estudios han sido realizados de los campos en la región de los militeslas, comparable a exposiciones industriales relativamente altas. Más recientemente con el advenimiento de la tecnología de magneto superconductivo y la MRI, los estudios del comportamiento, los efectos fisiológicos y reproductivos han sido realizados en densidades de flujo alrededor o excediendo 1 T. Pocos estudios sin embargo, han examinado los posibles efectos de la exposición crónica, particularmente en relación a la carcinogénesis.

Las respuestas más consistentes encontradas en los estudios neurológicos del comportamiento sugirieron que el movimiento de los roedores de laboratorio en campos magnetostáticos iguales o mayores que 4 T podrían ser torpes, induciendo respuestas de aversión y evitamiento condicionado. Se piensa que tales efectos son consistentes con los efectos magnetohidrodinámicos sobre la endolinfa del aparato vestibular. Por otro lado, los datos son variables.

Existe alguna evidencia que varias especies vertebradas e invertebradas pueden utilizar los campos magnetostáticos, en niveles tan bajos como las intensidades del campo geomagnético, para orientación, sin embargo, no se piensa que estas respuestas tengan algún significado para la salud.

Existe buena evidencia de que la exposición a campos mayores que 1T (0.1 T en grandes animales) inducirán potenciales de flujo alrededor del corazón y principales vasos sanguíneos, pero las consecuencias fisiológicas de esto permanecen sin aclararse. Varias horas de exposición a densidades de flujo muy altas de hasta 8 T en la región del corazón no resultaron en ningún efecto cardiovascular en cerdos. En conejos, exposición de corto y largo plazo a campos en el rango desde los niveles geomagnéticos hasta los militeslas se reportaron que afectan el sistema cardiovascular, aunque la evidencia no es fuerte.

Los resultados de un grupo sugieren que los campos magnetostáticos de intensidades de mT podrían suprimir la elevación temprana de la presión de sangre a través del sistema regulatorio hormonal. El mismo grupo ha reportado que campos magnetostáticos de baja intensidad de hasta 0.2 T podrían inducir efectos locales sobre el flujo de sangre que podría conducir a la mejora de la microcirculación. Además, otro grupo reportó que densidades altas de flujo del campo magnetostático de hasta 10 T podrían llevar a reducir el flujo de sangre de la piel y la temperatura. En todos estos casos, sin embargo, los criterios de valoración son muy débiles, una situación que podría haber sido complicada por la manipulación farmacológica, incluyendo la anestesia en algunos casos, y la inmovilización. En general, es difícil alcanzar alguna conclusión firme sin alguna replicación independiente.

Existen varios estudios que describen los posibles efectos de exposición al campo magnético sobre las células de sangre y el sistema hematopoyético. Sin embargo, los resultados son equívocos, limitando las conclusiones que se pueden obtener. La evidencia disponible respecto de los efectos de la exposición al campo magnetostático sobre los constituyentes enzimáticos e iónicos del suero que viene primeramente de un laboratorio. Estos hallazgos necesitan ser confirmados por laboratorios independientes antes de sacar conclusiones.

Respecto a los efectos sobre el sistema endocrino, varios estudios provenientes de un laboratorio sugieren que la exposición al campo magnetostático puede afectar la síntesis pineal y el contenido de melatonina. Sin embargo, algunos estudios realizados en otros laboratorios no han podido demostrar ningún efecto. El hallazgo de un efecto supresivo sobre la producción de melatonina de la exposición al campo magnetostático necesita ser confirmada con mayor investigación antes de que puedan obtenerse conclusiones firmes. En general, pocos estudios han investigado los efectos del campo magnetostático sobre los sistemas endocrinos diferentes del pineal; ningún o efecto consistente emerge.

La reproducción y el desarrollo son temas muy importantes en la exposición proveniente de la MRI de los pacientes y del personal clínico. Al respecto solamente pocos buenos estudios de los campos magnetostáticos están disponibles para valores del campo por encima de 1 T. Los estudios de MRI per se no son informativos porque el efecto del campo estático no puede ser distinguida de los posibles efectos de los campos de radiofrecuencia y gradientes de pulsos en general. Para evaluar el riesgo a la salud se necesita urgentemente una mayor revisión.

En general, con respecto a la genotoxicidad y el cáncer, se han realizados tan pocos estudios que no es posible obtener ninguna conclusión firme.

15.1.5 Estudios de laboratorio en seres humanos

Los campos electrostáticos no penetran los objetos eléctricamente conductivos tales como el cuerpo humano; el campo induce una carga eléctrica superficial y siempre es perpendicular a la superficie del cuerpo. Una densidad de carga superficial suficientemente grande podría ser percibida a través de su interacción con el pelo del cuerpo y por otros efectos tales como descargas tipo chispas (microshocks). La percepción del umbral en las personas depende de varios factores y puede estar en el rango entre 10-45 kV m^{-1}. Los umbrales de sensaciones molestas son probablemente igualmente variables, pero no han sido sistemáticamente estudiados. Microshocks dolorosos se pueden esperar cuando una persona bien aislado de tierra toca un objeto puesto a tierra o cuando una persona conectada a tierra toca un objeto conductivo que esta bien aislado de la tierra; sin embargo, los valores del umbral del campo eléctrico estático variarán dependiendo del grado de aislamiento y otro factores.

En estudios experimentales con seres humanos los criterios de valoración investigados han sido la función nervioso periférica, la actividad del cerebro, la función neuroconductual y cognitiva, la percepción sensorial, la función cardiaca, la presión sanguínea, el ritmo del corazón, los niveles de las proteínas del suero y hormonas, la temperatura del cuerpo y la piel, y efectos terapéuticos. Niveles de exposición de hasta 8 T han sido investigados, y los campos estáticos puros y de imaginología MRI han sido estudiados. La duración de la exposición esta en el rango de pocos segundos hasta nueve horas, pero usualmente fue menos de una hora. Los datos disponibles son limitados por varias razones; generalmente muestras convenientes de pacientes o voluntarios saludables han sido estudiadas, y el número de los sujetos ha sido usualmente pequeño.

Los resultados no indican que exista efectos de la exposición a los campos magnetostáticos sobre las respuestas neurofisiológicas y funciones cognitivas en voluntarios estacionarios; pero tampoco se pueden descartar tales efectos. Una inducción dependiente de la dosis de vértigo y nauseas se encontró en los trabajadores, pacientes u voluntarios durante el movimiento dentro campos estáticos mayores que 2 T. Un estudio sugiere que la coordinación de ojo-mano y la sensibilidad del contraste visual cercano se reducen para campos adyacentes a una unidad MRI de 1.5 T. La ocurrencia de estos efectos es probable que sea dependiente del gradiente del campo y el movimiento del sujeto. Un pequeño cambio en la presión sanguínea y el ritmo del corazón se observó en algunos estudios, pero estuvieron en el rango de variabilidad fisiológica normal. No existe evidencia de efectos de los campos magnetostáticos sobre otros aspectos de la fisiología cardiovascular, o sobre las proteínas del suero y hormonas. La exposición a los campos magnetostáticos de hasta 8 T no parece inducir cambios de temperatura en los seres humanos.

Note sin embargo, que muchos de los estudios fueron muy pequeños, estuvieron basados en muestras de conveniencia, y con frecuencia incluyeron grupos no comparables. Además, no es posible obtener algunas conclusiones con respecto a la amplia variedad de criterios de valoración examinados en este reporte.

15.1.6 Estudios epidemiológicos

Los estudios epidemiológicos han sido realizados casi exclusivamente en trabajadores expuestos a campos magnetostáticos generados por equipamiento que utilizo grandes corrientes DC. Muchos trabajadores estuvieron expuestos a campos magnetostáticos moderados de hasta varias decenas de mT como soldadores, fundidores de aluminio, o trabajadores en varias plantas industriales que utilizaron grandes celdas electrolíticas en procesos de separación química. Sin embargo, tal trabajo también es probable que haya involucrado la exposición a una variedad de gases y aerosoles potencialmente peligrosos; confundiendo la interpretación. Los criterios de valoración de la salud en estos trabajadores incluyen el cáncer, cambios hematológicos y resultados relacionados, la frecuencia de aberración de los cromosomas, resultados reproductivos, y desórdenes muscoesqueléticos. Además, unos pocos estudios examinaron la fertilidad y el resultado de los embarazos de operadoras de MRI, donde el potencial de haber sido expuesto a campos estáticos relativamente grandes de hasta ~ 1T podría haber existido. Dos estudios examinaron los resultados del embarazo en voluntarias saludables expuestas a exámenes de MRI durante el embarazo.

El incremento de los riesgos de varios cánceres fueron reportados por ej. cáncer al pulmón, cáncer pancreático y malignidades hematológicas, pero los resultados no fueron consistentes a través de los estudios. Los pocos estudios epidemiológicos publicados hasta la fecha dejan un número de temas sin resolver concerniente a la posibilidad del incremento del riesgo de cáncer provenientes de la exposición a los campos magnetostáticos. La evaluación de la exposición ha sido pobre, y el número de participantes en algunos de los estudios ha sido muy pequeño, por lo que estos estudios son capaces de detectar solo riesgos muy grandes para estas raras enfermedades. La incapacidad de estos estudios para proporcionar informaciones útiles es apoyada por la falta de una evidencia clara para otros, factores carcinogénicos más establecidos presentes en algunos de los ambientes de trabajo. Otros efectos a la salud que no sean cáncer han sido considerados aún más esporádicamente. Muchos de estos estudios se basan en números muy pequeños y tienen numerosas limitaciones metodológicas. Otros ambientes con un potencial para campos altos no han sido adecuadamente evaluados, ej. Los operadores MRI. En el presente existen datos inadecuados para una evaluación de la salud.

15.1.7 Evaluación del riesgo a la salud

Campos electrostáticos

No existen estudios sobre exposición a campos electrostáticos de los cuales se obtengan alguna conclusión sobre los efectos crónicos o retardados. La IARC (IARC 2002) notó que existía una evidencia insuficiente para determinar la carcinogenicidad de campos electrostáticos.

Pocos estudios de los efectos agudos del campo eléctrico estático han sido realizados. En general, los resultados sugieren que el único efecto agudo adverso a la salud esta asociado con la percepción directa de los campos y las molestias de los microshocks.

Con respecto a los efectos crónicos y retardados, la evidencia disponible de los estudios epidemiológicos y de laboratorio no es suficiente para obtener algunas conclusiones. La IARC (IARC, 2002) concluyó que existía inadecuada evidencia en seres humanos para la carcinogenicidad de los campos magnetostáticos y ningún dato relevante disponible proveniente de experimentos en animales. Por consiguiente, en el presente, no son clasificables como carcinogénicos para los seres humanos.

La exposición de corto plazo a los campos magnetostáticos en el rango de los teslas y a las gradientes de campo indican un número de efectos agudos.

Las respuestas cardiovasculares, tales como los cambios en la presión de sanguínea y el ritmo cardiaco, han sido ocasionalmente observados en voluntarios humanos y estudios en animales. Sin embargo, estos estuvieron dentro del rango fisiológico normal para exposición a campos magnetostáticos de hasta 8 T.

Aunque no verificada experimentalmente, es importante notar que los cálculos sugieren tres posibles efectos de los potenciales de flujo inducidos: cambios menores en el ritmo de latidos del corazón (que podrían ser considerados sin consecuencias a la salud), la inducción de latidos ectópicos del corazón (que podrían ser fisiológicamente más significativos), y un incremento de la probabilidad de arritmia reentrante (posiblemente conduciendo a la fibrilación ventricular). Se piensa que los primeros dos efectos tienen umbrales por encima de 8 T, y los valores de umbral para el tercero son difíciles de evaluar en el presente por causa de la complejidad del modelamiento. Algo de 5-10 por 10,000 personas son particularmente susceptibles a la arritmia reentrante, y el riesgo para tales personas podría ser incrementado por exposición al campo magnetostático y la gradiente de los campos.

Las limitaciones de los datos disponibles son tales, que sin embargo, tomados en forma integral no es posible sacar conclusiones firmes acerca de los efectos de los campos magnetostáticos sobre los criterios de valoración considerados anteriormente.

El movimiento físico dentro de una gradiente de campo estático se reporto que induce sensaciones de vértigo y nauseas, y algunas veces fosfenos y un sabor metálico en la boca para los campos estáticos en exceso de alrededor de 2-4 T. Aunque solamente transitorios, tales efectos podrían afectar adversamente a las personas. Junto con los posibles efectos sobre la coordinación ojo-mano, la ejecución óptima por parte de los trabajadores de procedimientos delicados (ej. cirujanos) podría verse reducida con un impacto concomitante sobre la seguridad.

Efectos sobre otras respuestas fisiológicas han sido reportados, pero es difícil llegar a alguna conclusión firme sin una replicación independiente.

15.1.8 Recomendaciones para las autoridades nacionales

Se recomienda a las autoridades nacionales implementar programas que protejan al público y los trabajadores de algunos efectos desfavorables de los campos estáticos. Sin embargo, dado que el principal efecto de campos electrostáticos es la incomodidad proveniente de la descarga eléctrica sobre los tejidos del cuerpo, el programa de protección podría ser simplemente la provisión de información sobre situaciones que podrían llevar a exposición a grandes campos eléctricos y el como evitarlos. Se necesita un programa para campos magnetostáticos, para proteger contra los efectos agudos establecidos. A causa de la insuficiente información actualmente disponible sobre los posibles efectos de largo plazo o retardados de la exposición, medidas precautorias costo/efectivas, como las que están siendo desarrolladas por la OMS (www.who.int/emf) podrían necesitarse para controlar las exposiciones de los trabajadores y el público.

Las autoridades nacionales deberían adoptar estándares basados en ciencia sólida que limiten la exposición de las personas a campos magnetostáticos. La implementación de los estándares basados en la salud proporciona la medida precautoria primaria para los trabajadores y el público. Estándares internacionales existen para los campos magnetostáticos (ICNIRP, 1994) y son descritos en el Apéndice 1. Sin embargo, la OMS recomienda que estos deban revisarse a la luz de la evidencia más reciente proveniente de la literatura científica.

Las autoridades nacionales deberían establecer o complementar los programas existentes que proporcionan protección contra los posibles efectos de exposición a campos magnetostáticos. Las medidas protectoras para el uso industrial y científico de campos magnéticos puedan ser categorizadas como controles de diseño de ingeniería, el uso de una distancia de separación, y los controles administrativos. Las medidas protectoras contra los peligros secundarios provenientes de la interferencia magnética con equipamiento electrónico de emergencia o médico y con implantes quirúrgicos y dentales son un área especial de preocupación con respecto a los posibles efectos adversos a la salud de los campos magnetostáticos. Las fuerzas mecánicas impartidas a los implantes ferromagnéticos y los objetos flojos en instalaciones con campos altos requieren que se tomen precauciones.

Las autoridades nacionales deberían considerar el uso bajo licencia de las unidades de MRI para asegurar que las medidas precautorias sean implementadas. Esto también permitiría requerimientos adicionales a cumplir por las unidades de MRI con intensidades en exceso de los estándares locales nacionales ó 2T. Tales requerimientos se relacionan al suministro de información de los pacientes, trabajadores y de cualquier incidente o lesión resultante de los campos magnéticos fuertes.

Las autoridades nacionales deberían proveer financiamiento para la investigación a fin de llenar los grandes vacíos en el conocimiento que conciernen a la seguridad de las personas expuestas a campos magnetostáticos. Recomendaciones para mayor investigación forman parte de este documento (ver a continuación) y son colocados la página web de la OMS: www.who.int/emf. Los investigadores deberían ser financiados para realizar los estudios recomendados en esta agenda de investigación de la OMS.

Las autoridades nacionales deberían financiar unidades MRI para recolectar información sobre la exposición del trabajador a campos magnetostáticos y la exposición del paciente a MRI y hacerlo disponible para estudios epidemiológicos futuros. Ellos también deberían financiar bases de datos que recolecten información sobre exposiciones a los trabajadores donde exposiciones altas de largo plazo ocurran, tales como aquellas involucradas en la fabricación de MRI o similarmente de magnetos de alta intensidad y nuevas tecnologías tales como los trenes MagLev.

15.2 Recomendaciones para mayor estudio

Identificar los vacíos en nuestro conocimiento de los posibles efectos a la salud de la exposición al campo estático es una parte esencial de esta evaluación de riesgo a la salud y las siguientes recomendaciones se realizan para mayor investigación.

15.2.1 Campos electrostáticos

Parece haber poco de beneficio de continuar la investigación relacionada con los efectos a la salud concernientes a los campos electrostáticos. Ninguno de los estudios conducidos hasta la fecha sugieren algún efecto adverso a la salud, excepto al posible estrés resultante de la prolongada exposición a los microshocks. Por consiguiente no existen recomendaciones de mayor investigación concerniente a los efectos biológicos de exposición a campos electrostáticos. Además, solamente existe oportunidad limitada para exposición significativa a estos campos en el lugar de trabajo o el ambiente en el que vivimos y por consiguiente no garantiza ningún estudio epidemiológico.

15.2.2 Campos magnetostáticos

En términos generales, la investigación realizada hasta la fecha no ha sido sistemática y ha sido con frecuencia realizada sin una metodología apropiada e información de la exposición. Programas de investigación coordinados son recomendados como una ayuda a un enfoque más sistemático. Existe también la necesidad de investigar la importancia de los parámetros físicos como la intensidad, duración y la gradiente del resultado biológico.

Siguiendo una discusión de las limitaciones de los estudios existentes, se recomienda una mayor investigación que cubra epidemiología, estudios voluntarios, biología animal e in vitro, y estudios de los mecanismos de interacción, e investigaciones teóricas y computacionales. Estas recomendaciones están resumidas en la Tabla 1

15.2.2.1 Estudios teóricos y computacionales

La dosimetría computacional proporciona en vínculo entre un campo magnético externo y los campos eléctricos internos y las corrientes inducidas causadas por el movimiento de los tejidos vivos en el campo. Tales técnicas teóricas permiten que los campos sean caracterizados en tejidos y órganos específicos. Para buenas resoluciones, anatómicamente realistas, fantomas basados en voxels de adultos varones están disponibles, y han sido ampliamente utilizados en estudios con campos electromagnéticos variables en el tiempo. Sin embargo, se ha realizado muy poco trabajo con los campos estáticos, y se considera necesario un mayor trabajo utilizando estos modelos. En particular, el uso de fantomas de diferentes tamaños, y el uso de fantomas femeninos se considera importante, como es el uso de fantomas embarazadas con fetos de diferentes edades. Podrían ser presentados estudios similares con fantomas de animales preñadas para ayudar a la interpretación de los resultados de los estudios en desarrollo con estos modelos (**prioridad media**).

Debería desarrollarse un fantoma de cabeza y hombros de muy buena resolución y utilizarlo para investigar los campos eléctricos y las corrientes asociadas con los fosfenos visuales y vértigo. Este modelo podría también ser utilizado para investigar los campos y corrientes generadas por los movimientos de la cabeza y el ojo en un campo magnetostático. Lo último es considerado de particular relevancia a los procedimientos de MRI intervencional donde los movimientos reducidos de la cabeza de los cirujanos y otro personal clínico podrían necesitar un movimiento incrementado de los ojos. El movimiento brusco del cuerpo del personal alrededor del sistema intervencional tiene que ser también simulado (**alta prioridad**).

Los cómputos que utilizan un modelo detallado del corazón y el modelamiento de las patologías cardiacas comunes son considerados importantes. Este modelo debería incluir la microarquitectura del corazón así como de los vasos sanguíneos más pequeños dentro del corazón que podrían producir campos y corrientes con alguna influencia sobre la generación del ritmo del marca pasos y la propagación de depolarización. Además, son necesarios cálculos para estimar la magnitud y la distribución espacial de las corrientes que son inducidas en el corazón como consecuencia del campo y la exposición a la gradiente del campo. Múltiples orientaciones del campo deberían ser estudiados. Esto permitiría la comparación con las corrientes que han sido calculadas para inducir los efectos cardiacos. Se recomienda estudios experimentales y de laboratorio que soporten estos cálculos (**alta prioridad**).

Aunque haya una resistencia al uso de MRI de campo alto sobre mujeres embarazadas en la actualidad, se reconoce que esta situación podría cambiar. Por consiguiente, sería recomendable realizar los estudios de modelamiento investigando las corrientes inducidas en un feto por el movimiento maternal o intrínseco fetal en un campo alto. Estos cálculos (y estudios similares con gradiente y campos de radiofrecuencia) permitirían realizar una estimación de la probabilidad de los posibles efectos sobre el feto (**alta prioridad**).

15.2.2.2 Estudios in Vitro

Los campos magnetostáticos podrían interactuar con los sistemas biológicos en un número de formas, aunque el más probable medio para causar efectos a la salud es a través de los efectos de campo inducido sobre moléculas cargadas y alteraciones en la tasa de las reacciones bioquímicas.

Se necesitan mayores estudios sobre los posibles mecanismos y los órganos blanco de los efectos biológicos de campos magnetostáticos. Se recomienda investigar los efectos de campos magnetostáticos de 0.01-10 T sobre la interacción de los iones (ej. Ca^{2+} o Mg^{2+}) con formación de enzimas y pares radicales. Aunque se considera difícil hacerlo, es conveniente buscar más reacciones enzimáticas que procedan a través de los mecanismos de pares radicales en sistemas modelos que son relevantes para la salud humana. Otra sugerencia es concentrarse sobre las especies de radical tóxico, tales como el superoxido que son conocidos por ser dañinas y ser producidas por los mecanismos de radical libre (**prioridad media**).

Los reportes de un efecto comutagénico en varias células son de particular interés con respecto al potencial carcinogénico de campos magnetostáticos. Este tipo de estudios deben ser presentados utilizando células primarias de seres humanos y extendidas para incluir sistemas transformados y genéticamente modificados (**alta prioridad**).

Los campos magnetostáticos podrían afectar la expresión del gen y varias de las funciones pertinentes en células de seres humanos y de mamíferos bajo condiciones específicas de exposición, pero se tiene poca información disponible sobre esto. Estudios con técnicas tales como proteómica y genómica deberían ser realizados con las células humanas primarias para buscar posibles marcadores moleculares para los efectos de campos magnetostáticos relevantes a los temas de salud humana (**baja prioridad**).

15.2.2.3 Estudios experimentales en animales

Lo efectos de exposición de largo plazo a campos magnetostáticos pueden ser enfocados utilizando modelos de animales. En ausencia de información específica con respecto al potencial carcinogénico de los campos magnetostáticos, se recomienda estudios de largo plazo (incluyendo estudios de por vida). Animales normales y genéticamente modificados podrían ser utilizados. Por ejemplo, si una amplificación de los radicales libres fuese considerada una ruta posible por la cual el riesgo de cáncer podría ser incrementado, podría ser utilizado un modelo de ratón con supresión del gen superoxido dismutasa. En este modelo, la susceptibilidad a los tumores y otros enfermedades relacionadas a los radicales libres es muy elevada. El uso de las técnicas de microarreglos permiten que los efectos de muchos parámetros diferentes de exposición sean fácilmente evaluados y cuantificados sobre el genoma y proteoma (**alta prioridad**).

La posibilidad del aumento de riesgo de anormalidades en el desarrollo y efectos teratológicos necesitan ser enfocadas de modo sistemático. El desarrollo del cerebro podría ser particularmente susceptible a los efectos de las corrientes inducidas por movimiento: los efectos de orientación son muy importantes para guiar el crecimiento normal de las dendritas neuronales. También es posible que cambios duraderos podrían ser inducidos por exposiciones relativamente cortas. El estudio de los parámetros neuroconductuales pueden proporcionar un ensayo rápido y sensible para explorar los efectos de exposición sobre el desarrollo de la función del cerebro, y se recomienda tales estudios. Los estudios para registrar los sutiles cambios morfológicos que ocurren durante el desarrollo de regiones específicas del cerebro, tales como al corteza o el hipocampo también son del valor. El uso de los modelos trasngénicos apropiados debería ser considerado (**alta prioridad**).

Aunque haya datos que indiquen que la exposición de animales (y seres humanos) a los campos alrededor de 2 T no causan efectos electrofisiológicos, sería útil conocer los efectos de los campos más altos. Además los efectos de exposición de hasta y por encima de 10 T podrían ser provechosamente explorados en animales (**prioridad media**).

Una variedad de otros criterios de valoración han sido investigados en animales que proporcionan en el mejor de los casos solo información limitada. Mientras que una serie estudios individuales para cada uno de estos criterios de valoración podría no ser costo-efectivos, un amplio estudio animal para cubrir diferentes criterios de valoración sería valioso (**baja prioridad**).

15.2.2.4 Estudios experimentales en seres humanos

Los efectos cognitivos y conductuales de los campos magnetostáticos deberían de investigarse más, aunque los datos disponibles no sugieren riesgos particulares para aspectos específicos de cognición ni sirven para sugerir que parámetros deberían ser evaluados en el laboratorio. En la ausencia de una dirección clara un enfoque posible sería investigar los efectos de exposición sobre la realización de una batería de tareas cognitivas, que incluyan evaluaciones estándares de atención, tiempo de reacción y memoria, solamente para actuar como un tamiz inicial dejando pendiente trabajo más enfocado. El trabajo inicial podría ser realizado con voluntarios como parte de los estudios experimentales (**prioridad media**).

Con una utilización más amplia de los estudios de MRI donde el personal de apoyo esta en una proximidad cercana a pacientes dentro de un magneto, tal como en los procedimientos de MRI intervencional, se necesitan estudios adicionales de la coordinación de la cabeza y la vista, función cognitiva y del comportamiento en una gradiente de campo. Se considera de especial interés una mayor investigación de los mecanismos y la intensidad de disfunción vestibular inducida por el campo incluyendo el vértigo debido al incremento de la probabilidad que el personal médico estará realizando tareas complicadas dentro de un campo magnético por largos periodos de tiempo (**alta prioridad**).

Similarmente, estudios adicionales sobre la función cardiaca serían útiles y podrían investigar los efectos sobre el sistema cardiovasculatorio. Estos estudios podrían necesitar ser completados para niveles superiores a 3 T, para evaluar el riesgo potencial por encima del que existe en el ambiente clínico rutinario (**baja prioridad**).

15.2.2.5 Estudios epidemiológicos

Existe un número de categorías de trabajadores con exposiciones elevadas a campos magnetostáticos, por ejemplo los técnicos de MRI, los trabajadores en las plantas de fundición de aluminio, y ciertos trabajadores de transporte (metros, trenes MagLev, trenes conmutados, y trenes urbanos). Para las enfermedades crónicas raras como el cáncer, estudios de factibilidad son necesarios para identificar los grupos ocupacionales altamente expuestos que cuya participación sería posible asegurar en los estudios epidemiológicos. Los estudios de factibilidad también necesitan determinar que otras exposiciones están presentes en estas ocupaciones. Si números suficientes de trabajadores pueden ser identificados, un enfoque de caso control anidado es probablemente el más apropiado, ya que información detallada acerca de la exposición y factores importantes de confusión tales como la radiación ionizante necesitan obtenerse. Estudios de colaboración internacionales probablemente son necesarios para obtener números suficientes de personas expuestas (**alta prioridad**).

Para otros resultados de salud más comunes con periodos cortos de latencia grupos ocupacionales altamente expuestos específicos pueden ser identificados y seguidos en el tiempo, por ejemplo los trabajadores en industrias donde los sistemas de MRI son fabricados. Información acerca de diferentes resultados de salud podrían ya estar disponibles provenientes de los exámenes de salud realizados rutinariamente a estos trabajadores, pero solamente pueden ser utilizados si información similar también esta disponible para un grupo comparable no expuesto. Una encuesta de salud de cirujanos, enfermeras, y otros trabajadores que utilizan MRI intervencional proporcionaría información útil como los niveles, duraciones y frecuencia de las exposiciones de los trabajadores a campos estáticos en estos sistemas. Similarmente, el registros de pacientes podrían existir en algunos hospitales de los cuales sería posible obtener los datos de las personas que estuvieron expuestas pero cuyas condiciones fueron subsecuentemente encontrados ser benignas (**alta prioridad**)

También es considerado conveniente realizar un estudio prospectivo de los riesgos del embarazo asociados con la exposición ocupacional al campo magnetostático, así como también el seguimiento de los resultados del embarazo de las mujeres embarazadas que experimentaron exámenes MRI (**alta prioridad**).

La experiencia con otras frecuencias ha mostrado que obtener estimaciones confiables de la exposición a campos electromagnéticos para uso en estudios epidemiológicos puede ser muy difícil, y mediciones sustitutas de la exposición, tales el cargo en el trabajo o la distancia a una fuente en particular podrían no siempre proporcionar evaluaciones suficientemente exactas. Por consiguiente el uso de instrumentos específicos es requerido para medir la exposición. Los dosímetros personales relativamente pequeños han demostrado ser muy útiles en la investigación de los campos de ELF, de esta manera, los dosímetros personales mejorarían mucho la evaluación de la exposición en los estudios epidemiológicos. La validación numérica y experimental de los dosímetros debería ser realizada. La intensidad del campo magnético, las gradientes del campo magnético, las duraciones de las exposiciones e idealmente la tasa de cambio magnético debido al movimiento debería ser registrada (**alta prioridad**).

Tabla 1. Recomendaciones para la investigación

Mecanismos de interacción
Química de las reacciones de pares radicales (0.1-10T)
Efectos comutagénicos utilizando células humanas

Estudios teóricos y computacionales
Estudios dosimétricos con fantomas voxel masculino/femenino/ embarazada
Corrientes inducidas en el ojo
Potenciales de flujo en el corazón

Estudios in Vitro
Mecanismos de interacción: reacciones de pares de radicales y actividad enzimática
Influencia de parámetros físicos (intensidad, duración, recurrencia, gradientes de SMF
Mutagenicidad y transformación en células primarias de seres humanos
Expresión del gen en células primarias de seres humanos

Estudios experimentales en animales
Cáncer
Efectos en desarrollo/neuroconductuales
Función cardiaca (~20 T)

Estudios experimentales en voluntarios
Función vestibular, coordinación de cabeza y ojos
Función cognitiva y del comportamiento
Efectos cardiovasculares

Estudios epidemiológicos
Estudio de factibilidad de fuentes de exposición, factores de confusión, número de personas expuestas
Estudio de caso control anidado de enfermedad crónica ej. cáncer (si es factible)
Resultados del embarazo en relación a la exposición ocupacional y exámenes MRI
Estudio cohorte de efectos de corto plazo en ocupaciones altamente expuestas

APPENDIX 1: INTERNATIONAL GUIDELINES ON EXPOSURE TO STATIC MAGNETIC FIELDS

International exposure guidelines are developed by the International Commission on Non-Ionizing Radiation Protection (ICNIRP). This independent scientific body is officially recognized by WHO and its exposure guidelines advice is based upon the health risk assessments published by WHO and cancer reviews and classifications carried out by IARC. National authorities are advised to adopt international standards, where they exist.

Exposure guidelines serve five main functions:

- a general framework for the protection of people who may be exposed to static electric or magnetic fields whether at work, in public spaces or in the home;

- a tool for the practical safety assessment of exposures in relation to recommended exposure restrictions (compliance assessment);

- a basis for national standards and regulations on limiting exposure;

- a basis for the development of technical standards pertaining to equipment design, device emissions and measurement procedures;

- a basis for operational procedures at workplaces and facilities, especially if exposure to high field strengths are required for short periods of time in occupational settings.

The basis for exposure guidelines is the health risk assessment. From this, exposure restrictions are recommended below which acute adverse health effects will not occur. In specifying restrictions on exposure, it is important to note any uncertainties in the scientific evidence as presented in the health risk assessment. This may be particularly important in considering the evidence for adverse health effects due to long-term exposure at levels lower than those that cause acute adverse effects. It is also important that caution is exercised, to ensure the adequate protection of all members of the community. For the general public, those exposed include people who, for a variety of reasons, might be especially susceptible to adverse health effects. In this respect, it is important to consider the evidence, if any, of effects in children, neonates and the unborn child, older people and people taking prescribed medicines. In addition, possible effects of fields on medical implants should be addressed by competent technical bodies.

Exposure to static electric fields is addressed in the ICNIRP exposure guidelines (ICNIRP, 1998), although only in a general manner.

Only the indirect effects of electric discharge are considered. No quantitative restrictions on field strength are provided.

ICNIRP published its advice on limiting public and occupational exposure to static magnetic fields in 1994 (ICNIRP, 1994). This had the objective of protecting individuals from the direct effects of fields, from indirect effects on ferromagnetic objects, and on implanted devices such as pacemakers, aneurism clips etc. ICNIRP's guidelines followed after the development of a few national exposure guidelines including those developed in the former USSR in 1978 (see WHO, 1987 for a review), the American Conference of Governmental Industrial Hygienists (ACGIH, 2001) and by the National Radiological Protection Board in the UK (NRPB, 1993). Elsewhere, guidelines recommending limits on occupational exposure to static magnetic fields were developed for specific laboratories/facilities such as in the US Department of Energy (Alpen, 1979), the Stanford Linear Accelerator (1970) and the Lawrence Livermore National Laboratory (Miller, 1987).

ICNIRP (1994) noted that the scientific knowledge existing at that time did not suggest any detrimental effect on major developmental, behavioural and physiological parameters following transient exposure to static magnetic flux densities up to 2 T. In the absence of knowledge on possible adverse health effects from long-term exposure, ICNIRP recommended a restriction of 200 mT on time-weighted exposure. In addition, the movement of a person in a magnetic field of 200 mT was thought to result in a current density of between 10 and 100 mA m^{-2}, which was considered not to result in adverse effects on the function of the central nervous system at frequencies of less than 10 Hz. ICNIRP calculated the maximum electric current density induced in the aorta by the flow of blood in the magnetic field to be about 40 mA m^{-2} and concluded that this would not be harmful. In addition, the magnetohydrodynamic effects at this flux density were also considered to be of negligible consequence.

Based on these considerations, ICNIRP (1994) recommended a time-weighted average exposure of 200 mT during the working day for occupational exposures, with a ceiling value of 2 T. A ceiling value of 5 T was considered acceptable for extremities, because they do not contain large blood vessels or critical organs.

A 'continuous exposure limit' of 40 mT was given for the general public. This is, in effect, a ceiling value, although "occasional access to special facilities where magnetic flux densities exceed 40 mT can be allowed under controlled conditions, provided that the appropriate occupational exposure limit is not exceeded."

ICNIRP suggested that wearers of cardiac pacemakers, ferromagnetic implants and implanted electronic devices might not be adequately protected by the exposure limits for direct effects. Therefore, ICNIRP recommended that people with cardiac pacemakers and implanted defibrillators should avoid locations where the magnetic flux density exceeds 0.5 mT. For other electronic devices, ICNIRP suggested that they 'may be susceptible' to magnetic flux densities exceeding a few mT. ICNIRP provided no specific quantitative restrictions on exposure levels to avoid such interference effects, but instead recommended that wearers of ferromagnetic implants, and specifically people with aneurism clips, should consult their physician for advice on whether environments with flux densities exceeding a few mT might pose a hazard. Finally, ICNIRP stated that precautions should be taken to prevent hazards from flying metallic objects if the magnetic flux density exceeded 3 mT.

Table 47. Limits of exposure to static magnetic fields (ICNIRP, 1994)

Exposure characteristics	Magnetic flux density
Occupational	
Whole work day (time-weighted average)	200 mT
Ceiling value	2 T
Limbs	5 T
General public	
Continuous exposure*	40 mT

*Occasional access for members of the public to special facilities where magnetic flux densities exceed 40 mT can be allowed under appropriately controlled conditions, provided that the appropriate occupational limit is not exceeded.

The ICNIRP exposure restrictions for the general public provided the basis for a Council of the European Union Recommendation on limiting public exposure to static magnetic fields throughout the European Community (CEU, 1999).